Nanotherapeutics for Inflammatory Arthritis

Nanotherapeutics for Inflammatory Arthritis: Design, Diagnosis, and Treatment highlights nanobiotechnology and its therapeutic applications in the field of inflammatory arthritis, the interaction of nanomaterials in the biological systems, and clinical development of nanomedicines. It also covers the discovery of personalized therapeutics, diagnostics, and nanoparticular delivery systems, and the role of bioinformatics nanobiotechnology in personalized oncology. The use of nanosensors for the detection and current challenges in the development of personalized medicine is explained including recent nanotechnology-based strategies.

Features:

- Covers all the fundamental information about nanotechnology and inflammatory arthritis.
- Highlights the interaction of nanomaterials in the biological systems, and the clinical development of nanomedicines for inflammatory arthritis.
- Explores the discovery of personalized therapeutics, diagnostics, and nanoparticle delivery systems.
- Reviews the current challenges in the development of personalized medicine as well as translation of nanomedicine with combination therapy.
- Discusses the toxicology of using nanomedicines and the risks associated with the use of these nanomedicines.

This book is aimed at researchers and professionals in nanotechnology, biomaterial, drug delivery, and inflammatory arthritis.

Advances in Bionanotechnology

Ravindra Pratap Singh, Department of Biotechnology, Indira Gandhi National Tribal University, Anuppur, Madhya Pradesh, India
Jay Singh, Department of Chemistry, Institute of Science, Banaras Hindu University, Varanasi, Uttar Pradesh, India
Charles Oluwaseun Adetunji, Department of Microbiology, Edo State University Uzairue, Iyamho, Edo State, Nigeria

Bionanotechnology is a multi-disciplinary field that shows immense applicability in different domains, namely chemistry, physics, material sciences, biomedical, agriculture, environment, robotics, aeronautics, energy, electronics, and so forth. This book series will explore the enormous utility of bionanotechnology for biomedical, agricultural, environmental, food technology, space industry, and many other fields. It aims to highlight all the spheres of bionanotechnological applications and its safety and regulations for using biogenic nanomaterials that are a key focus of the researchers globally.

Bionanotechnology towards Sustainable Management of Environmental Pollution
Edited by Naveen Dwivedi and Shubha Dwivedi

Natural Products and Nano-formulations in Cancer Chemoprevention
Edited by Shiv Kumar Dubey

Bionanotechnology towards Green Energy
Innovative and Sustainable Approach
Edited by Shubha Dwivedi and Naveen Dwivedi

Biotic Stress Management of Crop Plants Using Nanomaterials
Edited by Krishna Kant Mishra and Santosh Kumar

Bionanotechnology for Advanced Applications
Edited by Ajaya Kumar Singh and Bhawana Jain

Nanoarchitectonics for Brain Drug Delivery
Edited by Anurag Kumar Singh, Vivek K. Chaturvedi, and Jay Singh

Functional Fluorescent Materials: Applications in Sensing, Bioimaging, and Optoelectronics
Edited by Vivek Mishra, Syed Sibtay Razi, and Ajit Kumar

Nanotherapeutics for Inflammatory Arthritis
Design, Diagnosis, and Treatment
Edited by Vivek Mishra, Ramendra Pati Pandey, Anjali Priyadarshini, Chung-Ming Chang, and Elcio Leal

For more information about this series, please visit: www.routledge.com/Advances-in-Bionanotechnology/book-series/CRCBIONAN

Nanotherapeutics for Inflammatory Arthritis
Design, Diagnosis, and Treatment

Edited by
Vivek Mishra, Ramendra Pati Pandey,
Anjali Priyadarshini, Chung-Ming Chang,
and Elcio Leal

CRC Press
Taylor & Francis Group
Boca Raton London New York

CRC Press is an imprint of the
Taylor & Francis Group, an **informa** business

Designed cover image: shutterstock

First edition published 2025
by CRC Press
2385 NW Executive Center Drive, Suite 320, Boca Raton FL 33431

and by CRC Press
4 Park Square, Milton Park, Abingdon, Oxon, OX14 4RN

CRC Press is an imprint of Taylor & Francis Group, LLC

ISBN: 978-1-032-39163-2 (hbk)
ISBN: 978-1-032-39164-9 (pbk)
ISBN: 978-1-003-34867-2 (ebk)

DOI: 10.1201/9781003348672

Typeset in Times
by MPS Limited, Dehradun

Contents

v

Preface

Inflammation, a common feature of many diseases, is an essential immune response that enables survival and maintains tissue homeostasis. However, in some conditions, the inflammatory process becomes detrimental, contributing to the pathogenesis of a disease. Targeting inflammation by using nanomedicines (i.e., nanoparticles loaded with a therapeutic active principle), either through the recognition of molecules overexpressed onto the surface of activated macrophages or endothelial cells, enhanced vasculature permeability, or even biomimicry, offers a promising solution for the treatment of inflammatory diseases. Applications of nanotechnology are gaining attention worldwide for the treatment of inflammatory and complex diseases such as AIDS (acquired immune deficiency syndrome), cancer, and rheumatoid arthritis. Nanomedicine, which is being used for diagnosis, and treatment of the disease, is a very important application of nanotechnology. Nanomedicine confers a unique technology against complex diseases which includes early diagnosis, prevention, and personalized therapy. Besides diagnosis and treatment, nanomedicine is also being used for drug delivery using nanocarriers, nanotheranostics, and nanovaccinology. Nanocarriers may be used to deliver drugs and biomolecules like proteins, antibody fragments, DNA fragments, and RNA fragments as the basis of cancer biomarkers. The most common nanocarriers used globally are liposomes, polymeric nanoparticles, dendrimers, metallic nanoparticles, magnetic nanoparticles, solid lipid nanoparticles, polymeric micelles, and nanotubes among others.

Nanosystems promise specific and localized delivery of drugs while minimizing the quantity of drugs used, thus limiting potential off-target unwanted effects. These systems may allow the prolonged use of NSAIDs and GCs in high-risk patient populations, such as the young and the elderly. The versatility of the newer nanoplatforms also prompts investigators to reconsider formerly established drugs that were considered too toxic or insoluble for systemic use. Nanotechnology-based gene therapy represents an alternative that may circumvent the oncogenic concerns pertaining to viral-based gene transfer methods. Targeted anti-angiogenic nanotherapy, as single or combination therapy, has been proven effective in animal models and awaits clinical trials. Nanoparticle-based targeted delivery systems therefore represent an ideal therapeutic approach to evaluate these signaling molecule inhibitors in the future, as they can potentially limit generalized immunosuppression.

Significant progress has been made in recent years in nanotechnology and nanomedicine. Nanotechnologies are used to deliver anticancer therapeutics, to perform minimally invasive image-guided delivery of plasmids and non-coding RNAs, and to facilitate the targeted delivery of conventional and biological drugs. The main benefit of employing nanocarriers in the therapeutics arena is to achieve targeted delivery using the optimum drug dosage, extend drug circulation, reduce side effects, and decrease the likelihood of developing drug resistance. Nanotechnologies provide new platforms for achieving sustained drug release, preventing "burst release" and countering drug resistance.

Biological systems operate at the nanoscale. Nanomedicine is the application of nanotechnology to monitor and treat biological systems in health and disease. This is accomplished by real-time monitoring of molecular signaling at the cellular and tissue levels. During the past decade, there has been an explosion in this field, resulting in revolutionary advances in determining the microstructure and function of living systems. These discoveries have led to the development of powerful tools for fundamental biological and medical research. Nanotechnology has been applied to targeted drug delivery to minimize side effects, creating implantable materials as scaffolds for tissue engineering, implantable devices, surgical aids, and nanorobotics, as well as throughput drug screening and medical diagnostic imaging. The aim of this book is to highlight opportunities for the application of nanotechnologies in diagnostics and treatment of inflammatory diseases.

Editors
Dr. Vivek Mishra
AMITY University Noida, Uttar Pradesh, India
Dr. Ramendra Pati Pandey
School of Health Sciences and Technology (SOHST),
UPES, Dehradun, India
Dr. Anjali Priyadarshini
SRM University, Delhi-NCR, Sonepat, India
Prof. Chung-Ming Chang
Chang Gung University, Taiwan
Prof. Elcio Leal
University of Para, Brazil

Editor Biographies

Dr. Vivek Mishra is currently working as an Assistant Professor (grade-III) in Amity Institute of Click Chemistry Research and Studies (AICCRS) under the umbrella of Amity University Noida Campus. Before this, he joined the Department of Chemistry as a DST SERB-National Post-Doctoral Fellow in July 2017 from the Science and Engineering Research Board, New Delhi, Government of India. Dr. Mishra completed his Ph.D. in Chemistry from the Institute of Science-Banaras Hindu University (BHU), Varanasi, UP, India in 2012. After that, he was offered three postdoctoral fellowships: one from the Indian Institute of Technology (IIT) Indore, MP, India, and the other two are from South Korea. He was a Post-doctoral Research Associate under Brain Korea-21 programme at University of Ulsan, Ulsan, South Korea, and as a Specialist (PDF) at Korea Institute of Industrial Technology, Cheonan-si, South Korea for two years. Dr. Mishra's research is mainly focused on synthesis and characterization of polymers with selected functionality, composition, and molecular architecture, Drug delivery, Hydrogel and nanogel synthesis, Stimuli-responsive polymers, Magnetic nanoparticles for water remediation, catalysis, and dye removal and degradation, biowaste/plastic waste utilization for fruitful by-products. He has published 50 papers in international journals of high repute with H index of 20 and i-10 index 25, 4 International Patents and 6 Indian Patents, also presented a dozen papers in national and international symposia/conferences.

Dr. Ramendra Pati Pandey is an Associate Professor, School of Health Sciences and Technology (SOHST), UPES, Dehradun, 248007, Uttarakhand, India. He has also served as an Associate Professor in the Department of Biotechnology/Microbiology/Biomedical Engineering at SRM University, Delhi-NCR, Sonepat. He was a FAPESP Post-Doctoral Fellow at the Department of Medicine-InCor/HC-FMUSP, University of Sao Paulo, School of Medicine, Brazil. He was also a Research Associate at the Translational Health Science and Technology Institute, Faridabad-Gurgaon Expressway, Faridabad Gurgaon, India. Prior to joining as a research scholar for his Ph.D., he got a fellowship of National Science Council of Taiwan to work at Chang Gung University for two years from March 2007 to March 2009. He did his Doctorate Degree (2014) from University of Delhi, New Delhi, India. During his PhD, he developed nanoparticles carrying two secretory proteins of *Mycobacterium tuberculosis* – CFP-10 and CFP-21 and evaluated their potential to invoke an immune response coupled with oxidative stress when encapsulated in nanoparticles. He did his M.Sc. in Biotechnology from the School of Biotechnology, Jawaharlal Nehru University (JNU), New Delhi, India. He was an executive council member of the Indian Immunology Society. He is an editorial board member of more than ten journals.

Dr. Anjali Priyadarshini is an Associate Professor of Biomedical Engineering at SRM University, Delhi-NCR, Sonepat, India. She obtained her M.Sc. degree in Biotechnology from Banaras Hindu University, Varanasi, and received a Ph.D.

degree in Biomedical Sciences from Post Graduate Institute of Medical Education & Research (PGI), Chandigarh. She has published several articles in international journals of high repute, books, and chapters, and also presented a dozen papers in national and international symposia/conferences. Her research interests are related to biotechnology and nanotechnology fields.

Prof. Chung-Ming Chang has a Ph.D. degree in Animal Genetics from Institut National Agronomique Paris-Grignon, France, and a Master's degree in Veterinary Medicine National Taiwan University, Taiwan. He is also a Doctor of Veterinary Medicine National License of Doctor Veterinary Medicine, Taiwan. His expertise areas are Virology and Human Molecular Genetics; Avian Influenza; Human endogenous retrovirus: Copy number and insertional polymorphism study of human endogenous retrovirus HERV-K in rheumatoid arthritis patients. He has published several articles and review papers in international journals of high repute and also presented a dozen papers in national and international symposia/conferences.

Prof. Elcio Leal graduated in Veterinary Medicine from the Federal University of Paraná (1994), a Master's in veterinary medicine (Virology) from the Federal University of Rio Grande do Sul/Porto Alegre Biotechnology Center (1998), and a Ph.D. in Biotechnology from the University of São Paulo (2004). Postdoctoral candidate at the University of Tokyo (Laboratory of Biometry and Bioinformatics Graduate School of Agriculture and Life Sciences) and Federal University of São Paulo (Retrovirology Laboratory). He is currently an Adjunct Professor at the Federal University of Pará, where he teaches evolution, virology, and genetics. He has experience in the field of viral evolution, with an emphasis on metagenomics and phylogenetic analysis. Acting on the following topics: RNA virus evolution, Phylogenetics, Population genetics, Bayesian methods, Structural biology, and Bioinformatics.

Contributors

Neha Aggarwal
Centre for Drug Design Discovery and
    Development (C4D)
SRM University, Delhi-NCR
Rajiv Gandhi Education City, Sonepat,
    Haryana, India

Amrendra Ajay
Department of Medicine
Harvard Medical School
Boston, MA, United States

Sandrine Auger
Micalis Institute, INRAE,
    AgroParisTech
Université Paris-Saclay
Jouy-en-Josas, France

Vivekanand Bahuguna
School of Biological Sciences
Doon University
Dehradun, Uttarakhand, India

Chung-Ming Chang
Master & Ph.D. program in
    Biotechnology Industry
Chang Gung University
Wenhua, Guishan Dist., Taoyuan City,
    Taiwan

Tanushri Chatterji
School of Bioscience
Institute of Management Studies
Adhyatmik Nagar, Ghaziabad,
    Uttar Pradesh, India

Hitesh Chopra
Chitkara College of Pharmacy
Chitkara University
Rajpura, Punjab, India

Srijita Chowdhury
Department of Biotechnology
National Institute of Technology
Rourkela, Odisha, India

Vandana Dahiya
Department of Biomedical Engineering
SRM University, Delhi-NCR
Rajiv Gandhi Education City, Sonepat,
    Haryana, India

Ruby Dhiman
Centre for Drug Design Discovery and
    Development (C4D)
SRM University, Delhi-NCR
Rajiv Gandhi Education City, Sonepat,
    Haryana, India

Sonal Gaur
Department of Ophthalmology
Medical University of South Carolina
Charleston, South Carolina, USA

Gunjan
Centre for Drug Design Discovery and
    Development (C4D)
SRM University, Delhi-NCR
Rajiv Gandhi Education City, Sonepat,
    Haryana, India

Archana Gupta
Department of Biotechnology
SRM University, Delhi-NCR
Rajiv Gandhi Education City, Sonepat,
    Haryana, India

Himanshu
Centre for Drug Design Discovery and
    Development (C4D)
SRM University, Delhi NCR
Rajiv Gandhi Education City, Sonepat,
    Haryana, India

Sakshi Kataria
Centre for Drug Design Discovery and
    Development (C4D)
SRM University, Delhi-NCR
Rajiv Gandhi Education City, Sonepat,
    Haryana, India

Namrata Khanna
Department of Biochemistry
M A Rangoonwala College of Dental
    Sciences and Research Centre
Maharashtra, India

Dheeresh Kumar
Department of Pulmonary Medicine
Vallabhbhai Patel Chest Institute
University of Delhi
Delhi, India

Manoj Kumar
Department of Pulmonary Medicine
Vallabhbhai Patel Chest Institute
University of Delhi
Delhi, India

Umesh Kumar
Department of Bioscience
Institute of Management Studies
Adhyatmik Nagar, Ghaziabad,
    Uttar Pradesh, India

Jyoti Kumari
Pranveer Singh Institute of Technology
    (Pharmacy)
Bhisi Jargaon, Kanpur, Uttar Pradesh,
    India

Mansi Kumari
Department of Bioscience
Institute of Management Studies
Adhyatmik Nagar, Ghaziabad,
    Uttar Pradesh, India

Anil Kumar Mavi
Department of Botany & Life Science
Sri Aurobindo College
University of Delhi
Delhi, India

Vivek Mishra
Amity Institute of Click Chemistry
    Research and Studies
Amity University
Noida, Uttar Pradesh, India

Riya Mukherjee
Master & Ph.D. program in
    Biotechnology Industry
Chang Gung University
Wenhua, Guishan Dist., Taoyuan City,
    Taiwan

Ramendra Pati Pandey
School of Health Sciences and
    Technology (SOHST)
UPES
Dehradun, Uttarakhand, India

G D Ghouse Peer
Centre for Drug Design Discovery and
    Development (C4D)
SRM University, Delhi-NCR
Rajiv Gandhi Education City, Sonepat,
    Haryana, India

Keshva Sai Pentapati
Department of Biotechnology
GITAM School of Sciences
Gandhi Institute of Technology and
    Management (Deemed to be
    University)
Bangalore, Karnataka, India

Anjali Priyadarshini
Centre for Drug Design Discovery and
  Development (C4D)
SRM University, Delhi-NCR
Rajiv Gandhi Education City, Sonepat,
  Haryana, India

V. Samuel Raj
Centre for Drug Design Discovery and
  Development (C4D)
SRM University, Delhi-NCR
Rajiv Gandhi Education City, Sonepat,
  Haryana, India

Neeraj Rajdan
Department of Pharmacology
Government Medical College
Haldwani, Uttarakhand, India

Monika Rani
Department of Mechanical and
  Industrial Engineering
University of Brescia
Piazza del Mercato, Brescia BS, Italy

Kumar Rakesh Ranjan
Amity Institute of Applied Sciences
Amity University
Noida, Uttar Pradesh, India

Krislay Rathour
Pranveer Singh Institute of Technology
  (Pharmacy)
Kanpur, Uttar Pradesh, India

Bhupendra Sahu
Department of Bioscience
Institute of Management Studies
Adhyatmik Nagar, Ghaziabad,
  Uttar Pradesh, India

Anu Saini
Centre for Drug Design Discovery and
  Development (C4D)
SRM University, Delhi-NCR
Rajiv Gandhi Education City, Sonepat,
  Haryana, India

Yashendra Sethi
Government Doon Medical College
Dehradun, Uttarakhand, India

Gaurav Sharma
Department of Translational &
  Regenerative Medicine
Postgraduate Institute of Medical
  Education & Research
Chandigarh, India

Kunal Sharma
Department of Pharmacology
Government Medical College
Haldwani, Uttarakhand, India

Avanish Kumar Shrivastav
Department of Biotechnology
Delhi Technological University
Delhi, India

Vikas Shukla
Department of Zoology
University of Delhi
Delhi, India

Arun Kumar Singh
School of Bioscience
Institute of Management Studies
Adhyatmik Nagar, Ghaziabad,
  Uttar Pradesh, India

Mamata Singh
Department of Chemistry
GITAM School of Sciences
Gandhi Institute of Technology and
  Management
Bangalore, Karnataka, India

N.P. Singh
Center for Nano science and
  Engineering (CeNSE)
Indian Institute of Science
Bangalore, Karnataka, India

Tanya Singh
Department of Botany
TPS College, Patliputra University
Mithapur, Patna, Bihar, India

Amrita Soni
Department of Biomedical Engineering
SRM University, Delhi-NCR
Rajiv Gandhi Education City, Sonepat,
  Haryana, India

Bhavana Srivastava
Department of Pharmacology
Government Medical College
Haldwani, Uttarakhand, India

Neelam Thakur
Department of Zoology
Sardar Patel University
Vallabh Government College Campus,
  Paddal, Kartarpur, Mandi, Himachal
  Pradesh, India

Devika Tripathi
Pranveer Singh Institute of Technology
  (Pharmacy)
Kanpur, Uttar Pradesh, India

Arpana Vibhuti
Centre for Drug Design Discovery and
  Development (C4D)
SRM University, Delhi-NCR
Rajiv Gandhi Education City, Sonepat,
  Haryana, India
and
Department of Biomedical Engineering
SRM University, Delhi-NCR
Rajiv Gandhi Education City, Sonepat,
  Haryana, India

Jasmina Vidic
Micalis Institute, INRAE,
  AgroParisTech
Université Paris-Saclay
Jouy-en-Josas, France

Daanish Vij
Department of Bioscience
Institute of Management Studies
Adhyatmik Nagar, Ghaziabad,
  Uttar Pradesh, India

Lakshay Virmani
Department of Bioscience
Institute of Management Studies
Adhyatmik Nagar, Ghaziabad,
  Uttar Pradesh, India

Manoj K. Yadav
Department of Biomedical Engineering
SRM University, Delhi-NCR
Rajiv Gandhi Education City, Sonepat,
  Haryana, India

1 Personalized Therapeutics

G D Ghouse Peer, Anu Saini, Arpana Vibhuti, and Amrendra Ajay

1.1 INTRODUCTION

Many drugs are designed and developed in such a way that they can be helpful to a vast population, as this is considered "one-drug-fits-all," but it may not be efficient for some people, as in the clinical trials, a few individual patients show no response and others show some drastic changes. Here, the statement "one drug fits for all" is wrong (Jain, 2021a). So personalized solutions for individual patients must be needed and an individualized approach is a must. Each individual has their own unique molecular and genetic profile, which makes them susceptible to certain diseases as a result of this, individuals are considered more prone to some diseases (Per. Med., n.d.). Alteration of the medical treatment for each patient by their characteristic is considered Personalized Therapeutics.

Many reasons contribute to the development of personalized medicine but advances in molecular biology have been particularly significant. The whole set of human chromosomes is made up of a collection of lengthy DNA polymers that make a complete human genome. Up until 2003, when the complete human genome DNA sequence was discovered by the "Human Genome Project", the entire sequence was unknown (*Human Genome – Origins of the Human Genome/Britannica*, n.d.). Human chromosomes, genes, genetic coding, gene expression, DNA sequencing, and their structure have all been the subject of much research over the past two decades. This research has had a substantial impact on the development of personalized medicine. Pharmacogenomics and pharmacogenetics are the two important studies where this personalization process is based and begins during the drug development stage. They are commonly acknowledged as the first stages in personalized medicine. They have the potential to completely change how drug design is applied. Additionally, the use of pharmacogenetics and pharmacogenomics are the development and treatment of many diseases (Figure 1.1). Medicine will transition to a new era of customized medicine and stop concentrating, as it has previously done, on symptomatic disease management and empirical drug-prescribing regimens (Mini & Nobili, 2009a).

The development of personalized medicines has been aided by genomics, proteomics, and metabolomics technology (Jain, 2021g, 2021f). Before the human genome was sequenced, biological treatments were personalized. The ideal way to incorporate emerging biotechnologies into medical practice to enhance patient care

DOI: 10.1201/9781003348672-1

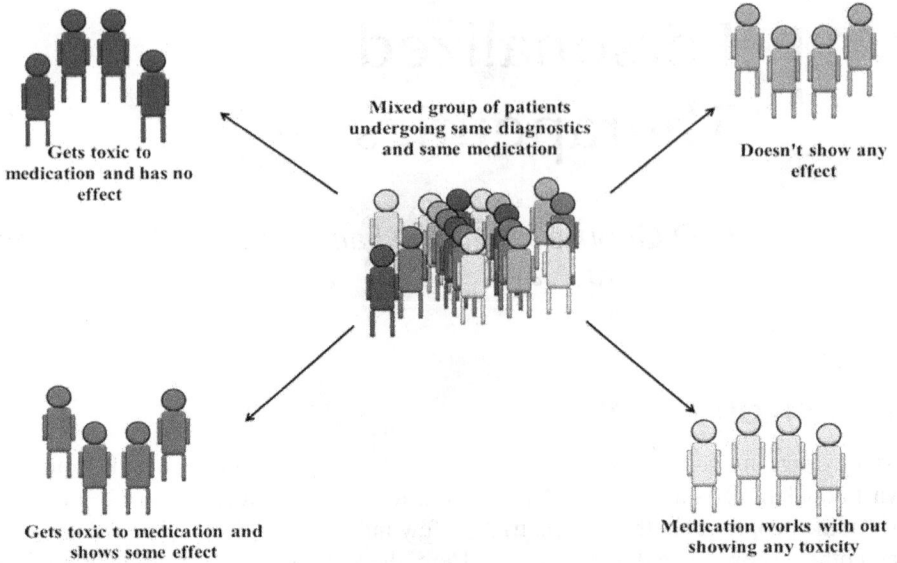

FIGURE 1.1 Representation of how medication and diagnosis differ for each individuals (*The Role of Pharmacogenomics in Precision Medicine/Medical Laboratory Observer*, n.d.).

is through personalized medicine. Previously, because they were designed for each patient, blood transfusion and organ transplantation were the first personalized medicines. Vaccines made from a patient's unique tumor cells are among the cell therapies that use the patient's cells and are regarded as personalized medicines. Recombinant human proteins have made it possible to personalize treatments more recently. Recent scientific and technical developments have increased our knowledge of illness causation, altered how diseases are diagnosed, and modified how they are treated, making it possible to provide each patient with more precise, powerful, and individualized healthcare. There seems to be a connection between certain diseases and genetic, genomic, and epigenetic changes. The development of causal network models in which a genomic region is postulated to influence the quantities of transcripts, proteins, and metabolites is made possible by deep clinical phenotyping in conjunction with sophisticated molecular phenotypic profiling. To understand the pathophysiology of networks at the molecular and cellular level, phenotypic analysis is crucial (Seyhan & Carini, 2019).

Different names for personalized medicine include customized drug therapy, genomic medicine, molecular medicine, integrated healthcare, individually tailored medicine, and precision medicine (Figure 1.2). Personalized medicines, also known as genomic medicine where each patient's unique genome will assist in determining the best course of treatment, whether it is preventive, diagnostic, or therapeutic. For the term precision medicine diagnostic, prognostic, and therapeutic approaches are precisely customized to each patient's needs; the term "precision medicine" is frequently used for the personalized medicine (Lamberti et al., 2012). The high rate of adverse medication reactions and their lack of efficacy in many people, which

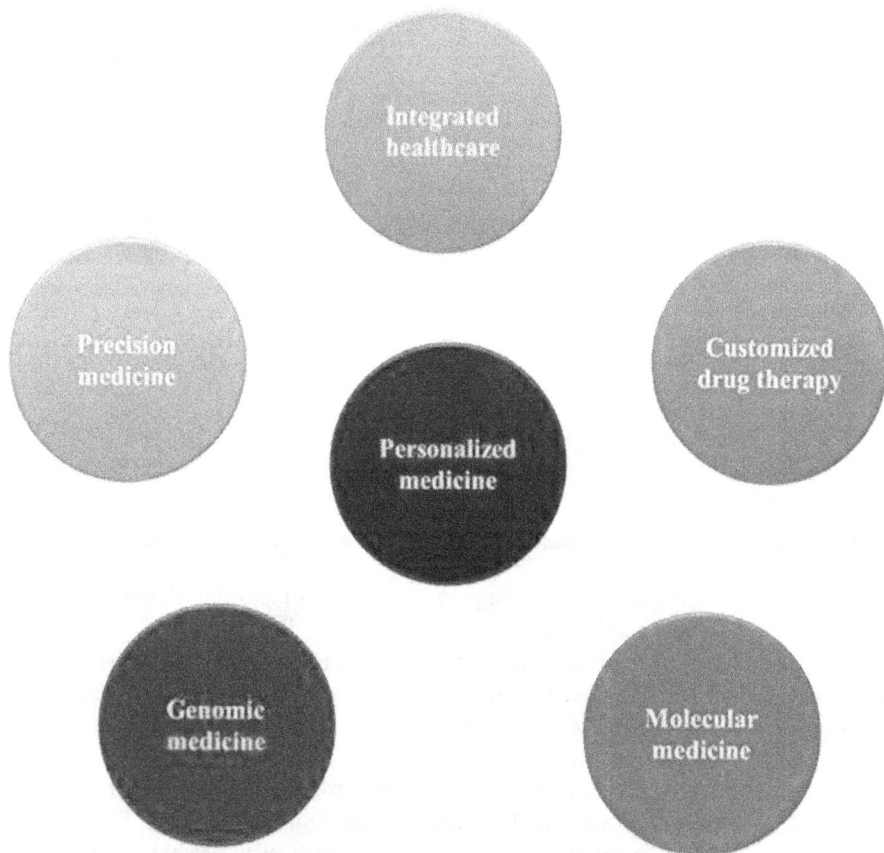

FIGURE 1.2 Terms that represent personalized medicines.

can be predicted by knowledge of their specific genetic makeup, is the clinical need for novel techniques to better drug therapy (Wilke et al., 2007).

1.2 DEVELOPMENT OF PERSONALIZED MEDICINE

The development of contemporary molecular biology technology has led to a paradigm change in the life sciences. The sequencing of the human genome has been the most significant development in this area. There are different biological treatment functions in the advancement of personalized medicine. Recombinant proteins, vaccinations, RNAi, and cell and gene therapies, in particular vaccines generated from the patient's tumor cells, are key components of personalized medicine (Figure 1.3).

One of the biological treatments for personalized medicine is recombinant human proteins. Many diseases are treated with recombinant human proteins and other protein-based products. They are used widely because they are believed to be structurally and biologically identical to their endogenous counterparts and because

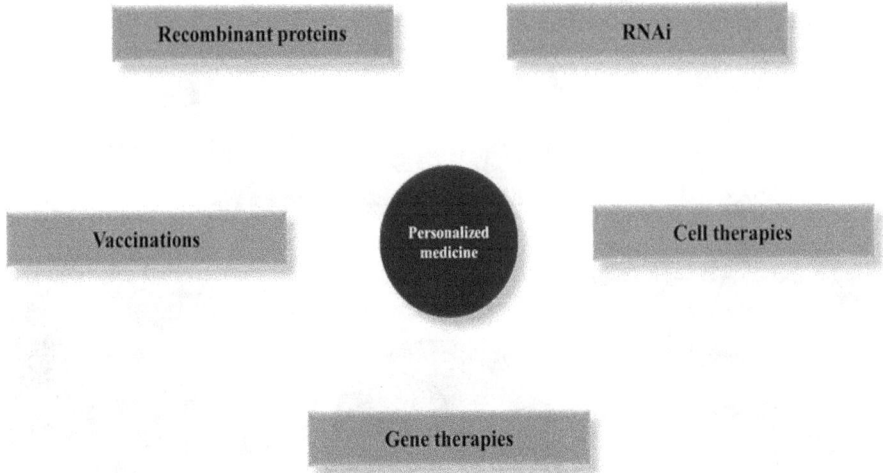

FIGURE 1.3 Various technologies combined to develop personalized medicine.

they are biologically safe when compared to items of animal or human origin. However, the production of antibodies against these medications could make the use of recombinant proteins more challenging (Schellekens & Casadevall, 2004). Most of these proteins are recombinant human or "humanized" molecules. The immunogenicity of therapeutic proteins can have negative effects, and the antibody reaction to therapeutic proteins in traditional animal models is typically not indicative of the reaction in humans. Accurate detection, characterization, and evaluation of antibody responses are required to evaluate these compounds' immunogenicity. The development of computational techniques for predicting the epitopes in protein molecules that may trigger an immunological response in a recipient has advanced significantly, which produces therapeutic proteins. To restrict the use of recombinant proteins in patients where they are not only beneficial but also unlikely to trigger immunological reactions, they can be developed in conjunction with diagnostic assays. Another strategy for protein treatment is in vivo protein production using genetically modified cells, where protein administration can be tailored to the demands of the patient. This contribution can be used to develop a personalized medicine (Jain, 2011).

1.2.1 Recombinant Technology for the Development of Personalized Medicine

Recombinant technology can now be used to create biological therapies with therapeutic potential for personalized medicine. Monoclonal antibodies (mAb) are immune system defenses made by a single B cell clone. Unlike polyclonal antibodies, which are heterogeneous and monospecific, monospecific antibodies (mAb) are useful tools for developing treatments and diagnostics for personalized medicine (Breedveld, 2000). mAbs are therapeutic proteins that differ from chemical medications like aminosalicylates, antimetabolites, and immunosuppressants due to their distinctive pharmacokinetic properties (Di Paolo & Luci, 2021). mAbs are far more selective than small-molecule medications and are less likely to be hazardous due to causes other than their mode of action. Small compounds that can be taken orally have a wide range of targets, but they also have the potential to be hepatotoxic and interact with other drugs. mAbs have an excellent safety profile, which makes them very appealing. They can be made to be very specialized and responsive to the target. For many years, mAbs have been considered the best molecules for cancer therapy. The utility of mAbs in molecular targeting therapeutics has been significantly increased by genetic engineering them to create chimeric or humanized mAbs. The use of monoclonal antibodies (mAbs) alone or in conjunction with immunoconjugates or current standard chemotherapy has shown promise in numerous clinical trials for the treatment of particular disorders, such as cancer (Zahavi & Weiner, 2020).

1.2.1.1 Cell-Based Therapies

Personalized medicine will greatly benefit from the use of **cell therapies**. In addition to avoiding some of the ethical concerns associated with the use of embryonic stem cells, adult stem cells from a specific patient are better suited for personalized therapy. The possibility of personalized cell-based therapy will increase with the development of technology to produce induced pluripotent stem cells from adult somatic cells. It is possible to mobilize a patient's stem cells in vivo for therapeutic purposes, and numerous medications, including biological agents, are being researched for personalized medicine (K. K. Jain, n.d.).

1.2.1.2 Gene Therapy

The use of **gene therapy** to tailor cancer treatment will increase. Gene-expression signatures and imaging technologies have the potential to play significant roles as biomarkers in the future, even though single-gene mutation-based diagnostics are often utilized in clinical oncology treatment now (Wistuba et al., 2011). Since the gene was identified as the fundamental component of heredity, the capacity to alter the human genome at precise sites has been a goal in medicine. Gene therapy is thus defined as the ability to change a person's genetic makeup through the correction of altered (mutated) genes or site-specific alterations that are intended to treat a medical condition. The development of genetics and bioengineering, which allowed for the manipulation of vectors for the transfer of extrachromosomal material to target cells, made this therapy possible. The optimization of delivery vehicles (vectors), which are mostly plasmids, nanostructured materials, or viruses, is one of this technique's primary areas of interest (Gonçalves & Paiva, 2017). Genetically altered cells can secrete therapeutic compounds like neurotrophic factors. Ex vivo gene therapy is genetically altering patient cells in vitro, typically using viral vectors, before reinjecting these cells back into the patient's body tissues. It is possible to use additional DNA components to activate the healthy gene in the appropriate cells and concentrations. This is an instance of personalized therapy.

1.2.1.3 Personalized Vaccinations

A growing understanding of immune response phenotype/genotype information has been a foundation for the development of **personalized vaccinations**, thanks to the use of various "omics" technologies. When referring to vaccines, the term "personalized" means "targeting" vaccine antigens to achieve the best possible result, which is to maximize immunogenicity while minimizing the risk of vaccine failure or reactogenicity and side effects in a host at risk for serious illness or complications. In terms of the objectives of immunization provision, it refers to an improved set of results. Personalized might relate to the individual level, the gender level, the racial/ethnic level, or the subpopulation level. This is an instance of personalized therapy (Poland et al., 2008). Cancer and viral diseases are two crucial areas where personalized vaccinations might be used. Vaccines against cancer make an effort to take advantage of the immune system's capacity for resistance and specificity. Cancer vaccines work to activate the immune system to find, target, and eliminate tumor cells. Cancer vaccines are therapeutic, as opposed to vaccinations used to prevent infectious diseases, and the majority of personalized cancer vaccines are cell-based (Jain, 2005).

1.2.1.4   RNA Interference (RNAi)

A crucial physiological process for suppressing gene expression, RNA interference (**RNAi**), can be used to develop novel medications (Dykxhoorn et al., 2006; Dykxhoorn & Lieberman, 2006). Antisense therapy is regarded as a type of gene therapy since it modifies gene function for therapeutic purposes by using antisense oligonucleotides (AOs) to block aberrant disease-related proteins. However, AOs are different from conventional gene therapies in that they cannot produce proteins; instead, they can only prevent the expression of genes that are already present. Therapeutic applications are increasingly potential for personalized medicine as new technologies are solving some of the AOs' drug delivery issues. Antisense has been improved into RNA interference (RNAi), which is used to control gene expression. siRNAs may be employed as genotype-specific medications to mediate allele-specific inhibition in addition to being a tool for studying gene activity. By focusing on an SNP in POLR2A (the major subunit of RNA polymerase II situated adjacent to the tumor suppressor gene p53, which typically exhibits loss of heterozygosity in cancer cells), siRNA has been demonstrated to provide genotype-specific suppression of tumor development in vivo. Consequently, RNAi may be crucial to the practice of personalized medicine.

1.3   BIOMARKERS

Free radical biologists have adopted the word "biomarker" from molecular epidemiology to designate a molecular alteration in a biological molecule that results from an attack by reactive oxygen, nitrogen species (*Markers of Oxidative Damage and Antioxidant Protection: Current Status and Relevance to Disease/ Request* PDF, n.d.). It relates to products made from lipids, DNA, proteins, and antioxidant consumption, with the type of reaction being either direct addition, proton abstraction, or electron transfer. Biomarkers are a large group of signs that can be tested precisely and repeatedly. They are objective indicators of a patient's health as seen from the outside. Medical symptoms, on the other hand, are only those markers of health or illness that patients themselves may perceive (Strimbu & Tavel, 2010). The improvement of the drug development process as well as the overall biomedical research sector depends heavily on biomarkers. Expanding our toolbox of treatments for all diseases and improving our comprehension of typical, healthy physiology depends on our ability to relate quantifiable biological processes to clinical outcomes. The necessity of utilizing biomarkers as surrogate outcomes in sizable trials of serious diseases, including cancer (Ellenberg & Hamilton, 1989) and heart disease (Wittes et al., 1989), has been heavily disputed at least since the 1980s. The FDA continues to support research on potential new biomarkers that could be used as surrogates in upcoming trials as well as the use of biomarkers in fundamental and clinical research.

Early clinical studies using biomarker techniques have begun, and they are rapidly being employed to provide new diagnoses that help to stratify or distinguish the expected effects of therapeutic intervention. To date, a great deal of work has gone into finding new biomarkers that can be applied in clinical settings. However, there are not many markers that are used in clinical practice.

1.3.1 DIAGNOSTIC AND PREDICTIVE BIOMARKERS

The predictive and prognostic biomarker categories are particularly crucial for personalized therapy. Predictive biomarkers are baseline or pre-treatment data that reveal whether patients are more or less likely to benefit from a certain treatment. A predictive biomarker is frequently chosen to be a companion predictive biomarker in the development of a specific therapeutic medication. As a typical oncology example, a biomarker that detects over-expression of the growth factor protein Her-2, which transmits growth signals to breast cancer cells, maybe a predictive biomarker for the administration of trastuzumab (Herceptin), a drug that inhibits the effects of Her-2, to breast cancer patients. Prognostic biomarkers are measurements taken before therapy that reveal information about the long-term outcome of individuals who have not received treatment or those who have. Prognostic biomarkers, unlike predictive biomarkers, represent baseline risk and may not always signal responsiveness to a specific treatment, but they can nevertheless recommend a course of action for patients receiving routine care. Patients with a bad prognosis would need a more aggressive course of treatment, while those with a sufficiently favorable outlook would not need any more therapies (Matsui, 2013).

Biomarkers will help in early disease identification and therapeutic optimization. Combining diagnosis and treatment is a key component of personalized medicine, and biomarkers will play a significant part in this. As a result of the use of biomarkers, there will be a rise in the number of new pharmaceuticals that are appropriate for personalized treatment. Validated biomarkers will become more important in clinical trials for personalized therapy. Personalized care of numerous diseases will be aided by biomarker-based drug efficacy monitoring (Jain, 2021e).

1.3.2 BIOMARKER VALIDATION CRITERIA

A biomarker's intended usage should determine the criteria for verifying the biomarker. For predictive and prognostic biomarkers, three distinct methods of validation have been proposed: Analytical or quantitative validation is the process of determining the assay's robustness, repeatability, and accuracy of measurement in comparison to a gold standard test, if one is available. The other one is clinical validation, which is the determination of a biomarker's capacity to forecast treatment outcomes or prognosis in a given patient. A prognostic biomarker's clinical validity may be indicated by a correlation between its status and a clinical outcome. A randomized clinical study would be necessary to accurately quantify treatment effects and determine whether the treatment effects vary based on the status of the biomarker, or whether there is a treatment-by-biomarker interaction. The last one is the clinical significance or clinical utility (Simon, 2010; Hunter et al., 2008), where the biomarker is used in clinical settings, that it enhances patient outcomes, and that it benefits patients. Therefore, comparing the improved patient outcomes linked with the use of the established prognostic biomarker to those based on a standard of treatment without the biomarker is a crucial step in determining clinical value. Treatment outcomes related to the application of the created predictive biomarker will be assessed in the co-development of novel treatments and companion predictive biomarker (Simon, 2010).

1.3.3 BIOMARKERS PRESENT IMPACT ON PERSONALIZED MEDICINE

Expectations for how biomarkers might revolutionize clinical research and personalized therapy are very high. Within the past ten years, numerous biomarker techniques have started early clinical trials. To discriminate or stratify the anticipated results of therapeutic intervention, biomarkers are increasingly being used in diagnostics. However, the rate of adoption of personalized medicine is generally thought to have been slower than anticipated (Milne et al., 2014). There has not yet been much of an impact on personalized medicine and treatments. Although the subject is still in its early stages of development, the pharmaceutical and diagnostics industries anticipate tremendous growth based on the foundations already in place. In particular, the understanding of disease heterogeneity and therapeutic response is made possible by advances in genomes and proteomics. Over the past ten years, enormous efforts have been made to identify novel cancer biomarkers for use in clinical practice as well as to provide the necessary technology to support the clinical setting. However, there is a startling disparity between the amount of work put into finding biomarkers and the number of indicators with established therapeutic relevance.

1.4 PHARMACOGENOMICS AND PERSONALIZED THERAPEUTICS

It is commonly acknowledged that Pharmacogenetics and Pharmacogenomics are the first steps toward personalized treatment, which are acknowledged universally. They engage with variations in medication responses that are genetically determined in individuals and have the potential to transform drug therapy by modifying it to each person's genotype. Pharmacogenomics mainly deals with the examination of the variation in gene expression at the cellular, tissue, individual, or population level that affects medication response and disease susceptibility (*WORK PROGRAMME FOR THE EUROPEAN AGENCY FOR THE EVALUATION OF MEDICINAL PRODUCTS 2002*, n.d.).

1.4.1 Current Scenario of Pharmacogenomic Technology

Using high-throughput technology, pharmacogenomics examines how the entire genome or its byproducts connect to drug response. There are two key functions of pharmacogenomics in personalized medicine. It first directs pharmaceutical companies in drug development and discovery. Second, it helps doctors choose the best medication for patients based on their genetic makeup, avoid adverse drug reactions, and maximize drug efficacy by providing the appropriate amount. And recent technologies including the development of arrays for the concurrent evaluation of several genes have been the most significant modification. Initial research "printed" a sequence of gene clones onto a silicone-coated glass slide using robotics-based technologies. The fluorescence intensity emitted from each gene clone and the observed amount of gene expression were shown to be correlated by tagging the relevant mRNA with a fluorochrome. Large gene clones from the Human Genome Project, short oligonucleotides for particular genes, and cDNA produced from differential expression initiatives have all been added to this method (Eisen & Brown, 1999).

The advancement of pharmacogenomics has been greatly aided by computational biology or bioinformatics. In a single experiment, gene expression arrays, and high throughput genotyping techniques generate a lot of data, far more than can be analyzed manually or with readily accessible spreadsheets. As a result, software has been created that not only records experimental data but also compares the results with genome databases already in existence, generates dendrograms for sequence homology, and uses pattern recognition as part of the initial algorithm to group genes with similar patterns of expression. This gives the researcher a robust and thorough output that allows for quick data analysis and application (McLeod et al., 2001).

1.5 PHARMACOGENOMICS AND DRUG DESIGN

The use of genomic data for drug target identification and evaluation, lead optimization through high throughput screening, and evaluation of drug-metabolizing enzymes, drug transporters, and drug receptors using computer-assisted techniques and bioinformatics library database are all ways that pharmacogenomics, both structural and functional, can facilitate the drug discovery process (Gupta & Jhawat, 2017).

Initially, several precandidate genes that may be helpful for drug discovery have already been identified as a result of the analysis of single nucleotide polymorphism data. Drug development can make use of knowledge gained through research on the role of genes, their interactions, their function in biological processes, as well as their variation among the population. Possible targets for drug development can be found by examining how gene expression changes from healthy tissues through the course of disease development in various populations. Lead selection, which can be based equally on biomarkers of toxicity or biomarkers of efficacy, is another crucial stage in the drug discovery process. The ability to create expression Pharmacogenomics profiles of medication response for numerous classes of pharmaceuticals in target tissues is made possible by the use of mRNA transcript profiling techniques in conjunction with database searches. The analysis of these response profiles can reveal biomarkers that relate to toxicity or efficacy. These biomarkers can lower the cost of drug development by helping to prioritize response profiles such as cardiotoxicity and hepatotoxicity (Jain, 2021d).

The incidence of Adverse Drug reactions would decrease and the drug manufacturer would avoid lawsuits, bad press, and even the possibility of having to pull a drug off the market if genetic tests based on Pharmacogenomics were available to screen patients before drug administration to determine whether the given drug may or may not be suitable for a given patient. It might potentially aid in expanding the market for some pharmaceuticals (*Bernard: The Five Myths of Pharmacogenomics Prevailing ... - Google Schola*r, n.d.). In drugs, designing Pharmacogenomics has a wide range of possible uses, including techniques for forecasting efficacy or toxicity during clinical development and the identification of novel targets against which new medicines are developed (Evans & Relling, 1999). It offers the potential to speed up the medication development process by lowering the number of individuals needed for early clinical trials to demonstrate efficacy (Fijal et al., 2000).

Mouse and humans are used to identify particular genes or genomic locations connected to the disease of concern, single nucleotide polymorphism initiatives. Gene expression array research is being adopted similarly. To synthesize mRNA for comparison with normal reference tissue, disease tissue is employed. Gene hunting is the aim of this strategy, hence arrays that cover the most known and unknown genes are preferred. The search for novel therapeutic targets is one of the objectives of the SNP and gene array exercise. These may be potential modifiers of the disease phenotype or novel disease processes. Once the target has been identified, a significant amount of work must go into confirming its viability in terms of the frequency of expression in the diseased tissue, the pattern of normal tissue expression for toxicity prediction, and normal-disease tissue expression. This is regarded as a strategy in the early stages of drug development.

To specify the mode of action for novel drugs or to check for an agent's direct impact on a particular pathway, gene expression arrays are also used. During *in vivo* testing, even medicines created using the most mechanistically grounded method-ology can exhibit surprises (Rowinsky et al., 1999). A profile of the genes altered following drug exposure can be created using expression arrays, which may lead to a better understanding of the mechanisms of action. Gene expression arrays may also be applied for novel compound screening. Gene dynamics can be employed as a functional readout for drug activity *in vitro* or even *in vivo* by building arrays for the genes implicated in a pathway of interest (McLeod et al., 2001).

One such example is testing by thiopurine methyltransferase (TPMT) which is used on individuals who may benefit from treatment with thiopurine drugs. Some autoimmune diseases, such as Crohn's disease and rheumatoid arthritis, as well as some cancers, like leukemia, are treated using thiopurine medications. The TPMT enzyme aids in the degradation of thiopurine medications. People with TPMT deficiencies have a slower rate of medication breakdown and elimination. As a result, there is an increased chance of adverse effects, such as bone marrow destruction, since the medication concentration in the body is too high (hematopoi-etic toxicity). Genetic testing can help diagnose TPMT deficiency so that a patient's doctor can limit the risk of major side effects by providing thiopurine medications at lower-than-usual doses or utilizing other medications (*Precision Medicine and Pharmacogenomics – Mayo Clinic*, n.d.).

1.6 PHARMACOGENETICS AND PERSONALIZED MEDICINE

The term "Pharmacogenetics" was first used by Friederich Vogel in 1959 (Vogel, 1959) to describe a brand-new field of study using genetic and pharmacological techniques to investigate the impact of hereditary variables on drug response variability (Mini & Nobili, 2009b). It is a branch of pharmacogenomics that aims to explain variations in drug absorption, distribution, metabolism, and excretion as well as pharmacological action using DNA-based analyses. When it comes to the basics, Pharmacogenetics is the study of how genetic influences on medication action, as opposed to genetic causes of disease, affect health. This was used first during the pre-genomic period. This helps to understand the relationship between an individual's genotype and their capacity to metabolize a foreign substance. This is a gateway to studying the link between phenotypic and genotypic reactions during drug metabolism (Figure 1.4). When it comes to how people respond to drugs, demographic variances are frequently bigger than those found inside an individual. Inheritance as a factor in medication response is compatible with the presence of huge population differences and low interpatient variability. Genetics is thought to be responsible for close to 20% to 95% of the heterogeneity regarding drug metabolism and effects. There are interindividual variations in the effectiveness and toxicity of many drugs that have been connected to genetic variants in drug-metabolizing enzymes, transporters, receptors, and other drug targets (Jain, 2021c). Since genetic variations in medication responses, there have been significant advancements in Pharmacogenetics study.

The high occurrence of adverse medication reactions and their general lack of efficacy in many people, which may be predicted by Pharmacogenetics testing, has led to a therapeutic need for novel techniques to enhance drug therapy. Pharmacogenetics uses molecular data to more exactly categorize disease, enable the design and validation of new targeted medicines, treat patients with greater specificity and efficacy but fewer side effects, and more precisely identify disease propensity (Mini & Nobili, 2009a).

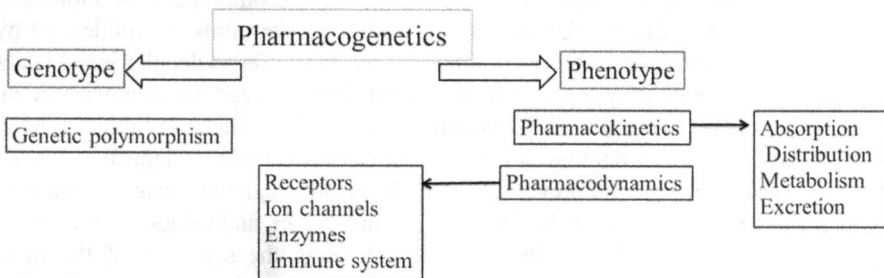

FIGURE 1.4 Using pharmacogenetics to connect genotype and phenotype (Jain, 2021c).

1.6.1 CLINICAL PHARMACOGENETICS AND THE POSSIBILITY OF PERSONALIZED MEDICINE

Pharmacogenetics aids in the understanding of interindividual variability in drug clearance and reactions in clinical practice and may be used in customized treatment via drug-metabolizing enzymes, drug transporters, and drug targets. Based on the genotypes of individuals, it is anticipated that personalized treatments will be made available shortly, optimizing dosage and reducing the frequency of negative medication reactions. A pharmaceutical, therapy, or preventative intervention that is specifically appropriate for a patient at the time of administration can be chosen using extensive information about that patient's genotype or level of gene expression as well as clinical data. This method has the advantages of accuracy, effectiveness, safety, and quickness. The phrase first appeared in the late 1990s as the Human Genome Project advanced (Zhou et al., 2008). Pharmacogenetics, in contrast to other genetic tests, characterizes a person based on their susceptibility to disease, risk of serious adverse effects, or even the effectiveness of specific medications (Grossman, 2007). A large portion of the uncertainty surrounding present pharmacotherapy can be eliminated by Pharmacogenetics testing, which can assess the expected effectiveness (Constable et al., 2006). The pharmacogenetic tests' ultimate objective is to help doctors prescribe the right medication at the right dose before therapy is started to reduce side effects and toxicity and maximize efficacy by excluding patients who are unlikely to benefit or who may be harmed (Grossman, 2007).

Pharmacogenetics may be able to pinpoint the ideal medicine and dosage for each patient. The use of pharmacogenetics attempts to develop better therapeutics and enhance the efficacy and safety of both upcoming and approved medications. All new drug applications submitted to the Food and Drug Administration must undergo minimal pharmacogenetic testing, which includes genotyping studies for drugs that are metabolized by enzymes whose genes have inactivating polymorphisms and prospective germline DNA collection from all subjects taking part in pre-approval clinical trials (Relling & Hoffman, 2007).

1.6.2 ROLE OF DIAGNOSIS IN PERSONALIZED MEDICINE

Delivering safe and efficient therapy for many diseases will depend heavily on molecular diagnostics, and the use of diagnostic testing to comprehend the molecular causes of a patient's disease. Up to 70% of healthcare decisions are influenced by diagnostics, and new generations of diagnostic tests that offer molecular insights are fulfilling the promise of personalized treatment. Personalized medicine relies on diagnostic tools in many ways. To decide which medical therapies will be most effective for each patient, doctors and medical researchers employ diagnostic tests. To better deliver therapeutic and preventive care, data from diagnostic tests is frequently coupled with an individual's medical history, circumstances, and values (*Personalized Medicine Focused on Diagnostics*, n.d.). By enabling the selection of the most appropriate treatment, assisting medical personnel in selecting the most effective preventative treatments, and providing crucial prognostic data that can optimize care pathways and management, diagnostics provide information that can benefit patients (Porter, 2010).

Early molecular diagnostic methods examined a single molecule, such as glucose, in the case of diabetes. However, "omics" technology has advanced significantly in the last ten years, making it possible to sequence a person's entire genome quickly, accurately, and affordably or to measure the concentrations of all proteins, metabolic by-products, or microbes in a sample of bodily fluid or tissue. Using the technology regularly has started to produce enormous data sets that artificial intelligence can mine to find new biomarkers helpful for medicine. With the ability to customize medicines to the molecular profiles of specific patients, high-throughput omics technology and artificial intelligence are ushering in a new era of enhanced diagnostics that will revolutionize how many diseases are understood and treated. For cancer, several cutting-edge diagnostics are already in use. One test, Oncotype DX (*Oncotype DX Tes*ts, n.d.), which screens 21 genes, showed that many breast cancer patients can forgo chemotherapy. Another, known as the Foundation One CDx test (*FoundationOne CDx/Foundation Medici*ne, n.d.), identifies specific gene-targeting medications that may be helpful for a certain patient by detecting genetic abnormalities in solid tumors in more than 300 genes. Unwanted uterine tissue grows in places other than the uterus in endometriosis, a painful condition. Surgery is frequently required for the diagnosis. Endometriosis can be detected with a new, non-invasive saliva-based test from DotLabs (*Could a Saliva Test Be the Future of Diagnosing Endo? A Q&A with D/EndoFound*, n.d.) by analyzing a panel of tiny molecules called microRNAs. Additionally, blood tests are being created to aid in the diagnosis of brain diseases, such as autism, Parkinson's disease, and Alzheimer's disease, which are currently identified by the subjective evaluation of symptoms by clinicians. Researchers are even examining whether whole genome sequencing, microbiome analysis, and measurements of hundreds of proteins and metabolites in healthy persons may provide personalized advice on how those people might prevent disease (*Advanced Diagnostics for Personalized Medicine – Scientific American*, n.d.).

Two test categories are important for personalized medication. One is the pharmacogenomics test, which is an assay designed to investigate interindividual differences in whole genome SNP maps, haplotype markers, or modifications in gene expression or inactivation that may be associated with pharmacological function and clinical intervention. Sometimes, the diagnosis depends more on the style or pattern of the change than it does on the specific biomarker. The other pharmacogenetic test is an analysis designed to examine interindividual differences in DNA sequence linked to drug absorption and disposition (pharmacokinetics), especially polymorphic differences in genes encoding the functions of transporters, involved in the metabolism of enzymes, receptors, and other proteins (Jain, 2021b).

1.6.3 CHALLENGES IN PERSONALIZED THERAPEUTICS

The multiple difficulties that scientists encounter impede the development of precision medicine, delaying its benefits and potential for patients. Absolute precision medicine requires the ability to pinpoint each patient's response, which is not straightforward from a research standpoint or workable from a pharmaco-logical, diagnostic, or prognostic standpoint. Before we are technologically and scientifically advanced enough to apply personalized medication, stratification of the patients' responses into groups may be more realistic and manageable first step to personalized medicine (Louca, 2012). For the effective implementation of this new healthcare system brought about by personalized medicine, various other issues must be addressed in addition to the scientific difficulties that scientists must overcome. These environments, which employ a completely new method for the drug development process and provide new and validated drug targets for the development of drugs with a much higher therapeutic success rate, safety, and cost efficiency, require well-trained and educated personnel to design, maintain, and education of medical professionals and the general public about these new advancements remains a significant challenge (Hudson, 2011). By providing patients with anticipatory and proactive knowledge, we are enabling them to take control of their health. They will be able to use the knowledge to maintain their health or benefit from treatments that are specifically suited to their genetic profile. However, because people will have the ability to forecast, based on their genetic profile, whether they are prone to specific diseases, they may decide that this is not an approach that is acceptable ("What Happened to Personalized Medicine?," 2012).

The ethics surrounding the use of patient information is a significant problem in the field of personalized medicine. First off, the discovery of diseases by accident raises a lot of ethical questions. While a patient is being examined for one disease, the existence of another, potentially fatal disease could be found. This is especially problematic if there are no viable options for therapy because it does nothing to improve the patient's outlook. Patients who learn they have a disease may also experience very profound psychological effects, raising additional ethical con-cerns. False-positive results happen when genetic factors are interpreted erro-neously, and a patient is found to have a condition they do not have. This could result in a wide range of moral and physiological problems. These include not just detrimental psychological impacts but also the use of ineffective therapies, which can harm the patient and add unnecessary costs to healthcare. Some people think that the family should be informed if they are at risk because genetic disorders are heritable and early management may prevent the development of the problem. To disclose their family or not would, however, currently be up to the patient. The stigmatization of those who have diseases is another problem that needs to be addressed. Many problems could arise if a patient's genetic information was compromised (*Personalized Medicine - Challenges for Industry*, n.d.).

1.7 CONCLUSION

Personalized medicine holds considerable promise and moves medical care toward determining disease risk and prevention. It may involve family history and genomic information. A patient's genomic information can now be used to inform important treatment decisions, thanks to genomic research, which serves as the foundation for genomic medicine. It is necessary to standardize and streamline the integration of genetic research into the clinic. The use of genomic techniques has improved patient care, and personalized medicine is already being applied in clinics, particularly in oncology and cardiology. Several barriers in education, accessibility, legislation, and reimbursement must be removed to better integrate personalized medicine into clinical workflow. Given that clinically significant inter-individual variation has been identified and will continue to be personalized medicine, on several levels that may shed light on their response to intervention, treating them accordingly is required. Modern biomedical technologies, like DNA sequencing, proteomics, and wireless monitoring tools, have made it possible to identify this diversity, thus revealing the need for some degree of personalization in medical care. Future challenges brought on by this reality will include enhancing the accuracy of how individuals are classified as well as the development and evaluation of tailored treatments to demonstrate their efficacy. Where they are regarded as acceptable, personalized approaches should be employed and are available. In conclusion, a more upbeat outlook is justified by the advancements in personalized medicine and related technology. Significant efforts in the clinical and biopharmaceutical industries will be related to personalized medicine.

REFERENCES

Advanced Diagnostics for Personalized Medicine—Scientific American. (n.d.). Retrieved August 10, 2022, from https://www.scientificamerican.com/article/advanced-diagnostics-for-personalized-medicine/

Bernard: The Five Myths of Pharmacogenomics Prevailing ... —Google Scholar. (n.d.). Retrieved August 6, 2022, from https://scholar.google.com/scholar_lookup?journal=Pharmaceutical+Executive&title=The+five+myths+of+pharmacogenomics&author=S+Bernard&publication_year=2003&pages=70-78&

Breedveld, F. C. (2000). Therapeutic monoclonal antibodies. *The Lancet*, *355*(9205), 735–740. 10.1016/S0140-6736(00)01034-5

Constable, S., Johnson, M. R., & Pirmohamed, M. (2006). Pharmacogenetics in clinical practice: considerations for testing. *Expert Review of Molecular Diagnostics*, *6*(2), 193–205. 10.1586/14737159.6.2.193

Could a Saliva Test Be the Future of Diagnosing Endo? A Q&A with D|EndoFound. (n.d.). Retrieved August 10, 2022, from https://www.endofound.org/could-a-saliva-test-be-the-future-of-diagnosing-endo-a-qa-with-dotlab-creator-heather-bowerman

Di Paolo, A., & Luci, G. (2021). Personalized medicine of monoclonal antibodies in inflammatory bowel disease: pharmacogenetics, therapeutic drug monitoring, and beyond. *Frontiers in Pharmacology*, *11*, 2503. 10.3389/FPHAR.2020.610806/BIBTEX

Dykxhoorn, D. & Lieberman, J. (2006). Running interference: prospects and obstacles to using small interfering RNAs as small molecule drugs. *Annual Review of Biomedical Engineering*. 10.1146/annurev.bioeng.8.061505.095848

Dykxhoorn, D., Palliser, D., & Lieberman, J. (2006). The silent treatment: siRNAs as small molecule drugs. *Gene Therapy*, *13*(6), 541–552. 10.1038/sj.gt.3302703

Eisen, M. B., & Brown, P. O. (1999). DNA arrays for analysis of gene expression. *Methods in Enzymology*, *303*, 179–205. 10.1016/S0076-6879(99)03014-1

Ellenberg, S. S., & Hamilton, J. M. (1989). Surrogate endpoints in clinical trials: cancer. *Statistics in Medicine*, *8*(4), 405–413. 10.1002/SIM.4780080404

Evans, W. E., & Relling, M. V. (1999). Pharmacogenomics: translating functional genomics into rational therapeutics. *Science*, *286*(5439), 487–491. 10.1126/SCIENCE.286.543 9.487/SUPPL_FILE/1044449.XHTML

Fijal, B. A., Hall, J. M., & Witte, J. S. (2000). Clinical trials in the genomic era: effects of protective genotypes on sample size and duration of trial. *Controlled Clinical Trials*, *21*(1), 7–20. 10.1016/S0197-2456(99)00039-2

FoundationOne CDx | Foundation Medicine. (n.d.). Retrieved August 10, 2022, from https://www.foundationmedicine.com/test/foundationone-cdx

Gonçalves, G. A. R., & Paiva, R. de M. A. (2017). Gene therapy: advances, challenges and perspectives. *Einstein*, *15*(3), 369. 10.1590/S1679-45082017RB4024

Grossman, I. (2007). Routine pharmacogenetic testing in clinical practice: dream or reality? *Pharmacogenomics*, *8*(10), 1449–1459. 10.2217/14622416.8.10.1449

Gupta, S., & Jhawat, V. (2017). Quality by design (QbD) approach of pharmacogenomics in drug designing and formulation development for optimization of drug delivery systems. *Journal of Controlled Release: Official Journal of the Controlled Release Society*, *245*, 15–26. 10.1016/J.JCONREL.2016.11.018

Hudson, K. L. (2011). Genomics, health care, and society. *The New England Journal of Medicine*, *365*(11), 1033–1041. 10.1056/NEJMRA1010517

Human Genome—Origins of the Human Genome|Britannica. (n.d.). Retrieved July 25, 2022, from https://www.britannica.com/science/human-genome/Origins-of-the-human-genome

Hunter, D., ... M. K.-N. E., & 2008, undefined. (2008). Letting the genome out of the bottle-will we get our wish? *Www-Management.Wharton.Upenn* .... http://www-management.wharton.upenn.edu/raff/documents/2009/Your_Genome.Hunter.pdf

Jain, K. K. (2005). Personalised medicine for cancer: from drug development into clinical practice. *Expert Opinion on Pharmacotherapy*, *6*(9), 1463–1476. 10.1517/14656566.6.9.1463

Jain, K. K. (2011). Role of biological therapies in the development of personalized medicine. *Expert Opinion on Biological Therapy*, *12*(1), 1–5. 10.1517/14712598.2012.641010

Jain, K. K. (2021a). Basic aspects. *Textbook of Personalized Medicine*, 1–37. 10.1007/978-3-030-62080-6_1

Jain, K. K. (2021b). Molecular diagnostics in personalized medicine. *Textbook of Personalized Medicine*, 39–101. 10.1007/978-3-030-62080-6_2

Jain, K. K. (2021c). Pharmacogenetics. *Textbook of Personalized Medicine*, 115–152. 10.1007/978-3-030-62080-6_4

Jain, K. K. (2021d). Pharmacogenomics. *Textbook of Personalized Medicine*, 153–166. 10.1007/978-3-030-62080-6_5

Jain, K. K. (2021e). Role of biomarkers in personalized medicine. *Textbook of Personalized Medicine*, 103–113. 10.1007/978-3-030-62080-6_3

Jain, K. K. (2021f). Role of metabolomics in personalized medicine. *Textbook of Personalized Medicine*, 177–183. 10.1007/978-3-030-62080-6_7

Jain, K. K. (2021g). Role of pharmacoproteomics. *Textbook of Personalized Medicine*, 167–175. 10.1007/978-3-030-62080-6_6

Jain, K. K. (n.d.). *Cell Therapy*. Retrieved August 5, 2022, from http://pharmabiotech.ch/reports/celltherapy/contents-2.pdf

Lamberti, M. J., Wilkinson, M., Peña, Y., Getz, K., & Beltre, C. (2012). Preparing for precision medicine. *The New England Journal of Medicine*, *366*(6). 10.1056/NEJMP1114866

Louca, S. (2012). Personalized medicine—a tailored health care system: challenges and opportunities. *Croatian Medical Journal*, *53*(3), 211. 10.3325/CMJ.2012.53.211

Markers of Oxidative Damage and Antioxidant Protection: Current Status and Relevance to Disease|Request PDF. (n.d.). Retrieved August 9, 2022, from https://www.researchgate.net/publication/12140337_Markers_of_oxidative_damage_and_antioxidant_protection_Current_status_and_relevance_to_disease

Matsui, S. (2013). Genomic biomarkers for personalized medicine: development and validation in clinical studies. *Computational and Mathematical Methods in Medicine*, *2013*. 10.1155/2013/865980

McLeod, H., toxicology, W. E.-A. review of pharmacology and, & 2001, undefined. (2001). Pharmacogenomics: unlocking the human genome for better drug therapy. *Iitk.Ac.In*, *41*, 101–122. http://home.iitk.ac.in/~sganesh/hmg/pdf/PHARMACOGENOMICS-Unlocking the Human Genome for Better Drug Therapy.pdf

Milne, C. P., Garafalo, S., Bryan, C., & McKiernan, M. (2014). Trial watch: personalized medicines in late-stage development. *Nature Reviews Drug Discovery*, *13*(5), 324–325. 10.1038/NRD4325

Mini, E., & Nobili, S. (2009a). Pharmacogenetics: implementing personalized medicine. *Clinical Cases in Mineral and Bone Metabolism*, *6*(1), 17. /pmc/articles/PMC2781211/

Mini, E., & Nobili, S. (2009b). Pharmacogenetics: implementing personalized medicine. *Clinical Cases in Mineral and Bone Metabolism*, *6*(1), 17. /pmc/articles/PMC2781211/

Oncotype DX Tests. (n.d.). Retrieved August 10, 2022, from https://www.breastcancer.org/screening-testing/oncotype-dx

Personalized Medicine. (n.d.). Retrieved July 22, 2022, from https://www.genome.gov/genetics-glossary/Personalized-Medicine

Personalized Medicine—Challenges for Industry. (n.d.). Retrieved August 10, 2022, from https://www.news-medical.net/health/Personalized-Medicine-Challenges-for-Industry.aspx

Personalized Medicine Focused on Diagnostics. (n.d.). Retrieved August 9, 2022, from https://www.natlawreview.com/article/personalized-medicine-2021-fda-guideposts-progress-focus-diagnostics

Poland, G. A., Ovsyannikova, I. G., & Jacobson, R. M. (2008). Personalized vaccines: the emerging field of vaccinomics. *Expert Opinion on Biological Therapy*, *8*(11), 1659. 10.1517/14712598.8.11.1659

Porter, M. E. (2010). What is value in health care? *The New England Journal of Medicine*, *363*(26), 2477–2481. 10.1056/NEJMP1011024

Precision Medicine and Pharmacogenomics—Mayo Clinic. (n.d.). Retrieved August 8, 2022, from https://www.mayoclinic.org/healthy-lifestyle/consumer-health/in-depth/personalized-medicine/art-20044300

Relling, M. V., & Hoffman, J. M. (2007). Should pharmacogenomic studies be required for new drug approval? *Clinical Pharmacology and Therapeutics*, *81*(3), 425–428. 10.1038/SJ.CLPT.6100097

Rowinsky, E. K., Windle, J. J., & Von Hoff, D. D. (1999). Ras protein farnesyltransferase: a strategic target for anticancer therapeutic development. *Journal of Clinical Oncology: Official Journal of the American Society of Clinical Oncology*, *17*(11), 3631–3652. 10.1200/JCO.1999.17.11.3631

Schellekens, H., & Casadevall, N. (2004). Immunogenicity of recombinant human proteins: causes and consequences. *Journal of Neurology*, *251*(2), ii4–ii9. 10.1007/S00415-004-1202-9

Seyhan, A. A., & Carini, C. (2019). Are innovation and new technologies in precision medicine paving a new era in patients centric care? *Journal of Translational Medicine*, *17*(1), 1–28. 10.1186/S12967-019-1864-9/FIGURES/4

Simon, R. (2010). Clinical trial designs for evaluating the medical utility of prognostic and predictive biomarkers in oncology. *Personalized Medicine*, *7*(1), 33–47. 10.2217/PME.09.49

Strimbu, K., & Tavel, J. A. (2010). What are biomarkers? *Current Opinion in HIV and AIDS*, *5*(6), 463. 10.1097/COH.0B013E32833ED177

The Role of Pharmacogenomics in Precision Medicine|Medical Laboratory Observer. (n.d.). Retrieved August 6, 2022, from https://www.mlo-online.com/continuing-education/article/13009247/the-role-of-pharmacogenomics-in-precision-medicine

Vogel, F. (1959). Moderne problem der humangenetik. *Ergeb Inn Med U Kinderheilk*, *12*, 52125.

What Happened to Personalized Medicine? (2012). *Nature Biotechnology*, *30*(1), 1. 10.1038/NBT.2096

Wilke, R. A., Lin, D. W., Roden, D. M., Watkins, P. B., Flockhart, D., Zineh, I., Giacomini, K. M., & Krauss, R. M. (2007). Identifying genetic risk factors for serious adverse drug reactions: current progress and challenges. *Nature Reviews Drug Discovery*, *6*(11), 904–916. 10.1038/NRD2423

Wistuba, I. I., Gelovani, J. G., Jacoby, J. J., Davis, S. E., & Herbst, R. S. (2011). Methodological and practical challenges for personalized cancer therapies. *Nature Reviews Clinical Oncology*, *8*(3), 135–141. 10.1038/nrclinonc.2011.2

Wittes, J., Lakatos, E., & Probstfield, J. (1989). Surrogate endpoints in clinical trials: cardiovascular diseases. *Statistics in Medicine*, *8*(4), 415–425. 10.1002/SIM.4780080405

WORK PROGRAMME FOR THE EUROPEAN AGENCY FOR THE EVALUATION OF MEDICINAL PRODUCTS 2002. (n.d.). Retrieved August 3, 2022, from http://www.emea.eu.int

Zahavi, D., & Weiner, L. (2020). Monoclonal antibodies in cancer therapy. *Antibodies*, *9*(3), 34. 10.3390/ANTIB9030034

Zhou, S.-F., Ming Di, Y., Chan, E., Du, Y.-M., Chow, V., Xue, C., Lai, X., Wang, J.-C., Li, C., Tian, M., & Duan, W. (2008). Clinical pharmacogenetics and potential application in personalized medicine. *Current Drug Metabolism*, *9*(8), 738–784. 10.2174/13892 0008786049302

2 Interactions of Nanomaterials in Biological Systems
Their Characteristics Influencing Interaction

Ruby Dhiman, Ramendra Pati Pandey, and Chung-Ming Chang

2.1 INTRODUCTION

The use of nanostructures and nanomaterials in a variety of scientific domains, particularly in nanomedicine and nano-based drug delivery systems, where such particles are of great interest, has demonstrated how nanotechnology may overcome the divide between biological and physical sciences. Nanomaterials may be described as substances with diameters ranging from 1 to 100 nm. They have a significant impact on the frontiers of nanomedicine influencing everything from biosensors, microfluidics, drug delivery, and biomedical engineering to microarray studies [1]. Nanomaterials are a set of atoms and molecules with beneficial chemical and physical characteristics that differ dramatically from their bulk counterparts. The transition state between bulk materials and molecular clusters is represented by nanomaterials. As a result, nanomaterials deviate significantly from standard macro- or micro-perspectives, exhibiting distinct optical, magnetic, electrical, chemical, and mechanical characteristics [2]. As a result, they have vast development potential and have been dubbed "the most promising materials" of the 21st century. The emergence of nanotechnology and nanomaterials has created a larger area for the development of bio-analytical chemistry; biosensors, in particular, have become one of the most promising applications for nanomaterials. Novel functional nanomaterials can effectively improve the immobilization of biomolecules (such as enzymes, antibodies, or DNA), label biomolecules, catalyze reactions, promote electron transfer, and facilitate electrochemical signal amplification due to their special structural features, strong adsorption capacity, reliable orientation performance, biocompatibility, and structural compatibility [3]. In the scientific literature, the term "smart material" (alternatively, "active," "adaptive," or "stimuli-responsive material") refers to a material that modifies some essential characteristics during

DOI: 10.1201/9781003348672-2

application and initiates certain functionalities in response to one or more external stimuli. Smart nanomaterials are employed as nano-encapsulates and nanocarriers in controlled-release technologies and medicine delivery systems. The current COVID-19 epidemic has fueled the desire for effective diagnosis and treatment tools, and the stimuli-responsive properties of smart nanomaterials are being investigated for the construction of specialized controlled drug delivery systems, enhanced antigen presentation, and immune regulation [4]. Nanomaterials-based drug delivery systems and their ability to overcome the biological obstacles presented by the Blood Brain Barrier as the advances in nanomaterials engineering and biomedical applications (i.e., nanomedicine) are enabling novel tactics that have the potential to improve our knowledge and treatment of various neurological illnesses [5]. Several recent advancements in nanotechnologies with distinct properties address various challenges linked to wound healing [6]. Using nanoparticles as scaffolds to improve the interface between orthopedic implants and natural bone etc. mechanisms have been created [7].

Nanomaterials can influence cell fate, induce, or prevent mutations, begin cell-cell communication, and change cell shape in ways that are essentially determined by processes at the nano-bio interface. Chemical synthesis breakthroughs have resulted in novel nanoscale materials with precisely specified biochemical properties and increasing analytical tools have shed light on subtle and context-dependent nano-bio interactions within cells [8]. This chapter focuses on several types of nanomaterials used in medical applications and their interactions with living organisms. We examine the features of nanomaterials that influence system interactions and beneficial qualities, as well as current breakthroughs with future properties that have been studied and addressed. The publication finishes by reflecting on several outstanding difficulties that scientists, doctors, and engineers must solve collaboratively.

2.2 NANOMATERIALS AND THEIR TYPES

2.2.1 POLYMER-BASED NANOMATERIALS

Polymers, which are long chains of repeating monomers, are commonly employed in nanomedicine because they are biocompatible and biodegradable. Polymeric nano-materials are essentially made of carbon, hydrogen, oxygen, and nitrogen and may be synthesized or obtained biologically and the structure of different possibilities of polymeric nanomaterials are shown in Figure 2.1 [9]. The most common biomaterials include natural polymers such as chitosan, gelatin, collage, and alginate, as well as synthetic polymers such as polylactide (PLA), poly(lactic-co-glycolic acid) (PLGA), polycaprolactone (PCL), poly(glycerol sebacate), and polyurethane (PU) [10].

The interest in the formulation of chitosan nanoparticles has grown substantially over the years, with researchers investigating novel and inventive production methods.

Chitosan, the only naturally occurring polymer with a positive charge, is an appealing polymer due to its ability to electro-statically interact with a wide spectrum of negatively charged polysaccharides to create PEC [11]. Suresh Kumar et al. claim that chitosan-derived nanomaterials have the potential to be used as drug carriers [12]. Chitosan is used in the formulation of several drug delivery systems,

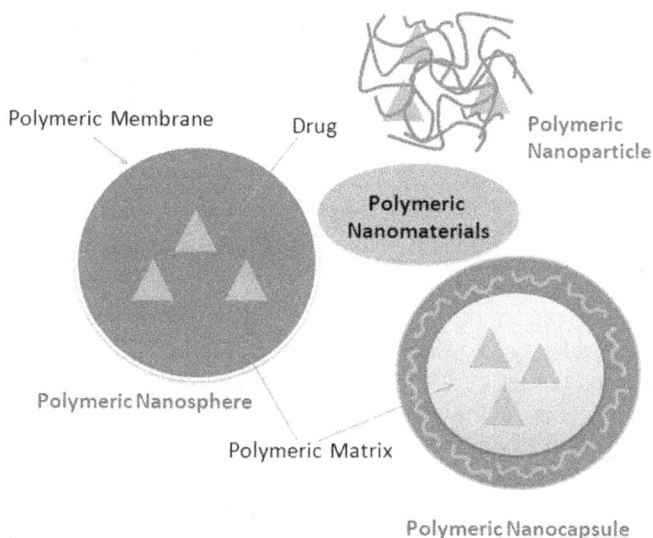

FIGURE 2.1 Schematic representation of the structure of different possibilities of polymeric nanomaterials.

including nanoparticles (NPs), nanofibers/nanoscaffolds (NFs), nanogels (NGs), and liposomes (LPs), with a focus on oral, transmucosal, pulmonary, and transdermal administration [13]. Chitosan may electrostatically attach to a negatively charged protein or plasmid DNA to generate polymer composites that preserve the protein and DNA from destruction. Chitosan derivatives have enormous promise in the biomedical area due to their strong intrinsic biological features, including antibacterial activity and non-toxicity [14]. Poly (L-glutamic acid) is a polymer that has been employed in conjugate production as well as evaluated for representing chemotherapeutics that are usually used in the clinic, and it has shown extraordinary skills and the ability to overcome the drawbacks of their free drug equivalents. Polymeric nanoparticles such as N-(2-hydroxypropyl) methacrylamide and PEG are commonly employed as anticancer agents. They have essentially demonstrated enormous success in chemotherapy and/or radiation testing [15].

As demonstrated by the synthesis of highly monodisperse PMMA particles by irradiation of MMA in an aqueous alcohol solution, dispersion polymerization is a straightforward single-step technique that results in the creation of micron- to sub-micron-size microbeads [16]. Essentially, these nanoentities enable the therapeutic value of numerous endowed biomolecules and medicines (B&D) to be used by directing the group transit of B&D at a certain pace or even on demand if an incentive is applied [17]. Furthermore, liposome and polymer-based NPs are now widely used as efficient adjuvants or immunomodulators in a variety of vaccinations [18]. In addition, water-soluble N-(2-hydroxypropyl) methacrylamide (HPMA) copolymers have been employed often in polymer-drug conjugates. Peptidyl linkers (Gly-Phe-Leu-Gly) are preferred for drug conjugation because they are stable in circulation but can be degraded by lysosomal proteases [19]. Researchers have recently focused on PPy (Polypyrrole) nanoparticles for photothermal cancer treatment due to their natural properties, which include strong electrical conductivity, outstanding optical stability, and good biocompatibility in biological studies. According to research, the PCE of PPy nanoparticles can reach 51% in vitro [20].

2.2.2 METAL-BASED NANOMATERIALS

Numerous nanoparticles and nanomaterials have developed from various bulk elements such as gold, silver, iron, copper, cobalt, platinum, and so on, as a result of recent advancements in nanotechnology and medical research and are manufactured either physiologically or physiochemically [21]. Metal-based nanoparticles have modest diameters ranging from 10 to 100 nm, which allows for their strong interaction with biomolecules both within and outside the cell. Their large surface area increases cell permeability. They may also be customized by conjugating particular ligands, proteins, antibodies, medicines, and enzymes with unique binding activity to specific target cells, enhancing their targeted drug delivery capabilities and therapeutic efficacy at the problematic location. The conjugation of medicines, antibodies, proteins, and other substances onto metal nanoparticles protects them from the body's immune system, increasing their blood circulation time [22].

Iron-based nanoparticles can be combined with various optical methods to create a commercially accessible toolbox that can be used to diagnose or treat cancer locally with more efficacy than more traditional medical treatments [23].

Another type of material is metal-organic frameworks (MOFs), which undergo thermal change, yielding a range of nanostructured materials such as carbon-based materials, metal oxides, metal chalcogenides, metal phosphides, and metal carbides. These MOF derivatives feature large surface areas, persistent porosities, and adjustable functionalities, allowing them to perform well in sensing, gas storage, catalysis, and energy-related applications [24]. AgS, CuS, FeS nanoparticles, Zn-based MOF, Cu-based, Mn-based MOF, and other nanoparticles, for example, are widely employed in medical applications such as drug transport and antibacterial properties [25]. Because of their size and shape-dependent electrical characteristics, Pt nanoparticles are appealing for in vivo use. Pt nanoparticles' fundamental characteristic is their intrinsic electrocatalytic activity. Pt has been shown to have good H_2O_2 electrocatalytic activity. Non-enzymatic detection of H_2O_2 can be accomplished using nanoporous gold created by dealloying Au-Ag. The perfect biocompatibility and durability of gold nanoparticles are further grounds for the current enthusiasm for gold nanoparticle research for in vivo use [26]. Based on these amazing features, the synthesis of nanostructured metal oxides, such as $NiCo_2O_4$, has previously been described employing a variety of traditional solvents, surfactants, and time-consuming procedures, as well as a post-thermal treatment at extremely high temperatures [27]. The hydrothermal process, which uses water as a solvent, has been used effectively to create a variety of 2D metal nanomaterials, including Ag nanoplates, Rh nanosheets, Co nanoplatelets, Co nanosheets, Ni nanoplatelets and nanobelts, Cu nanoplatelets, and Cu nanoplatelets, Nanoplates made of Ru [28,29].

2.2.3 CARBON-BASED NANOMATERIALS

Carbon-based nanomaterials (CBNs) have piqued the interest of researchers because of their unusual chemical and physical capabilities, which include thermal, mechanical, electrical, optical, and structural variety. CBNs, comprising carbon nanotubes (CNT), graphene oxide (GO), and graphene quantum dots (GQDs), have been intensively researched in biomedical applications due to their intrinsic features [30]. In terms of chemical composition and physical structure, carbon nanomaterials can provide a comparable milieu to a biological extracellular matrix, making them a suitable contender for the production of artificial scaffolds [31]. Carbon nanomaterials' infinite possibilities for modification and tailoring are associated with their small size, which is comparable to the size of many fundamental biomolecules, large specific surface area, high electrical and thermal conductivity, unique optical properties, and superior mechanical properties, which have paved the way for a wide range of applications. Different possibilities of carbon nanomaterials have been shown in Figure 2.2. Fullerene derivatives, in particular, have been used to capture solar energy, graphene has been widely used in flexible electronics, carbon nanotubes have been tailored to have molecular recognition capability, graphene quantum dots have been widely used for bio-imaging and sensing due to their photoluminescence properties, and nanodiamonds have been demonstrated to be useful in super-resolution imaging and nanoscale temperature sensing [32].

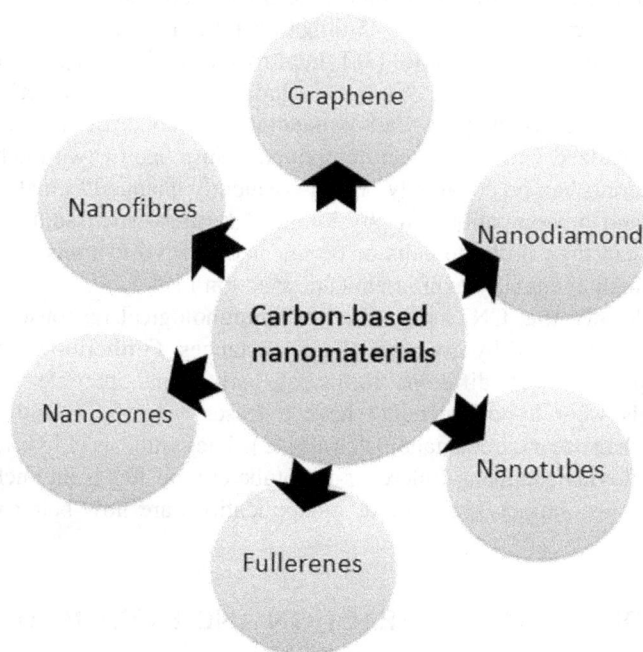

FIGURE 2.2 Schematic representation of different possibilities of carbon-based nanomaterials.

According to recent studies, the commercialization of nanomaterials as nanomedicine is ultimately dependent on establishing their advantage over existing techniques and verifying their safety [33]. CNMs with varying dimensionalities exhibit considerable changes in antibacterial activity and mode of action, according to Xin et. al. Similarly, antibacterial activities of CNMs of a certain dimension are shown to be impacted by other characteristics such as lateral size, shape, number of layers, surface charge, the presence and type of surface functional groups, and doping. These physicochemical parameters are also affected by the technique of production [34]. Research has determined that carbon-based nanomaterials often limit growth and cause cell death. Although carbon nanotubes are less poisonous than carbon fibers and nanoparticles, when carbonyl (CdO), carboxyl (COOH), and/or hydroxyl (OH) groups are present on their surface, their toxicity rises dramatically [35]. Furthermore, new research suggests that CBNs may be employed to modulate cellular activity [36]. Zhang et al. concluded that SPME fibers coated with graphene, carbon nanotubes, or carbon nanofibers displayed enhanced extraction efficiencies that were many times greater than a commercially available SPME fiber. These SPME fibers had better thermal and chemical stability, while the coatings demonstrated increased fiber lifespan. The nanodiamonds-based SPE materials were stable in very acidic and basic conditions, and the reusability of the columns was evaluated with positive results [37].

Carbon-based nanomaterials may also be combined with other types of nanoparticles to make nanocomposites, which combine various features into a single new material. When it comes to nanocomposites, the options are practically limitless: fullerene-Pd nanocrystals, poly (2, 5-dimethylaniline)-CNT, ceramic-CNT, and Teflon-CNT are just a few examples [38]. In vitro and in vivo, graphene compounds are biocompatible with several cell types (including human and bacterial cells) and exhibit antimicrobial effects [39]. Carbon nanotubes, nanohorns, and nanodiamonds can be functionalized with anticancer compounds using one of two methods. These new nanomaterials can be covalently or non-covalently changed to make them more manipulable and biocompatible. In physiological settings, such soluble/dispersible nano-objects can then infiltrate cells or be injected in vivo to transport their cargo molecules, which eventually exhibit anticancer action [40].

It is now known that CNTs may elicit an immunological response and that the interactions are regulated by a variety of circumstances. Furthermore, the immunological compatibility of different forms of carbon nanoparticles varies [41]. Nanodiamonds were hypothesized to have a lesser risk of generating oxidative stress in cells than other carbon nanomaterials [42]. The synthesis of hybrid/functional materials employing graphene-fullerenes-nanotube composites is an uncharted topic that merits further inquiry, and various bioapplications are now being investigated [43–45].

2.3 NANOMATERIALS INTERACTION AND ENTRY IN THE CELL

Mammalian cells have a lipid bilayer that divides the intracellular area from the outer environment and regulates the passage of chemicals in and out of cells. Small molecules, like ions and amino acids, can move freely through it or through particular transmembrane transporters and ion channels [46]. Nanoparticles (NPs) are frequently surface-coated with biopolymers or macromolecules, and bioconjugated with targeting ligands that bind precisely to the corresponding receptors on the cell membrane, to enable cell-type specific targeting [47]. Endocytosis is the primary mechanism by which cells internalize nanoparticles. Endocytosis is a key process for cellular food absorption, cell surface receptor modulation, cell polarity, motility, and signaling cascades [48]. Cell entrance is highly regulated at the plasma membrane. Small soluble compounds inside the lipid membrane can readily diffuse across passively, but polar molecules require active, energy-dependent activities to penetrate the membrane. This is accomplished by either protein transporters stuck inside the membrane or by causing membrane remodeling, which leads to the development of membrane-enclosed sacs known as vesicles [49]. Clathrin and caveolae-mediated endocytosis, phagocytosis, macropinocytosis, and pinocytosis are the most common endocytosis processes. Endocytosis mediated by clathrin and caveolae implies receptor-mediated endocytosis. Many types of cells employ clathrin and caveolae-mediated endocytosis to absorb nanoscale molecules such as viruses and nanoparticles [50].

Endocytosis is categorized into numerous kinds based on the cell type as well as the proteins, lipids, and other substances involved in the process. Endocytosis is characterized by five distinct mechanisms: Phagocytosis, caveolin-mediated endocytosis, Clathrin-mediated endocytosis, clathrin/caveolae-independent endocytosis, and macropinocytosis are all examples of endocytosis, also shown in Figure 2.3. The pictorial representation of various endocytic pathways is depicted in Figure 2.4 [8].

Phagocytosis (cell eating) is the process by which specialized mammalian cells called phagocytes consume debris, pathogens, or other massive solutes (i.e. monocytes, macrophages, and neutrophils). Phagocytosis is a complicated process that necessitates the coordinated activities of several receptors, ligands, and intracellular signals [51,52]. Opsonization, a process in which opsonins such as

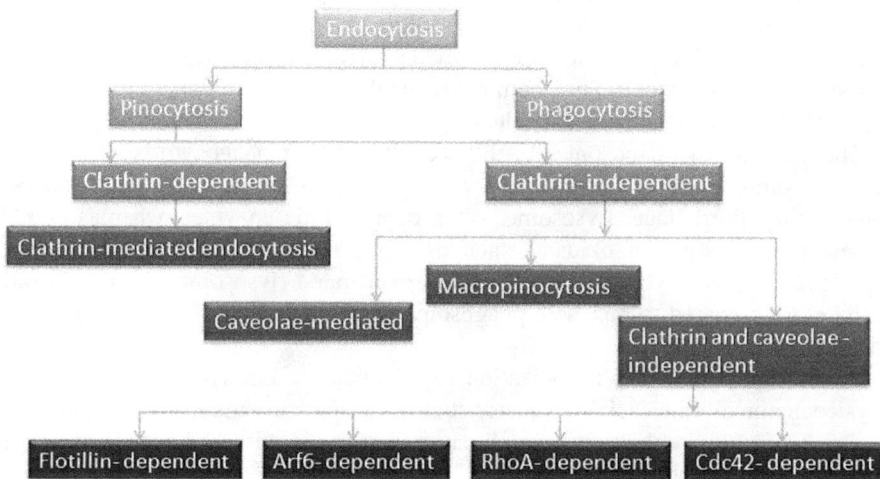

FIGURE 2.3   The flow chart showing endocytic pathway and its types.

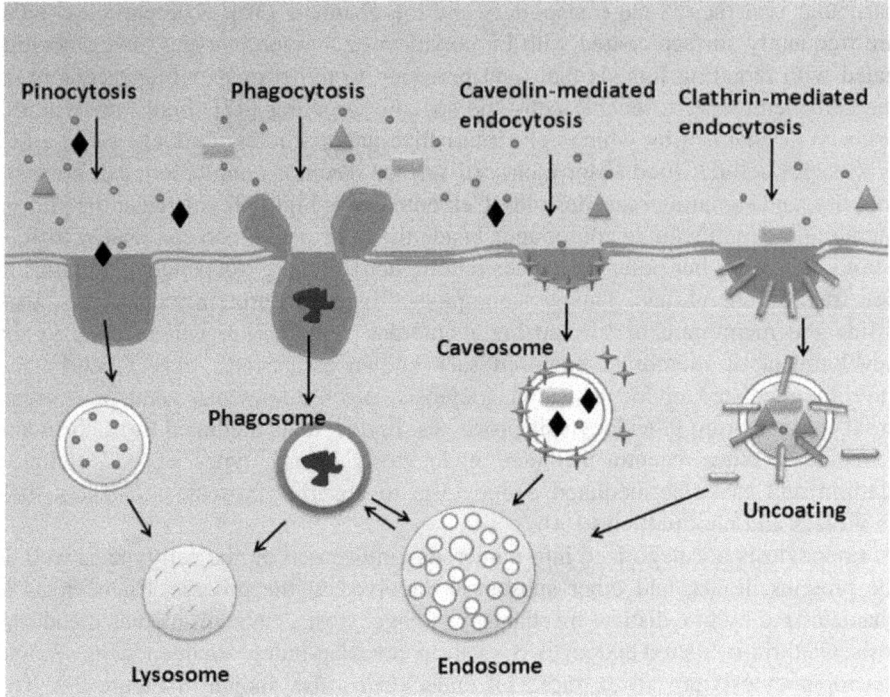

FIGURE 2.4 The pictorial representation of various endocytic pathways.

immunoglobulins and complement proteins wrap target materials to alert phagocytes to their existence and initiate phagocytosis activity, is essential to phagocytosis [52]. Qie et al. discovered increased nanoparticle absorption by activated
macrophages in research. More crucially, macrophage polarization toward the M1
phenotype resulted in increased nanoparticle absorption of all sizes [51]. Krpeti
et al. experimentally demonstrated the process with the help of gold particles, the
first stage in phagocytosis, i.e., chemotaxis. At this moment, the macrophage cell is
approaching nanoparticles while releasing pseudopodia.

The creation of phagosomes is the second stage in phagocytosis. Phagosome
vesicles combine with lysosomes and peroxisome vesicles to generate phagolysosomes in the third stage. Lysosomes often contain lytic enzymes, whereas peroxi-
somes include powerful oxidants such as H_2O_2, both of which are responsible
for digesting phagocytized material. As demonstrated, lysosome and peroxisome
vesicles are prepared to mix with phagosomes containing gold particles to generate
phagolysosomes [53].

Protein adsorptive and opsonization capabilities are known to be mediated by
physicochemical interfacial characteristics. Surface curvature, topography, and
surface energy/hydrophobicity can all cause changes in adsorbed protein structure.
To fully comprehend these implications on opsonization, every nanomaterial must
first be described in established surface composition and the precise surface
chemistry that interacts with biology. To comprehend the risks of nanomaterial

exposure, it is critical to comprehend how nanomaterials are recognized, internalized, trafficked, and distributed within various types of host macrophages, as well as how possible cell-based reactions resulting from nanomaterial exposures contribute to the inflammatory host response [54].

Caveolae are membrane invaginations 60–80 nm in diameter with a 10–50 nm diameter neck. They are found in numerous cell types, but endothelial cells in the artery wall lining monolayer are particularly common [55]. Caveolae-dependent endocytosis is another typical cellular entrance mechanism used by nanoparticles ranging in size from 20 to 100 nm. Caveolae-coated vesicles avoid fusion with lysosomes, resulting in higher quantities of targeted medicines in endosomes or caveosomes, and hence a better therapeutic impact [56]. Caveosomes encapsulating nanomaterials go to the ER through microtubules. Nanomaterials in the ER are hypothesized to enter the cytosol and subsequently enter the nuclear pore complex [56,57]. Caveolin-1, which is found in nearly all cells, there are additional isoforms such as caveolin-2 and caveolin-3 (specific for muscle). Caveolae are generated as a result of the oligomerization of caveolin-1 and 2 proteins, which are required for the establishment of membrane curvature, and caveolae play a role in endocytosis. Other caveolae endocytic machinery components include proteins such as cavin, which produces membrane curvature, dynamin, which allows vesicle scission, vesicle-associated membrane protein (VAMP2), and synaptosome-associated protein (SNAP), which influences subsequent vesicle fusion, and so on. Caveolae vesicles transport and fuse with caveosomes or MVBs with neutral pH after the plasma membrane budding [55,58]. Using Cy5-functional AuNPs with a size of around 4.5 nm as cell labels, Hao et al. revealed that the internalization of nanoscale AuNPs in Hela cells occurs via receptor-mediated endocytosis using a laser scanning confocal microscope. A series of control and block tests clearly suggested that endocytosis was mediated by caveolae. The majority of AuNPs were found in intracellular endocytic vesicles in the perinuclear area [59].

Caveolae's interior is around 50 nm in diameter and can only hold little cargo. Caveolae have been proposed to carry huge cargo, such as bacteria and larger nanoparticles, although it is unclear how the caveola structure might accept objects larger than the width of this channel. Because the structure of vesicles would have to be drastically altered to fit these particles, they should not be termed caveolae. Caveolar proteins, however, may still be hijacked to aid in the internalization process. If such processes are demonstrated, they should be clearly distinguished from genuine caveolar endocytosis, which should be limited to the budding of complete caveolae containing cargo [60].

The inward budding and creation of vesicles, as in clathrin-mediated endocytosis, is the most prevalent method for this sort of transport from the outside to the interior of the cell. Clathrin is a cytosolic protein that forms cage-like coated pits inside the cell membrane to promote membrane inward budding. The structure of clathrin-coated pits (CCPs), as well as their size distributions and lifespan, have been extensively studied and debated from biological and biochemical viewpoints in recent decades [61]. Experiments reveal that the cellular uptake of NPs entering via clathrin-coated vesicles (CCVs) is size-dependent, with an ideal NP size for maximal absorption. A theoretical model presented to explain this experimental fact ties size dependency to receptor diffusion rate on the plasma membrane. The protein coat, which causes the membrane to invaginate, has a natural curvature ranging from 1/80 to 1/40 nm. Banerjee et al. previously hypothesized that a CCV may hold cargo of comparable size and that the creation of a coat around a particle whose size falls outside of this range is energetically undesirable [62]. The NPs use both clathrin- and caveolae-mediated receptor-mediated endocytosis pathways to enter epithelial cells. The 50 nm NPs are the quickest to be absorbed, with clathrin-mediated endocytosis being the predominant pathway [63]. Smith et al.'s findings suggest that in the presence of serum, cellular entry of 20 nm nanoparticles is reduced primarily through inhibition of cell surface binding, that clathrin-mediated endocytosis is a significant route for nanoparticle uptake, and that these nanoparticles may have the ability to enter the cell directly through permeabilization of the plasma membrane. Furthermore, it was demonstrated that blocking the dynamin-dependent/clathrin-mediated endocytosis pathway significantly decreased nanoparticle penetration into cells. As a result, Clathrin-mediated endocytosis is an important method for nanoparticle endocytosis [64]. HyunJeong et al. revealed that the clathrin-mediated endocytosis route is a possible mechanism for SiNP intake in *Caenorhabditis elegans* [65]. Another research by Cheng Teng NG found that cellular import of AuNPs by lung fibroblasts and liver cells occurred via the clathrin-mediated endocytosis route [66]. Hua Deng showed the creation of new ligand-receptor interactions stimulates clathrin recruitment and accumulation in their model. Clathrin polymerization, which is triggered by ligand-receptor interactions, is principally responsible for membrane deformation and particle internalization [67].

Clathrin- and caveolae-independent endocytosis occurs in cells lacking clathrin and caveolae. Through additional channels, these cells take up various cargos such as cellular fluids, interleukin-2, and growth hormones, which need a certain lipid composition (mainly cholesterol) free of clathrin and caveolae [8,68].

This is a unique mechanism that is dependent on cholesterol and necessitates certain lipid compositions. Clathrin- and caveolae-independent endocytosis is categorized into different types based on GTPases that regulate the cellular entry pathway: Arf6-dependent, Cdc42-dependent, and Rho A-dependent [57], flotillin-assisted and fast endophilin-mediated endocytosis [48]. ARF6 Clathrin-independent endocytosis can be both dependent and independent of dynamin. Mechanisms relying on dynamin for vesicle formation include the RhoA-dependent system responsible for IL-2 absorption and tubule pinching caused by multivalent toxins such as Shiga toxins cross-linking glycolipids [68].

Pinocytosis is a much broader process that may be divided into two subtypes: macropinocytosis and micropinocytosis. Macropinocytosis is the non-selective intake of solute macromolecules with diameters more than 0.2 m, whereas micropinocytosis (clathrin-mediated, caveolae/lipid raft-mediated, and clathrin/caveolae-independent) occurs in all cell types for smaller particles. Given the size range of routinely utilized therapeutic NPs (10–200 nm), NPs are likely to enter cells mostly by micropinocytosis [69]. Macropinocytosis is characterized by the ingestion of fluids, macromolecules, and NPs through tiny vesicles. Although NPs have been demonstrated to be taken up by cells primarily by pinocytosis, various parameters such as cell type, surface charge, and NP size have been found to impact the interaction with cells [70]. It has been found that particles larger than 150 nm are more likely to be endocytosed by macropinocytosis [71]. Macropinosomes are generated when the expanded plasma membrane folds and fuses back with the plasma membrane, trapping extracellular fluid with the newly formed intracellular vacuoles [72]. Actin polymerization regulators, such as members of the Ras gene super family (e.g., Ras and Rac), are linked to macropinocytosis activity. Ras proteins encode tiny guanosine triphosphatases (GTPases), which act as molecular ON-OFF switches for numerous signaling pathways. Evidence shows that expression of Ras and phosphatidylinositol (3, 4, 5)-trisphosphate (PIP3) predominates in certain regions of the ruffles in the plasma membrane during early macropinosomes development and maturation. These substances are essential for the early development of macropinosomes since their ablation (either genetically or chemically) inhibits macropinosomes production [73].

Innate immune cells, such as macrophages and dendritic cells, experience a high rate of macropinocystosis to ingest antigens from their surroundings. Using macropinocytosis as the internalization method for NPs would have various benefits over conventional endocytic processes. First, its comparatively big and heterogeneous endocytic vesicles may contain a larger capacity of NPs of varied sizes and shapes than the CME or CavME pathways. Second, unlike phagocytosis, macropinocytosis offers a universal pathway into a considerably larger spectrum of cell types. Third, antigen-presenting immune cells and many cancer cells have a high rate of macropinocytosis, which can be helpful for specific NP applications. NP-based immunization is one such example [74].

2.4 NANOPARTICLES PROPERTIES INFLUENCING INTERACTION

2.4.1 SIZE

The precise definition of the NP is required to associate a specific physicochemical feature of an NP with biological responses and to ensure that these results are repeatable and relevant. The size of the NP is an important element (in the following, particle size always refers to the diameter). To maintain colloidal stability, many NPs are made of a "heavy" core (e.g., a metal or semiconductor nanocrystal) surrounded by tiny organic ligands. Transmission electron microscopy (TEM) and other electron microscopy methods may readily offer precise size measurements with sub-nanometer precision [75]. At the cellular level, the membrane prevents the release of complexes larger than 1 kDa, and the nuclear pore complex, which restricts material entry into the core, has a diameter of 10–25 nm. Internalized vesicles (endosomes) are 60–120 nm in size [76].

Experiments revealed that a ligand-coated nanoparticle with a diameter of 50 nm has the best cellular uptake. In experiments using HeLa cells, spherical mesoporous silica nanoparticles with a diameter of 50 nm demonstrated the greatest cellular uptake. Furthermore, research utilizing targeted gold nanoparticles found that 40–50 nm gold nanoparticles had the maximum cellular uptake in SKBR-3 cells. When the core was changed from gold to silver, the same pattern was seen [77]. Another study found that instilling Ir192-particles with diameters of 80 nm resulted in 0.1%

accumulation in the rat liver, whereas particles with diameters of 15 nm resulted in 0.3–0.5% accumulation. Furthermore, when smaller particles are maintained in the respiratory tract for a longer period of time, they enhance translocation to the pulmonary interstitium, impairing alveolar macrophage activity [78]. Research by Alaa Fehaid found that when cells were exposed to 10 and 200 nm AgNPs independently, the 200 nm AgNPs exhibited a lesser cytotoxic impact and a higher percentage of cellular uptake than the 10 nm AgNPs [79]. When compared to other sizes, 50 nm gold nanoparticles demonstrated the highest effective cellular uptake. A human colon adenocarcinoma cell line was also investigated for cellular absorption of polystyrene (PS) nanoparticles of various sizes [50].

For a study purpose, researchers were able to generate NPs varying in size from 50 to 250 nm by adjusting the procedure parameters in nanoprecipitation. The amount of encapsulated medicine per particle increased as particle size grew due to increasing capacity in the hydrophobic core. Cellular uptake, on the other hand, declines with increasing size. Internalization of the receptor-particle complex slows with increasing particle size, as evidenced by a threefold decrease in V_{max} as the size of folate-decorated NPs grows from 50 to 250 nm. The binding affinity of conjugated folate to cellular receptors increases as particle size increases [63]. The confocal microscope Z-scan picture series of one HeLa cell clearly demonstrated that SNPs-55.6 was carried not only into the cytoplasm but also into the nucleus. Recently, it was shown that SNPs with a diameter of 50 nm or smaller may successfully target the nucleus to deliver the active anticancer medicine and effectively destroy the cancer cell. The FCM data further revealed that cellular uptake is significantly size-dependent, with a size range of 55.64 > 167.84 > 307.6 nm [80].

Another Interesting study revealed that the endocytosis rate constant of SWNT (single-walled carbon nanotubes) (10^{-3} min^{-1}) is found to be over 1000 times that of Au nanoparticles (10^{-6} min^{-1}), although the recycling (exocytosis) rate constants are similar in magnitude (10^{-4} to 10^{-3} min^{-1}) across different cell lines. When scaled using an effective capture dimension for membrane diffusion, the overall absorption of both SWNT and Au nanoparticles is maximum at a common radius of 25 nm. Cells rapidly ingest AuNPs as small as 25 nm and AuNPs of 10 nm [81]. Another study revealed that DMAB-modified polymeric nanoparticles may improve medication oral bioavailability in cell types in vitro. In Caco-2 and HT-29 cells, cell absorption of modified polymeric nanoparticles was found to be size-dependent. Cellular absorption increased to maximum levels for 100 nm nanoparticles, which varied from the results for receptor-mediated endocytosis [82]. Xiaowei Ma et al. presented a histogram of the number of AuNPs per cell vs. AuNPs size. It suggests that cellular absorption of AuNPs is highly reliant on particle size, with 50 nm AuNPs being the most effective [83].

Qingxin Mu et al. used centrifugation to investigate the effect of particle size on cell intake quantity and internalization mechanisms. TEM and AFM were used to separate and analyze large (PCGO1) and tiny (PCGO2) protein-coated nanosheets. The researchers concluded that large nanosheets may preferentially translocate into the reticuloendothelial system, whereas tiny nanosheets can be dispersed in a variety of organs. The activity of GO nanosheets in vitro and in vivo may be controlled by varying their size. Recent research supports such a concept. In an in vitro investigation, little GO caused far higher cell viability loss than large GO [84].

2.4.2 SHAPE

As discussed in the previous subsection, the size of nanoparticles is critical in determining their interaction with biological systems. The shape of nanoparticles may also be essential in defining their biological activities. Recent tests have shown that the shape of the nanoparticle influences cellular absorption. Nanoscale rods had the highest absorption in human cervical cancer cells, followed by spheres, cylinders, and cubes, and cylindrical particle uptake is substantially influenced by their aspect ratio. However, when the aspect ratio of gold nanorods increased, so did their receptor-mediated endocytosis. Many different types of cells have been studied to compare the intracellular uptake efficiency of rod-shaped and spherical nanoparticles. Interestingly, the results showed that rod-shaped nanoparticles were more efficiently taken up by macrophages than spherical nanoparticles, whereas spherical nanoparticles were more efficiently taken up by cervical cancer cells and human lung epithelial cells than rod-shaped nanoparticles [50]. For high aspect ratios and "flat" particles, the membrane should wrap the highly curved tips or round edges to attain a totally wrapped condition, but no energy barrier occurs during spherical particle internalization [85].

Robert Vacha et al. performed molecular dynamics (MD) simulations on a coarse-grained model of phospholipids and different-shaped nanoparticles. They determined that bigger spherical particles endocytosed more easily than smaller ones due to a better combination of bending stiffness and surface adhesive energy. Finally, their simulations and elastic analysis indicate that the prolate form of spherocylinders can result in more efficient delivery than spheres of equal diameter. The reason for this is that while both forms appear to have the same kinetic barrier for absorption across a lipid membrane, spherocylinders have a bigger capacity [86]. Using endocytic inhibitors, Xie et al. investigated the role of distinct endocytic routes in the absorption of these three kinds of gold nanoparticles. According to their findings, gold nanotriangles had the highest cellular absorption, followed by gold nanorods and gold nanostars. They also looked into the potential processes of cellular absorption. Depending on the shape, gold nanoparticle uptake was promoted via diverse endocytosis processes. The clathrin-mediated endocytic route was used by all three forms [87]. Kim et al. investigated the influence of shape on the intracellular absorption of two MOF (metal-organic framework) nanoparticles. They did this by creating NH2-MIL-88(Fe) nanoparticles with the same composition but in two distinct shapes: rods and octahedrons. For the entire cell lines evaluated in this study (L929, HeLa, and MDA-MB231), the octahedrons outperformed the rods, probably because of the more sharp edges found in an octahedron nanoparticle. Thus, octahedrons were mostly endocytosed via a clathrin-mediated channel, whereas rods, which include a significant planar area in each particle, were absorbed into cells by both macropinocytosis and a clathrin-mediated pathway [88]. Increasing the size of nanoparticles promotes cellular uptake in cancer cells, independent of the kind of functional groups on the particle surface.

Carbon nanotube length, for example, influences cellular internalization capabilities. Submicron multiwall carbon nanotubes penetrate cells more effectively than longer ones [89]. Further research revealed that the critical wrapping fraction for the NP with a more irregular form is lower [90].

2.4.3 SURFACE CHEMISTRY

Significant computing research on cell nanoparticle interaction has been conducted, with a special emphasis on the influence of nanoparticle size, shape (discussed earlier), and surface chemistry. Endocytosis of nanoparticles is demonstrated to be followed by wrapping processes with the cell membrane, which include membrane-particle adhesion, elastic membrane deformation, and receptor diffusion on the membrane surface. All of these activities result in the nanoparticle size, shape, and surface chemistry [91]. Surface charge, among other physicochemical factors, is an important criterion to consider when applying a regulatory definition for nanomaterials. It has lately been identified as a crucial component in determining NP toxicity; however, a thorough understanding of the processes involved is still missing [92]. Hydrophobic nanoparticles, which favor lipid tails, may be put on the membrane but can't cross it. Charged nanoparticles, on the other hand, may pass the membrane via pore creation after wrapping with the membrane (Figure 2.5) [91].

Molecular dynamics simulations give an approach for controlling surface chemistry to enable varied uptake paths of nanomaterials. When designing nanoparticles with low charge densities, an energy-independent mechanism of translocation across the membrane may be favored in which cationic terminals anchored on the surface of the nanoparticle interact strongly with phosphate groups in both upper and lower membrane leaflets, resulting in the formation of a nanoscale pore on

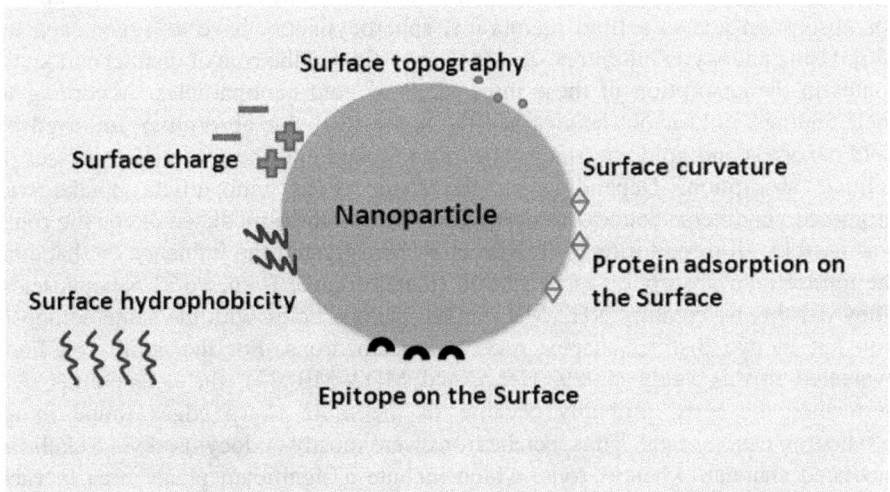

FIGURE 2.5 Schematic representation of different physicochemical properties of a nanoparticle.

the membrane surface. Higher charge densities may promote endocytic pathways, as indicated by structural differences in the lipid bilayer [93]. PLGA nanoparticles can be made more hydrophilic by adding an increasing proportion of PVA emulsifier to their surface had the same size and surface charge as more hydrophobic particles, but were taken up by smooth muscle cells substantially less. Positively charged nanoparticles are thought to perform better for in vitro cell transfection due to their improved binding to negatively charged proteoglycans on cell surfaces [94,95]. Many of the traditional endocytic ligands, such as EGF-modified PEI polyplexes and transferrin-modified lipoplexes targeted to clathrin-mediated endocytosis, have been added to the surface of DNA complexes to improve transfection efficiency [94].

Corona formation is important in NP-cell interactions and cell uptake because it modifies the nature and chemistry of the NPs surface. Because of its resistance to protein adsorption and low toxicity, methoxy-PEG modified with a thiol group (mPEG-SH) is recognized to be a highly favorable surface modification for NPs [95,96]. Coating NPs with certain proteins can aid in determining the patterns of adsorbed proteins on NPs. The interaction of nanoparticles with proteins provides a viable method for designing nanoparticulate drug delivery systems in which regulating protein and protein corona can obscure the NP surface while performing desirable biological activities [97].

2.5 CONCLUSION AND FUTURE PERSPECTIVE

To conclude, the use of nanomaterials in medicine has shown significant promise, from early illness detection to the development of extremely effective tailored treatments. The potential of nanomaterials to address the biological intricacies of illnesses will grow as our understanding of health and disease becomes more sophisticated at the molecular level. Similarly, possibilities will arise to develop patient- and disease-specific treatments or diagnostic techniques. Several years of research have resulted in the creation of a diverse range of nanomaterials originating from synthetic and natural sources. Several nanomaterial classes have also been shown in preclinical and early-stage clinical trials to be extremely successful in combating deadly illnesses, particularly malignancies. The most typically encountered obstacles in cancer therapy have been adequately handled by employing various nanoformulations, including the drug's hydrophobicity, quick clearance, hepatic and renal toxicity, and off-target toxicity.

The aspects of nanomaterials' cytotoxic processes remain unknown, making it challenging to properly inhibit/combat their harmful effects. It is consequently advised that more studies be conducted, as well as standard measures for their manufacturing and use are established. Nanomaterial discharges, both purposeful and unintentional, should be monitored and managed. However, for the vast majority of nanomaterials created in laboratories throughout the world, the transfer from benchtop to bedside is still a long way off. A few research on cell-nanoparticle interactions in the context of cell mechanics has been conducted. The effects of nanoparticles on the mechanobiological characteristics of cells can help us better comprehend nano-bio interactions. The perspective of intracellular interaction, as well as cell mechanics for nano-bio-interaction, needs to be explored.

The integration of nanotechnology into regular clinical practice will need a multidisciplinary approach guided by clinical, ethical, and social considerations. Given the enormous research findings committed to the topic, it is reasonable to anticipate that humans will considerably benefit from nanotechnology and nanomaterials in the very near future, particularly in tumor therapy. For more sophisticated future applications, nanolevel precision and research must be increased. Despite significant accomplishments, this discipline is still in its early stages. Because most previous results are based on in vitro tests, the heart of the research is to investigate the complicated endocytic process of nanomedicine entering cells in vivo. Furthermore, there are numerous contentious topics and undeclared fields. This field still requires much research. Researchers will devote significantly more work to studying the intracellular destiny of nanocarriers aimed at certain organelles.

REFERENCES

1. Patra, J. K., Das, G., Fraceto, L. F., Campos, E. V. R., Rodriguez-Torres, M. D. P., Acosta-Torres, L. S., Diaz-Torres, L. A., Grillo, R., Swamy, M. K., Sharma, S., Habtemariam, S., Shin, H. S. (2018 Sep 19). Nano based drug delivery systems: recent developments and future prospects. *J Nanobiotechnol*, 16(1), 71. doi: 10.1186/s12951-018-0392-8. PMID: 30231877; PMCID: PMC6145203.
2. Cheng, L.-C., Jiang, X., Wang, J., Chen, C., Liu, R.-S. (2013). Nano–bio effects: interaction of nanomaterials with cells. *Nanoscale*, 5(9), 3547. doi: 10.1039/c3nr34276j
3. Pan, M., Gu, Y., Yun, Y., Li, M., Jin, X., Wang, S. (2017 May 5). Nanomaterials for electrochemical immunosensing. *Sensors (Basel)*, 17(5), 1041. doi: 10.3390/s17051041. PMID: 28475158; PMCID: PMC5469646.
4. Gottardo, S., Mech, A., Drbohlavová, J., Małyska, A., Bøwadt, S., Riego Sintes, J., Rauscher, H. (2021 Jan). Towards safe and sustainable innovation in nanotechnology: state-of-play for smart nanomaterials. *NanoImpact*, 21, 100297. doi: 10.1016/j.impact.2021.100297. PMID: 33738354; PMCID: PMC7941606.
5. Furtado, D., Björnmalm, M., Ayton, S., Bush, A. I., Kempe, K., Caruso, F. (2018 Nov). Overcoming the blood-brain barrier: the role of nanomaterials in treating neurological diseases. *Adv Mater*, 30(46), e1801362. doi: 10.1002/adma.201801362. Epub 2018 Jul 31. PMID: 30066406.
6. Blanco-Fernandez, B., Castaño, O., Mateos-Timoneda, M.Á., Engel, E., Pérez-Amodio, S. (2021 May). Nanotechnology approaches in chronic wound healing. *Adv Wound Care (New Rochelle)*, 10(5), 234–256. doi: 10.1089/wound.2019.1094. Epub 2020 Jun 2. PMID: 32320364; PMCID: PMC8035922.
7. Smith, W. R., Hudson, P. W., Ponce, B. A., Rajaram Manoharan, S. R. (2018 Mar 2). Nanotechnology in orthopedics: a clinically oriented review. *BMC Musculoskelet Disord*, 19(1), 67. doi: 10.1186/s12891-018-1990-1. PMID: 29499666; PMCID: PMC5833027.
8. Behzadi, S., Serpooshan, V., Tao, W., Hamaly, M. A., Alkawareek, M. Y., Dreaden, E. C., Brown, D., Alkilany, A. M., Farokhzad, O. C., Mahmoudi, M. (2017 Jul 17). Cellular uptake of nanoparticles: journey inside the cell. *Chem Soc Rev*, 46(14), 4218–4244. doi: 10.1039/c6cs00636a. PMID: 28585944; PMCID: PMC5593313.
9. Kyriakides, T. R., Raj, A., Tseng, T. H., Xiao, H., Nguyen, R., Mohammed, F. S., Halder, S., Xu, M., Wu, M. J., Bao, S., Sheu, W. C. (2021 Mar 11). Biocompatibility of nanomaterials and their immunological properties. *Biomed Mater*, 16(4). 10.1088/1748-605X/abe5fa. doi: 10.1088/1748-605X/abe5fa. PMID: 33578402; PMCID: PMC8357854.

10. Guo, B., Ma, P. X. (2018 Jun 11). Conducting polymers for tissue engineering. *Biomacromolecules*, 19(6), 1764–1782. doi: 10.1021/acs.biomac.8b00276. Epub 2018 Apr 30. PMID: 29684268; PMCID: PMC6211800.

11. Bellich, B., D'Agostino, I., Semeraro, S., Gamini, A., Cesàro, A. (2016 May 17). "The good, the bad and the ugly" of chitosans. *Mar Drugs*, 14(5), 99. doi: 10.3390/md14050099. PMID: 27196916; PMCID: PMC4882573.

12. Kumar, S., Dhiman, R., Prudencio, C. R., da Costa, A. C., Vibhuti, A., Leal, E., Chang, C. M., Raj, V. S., Pandey, R. P. (2022 Jun 9). Chitosan: applications in drug delivery system. *Mini Rev Med Chem*. doi: 10.2174/1389557522666220609102010. Epub ahead of print. PMID: 35692143.

13. Iacob, A. T., Lupascu, F. G., Apotrosoaei, M., Vasincu, I. M., Tauser, R. G., Lupascu, D., Giusca, S. E., Caruntu, I. D., Profire, L. (2021 Apr 20). Recent biomedical approaches for chitosan based materials as drug delivery nanocarriers. *Pharmaceutics*, 13(4), 587. doi: 10.3390/pharmaceutics13040587. PMID: 33924046; PMCID: PMC8073149.

14. Han, J., Zhao, D., Li, D., Wang, X., Jin, Z., Zhao, K. (2018). Polymer-based nanomaterials and applications for vaccines and drugs. *Polymers*, 10(1), 31. 10.3390/polym10010031

15. Yadav, Hemant K. S. (2019). Polymer-based nanomaterials for drug-delivery carriers. In: Mohapatra, S. S., Ranjan, S., Dasgupta, N., Mishra, R. K., Thomas. S., editors. *Nanocarriers for drug delivery*, 531–556. Amsterdam: Elsevier.

16. Güven, O. (2021). Radiation-assisted synthesis of polymer-based nanomaterials. *Appl Sci*, 11(17), 7913. 10.3390/app1117791

17. Suriya Prabha, A. (2020). Recent advances in the study of toxicity of polymer-based nanomaterials. In: Rajendran, S., Mukherjee, A., Anh Nguyen, T. Godugu, C. Shukla, R. K., editors. *Nanotoxicity*, 143–165. Amsterdam: Elsevier.

18. Evelyn Roopngam, P. (2019). Liposome and polymer-based nanomaterials for vaccine applications. *Nanomed J*, 6(1), 1–10.

19. Tran, P. H-L., Tran, T. T-D., Vo, T. V. (2014). Polymer conjugate-based nanomaterials for drug delivery. *J Nanosci Nanotechnol*, 14(1), 815–827. doi: 10.1166/jnn.2014.8901

20. Yu, C., Xu, L., Zhang, Y., Timashev, P. S., Huang, Y., Liang, X-J. (2020). Polymer-based nanomaterials for noninvasive cancer photothermal therapy. *ACS Appl Polym Mater*. doi: 10.1021/acsapm.0c00704

21. Singh, P., Pandit, S., Mokkapati, V. R. S. S., Garg, A., Ravikumar, V., Mijakovic, I. (2018 Jul 6). Gold nanoparticles in diagnostics and therapeutics for human cancer. *Int J Mol Sci*, 19(7), 1979. doi: 10.3390/ijms19071979. PMID: 29986450; PMCID: PMC6073740.

22. Aderibigbe, B. A. (2017 Aug 18). Metal-based nanoparticles for the treatment of infectious diseases. *Molecules*, 22(8), 1370. doi: 10.3390/molecules22081370. PMID: 28820471; PMCID: PMC6152252.

23. Alphandéry, E. (2021 Apr 1). Light-interacting iron-based nanomaterials for localized cancer detection and treatment. *Acta Biomater*, 124, 50–71. doi: 10.1016/j.actbio.2021.01.028. Epub 2021 Feb 1. PMID: 33540060.

24. Dang, S., Zhu, Q. L., Xu, Q. (2018). Nanomaterials derived from metal–organic frameworks. *Nat Rev Mater* 3, 17075. 10.1038/natrevmats.2017.75

25. Yaqoob, A. A., Ahmad, H., Parveen, T., Ahmad, A., Oves, M., Ismail, I. M. I., Qari, H. A., Umar, K., Mohamad Ibrahim, M. N. (2020 May 19). Recent advances in metal decorated nanomaterials and their various biological applications: a review. *Front Chem*, 8, 341. doi: 10.3389/fchem.2020.00341. PMID: 32509720; PMCID: PMC7248377.

26. Zhang, L., Wang, J., Tian, Y. (2014). Electrochemical in-vivo sensors using nanomaterials made from carbon species, noble metals, or semiconductors. *Microchimica Acta*, 181(13-14), 1471–1484. doi: 10.1007/s00604-014-1203-z

27. Chen, J., Ali, M. C., Liu, R., Claude, M. J., Li, Z., Zhai, H., Qiu, H. (2019). Basic deep eutectic solvents as reactant, template and solvents for ultra-fast preparation of transition metal oxide nanomaterials. *Chin Chem Lett*. doi: 10.1016/j.cclet.2019.09.055

28. Chen, Y., Fan, Z., Zhang, Z., Niu, W., Li, C., Yang, N., Chen, B., Zhang, H. (2018). Two-dimensional metal nanomaterials: synthesis, properties, and applications. *Chem Rev*, 118(13), 6409–6455. doi: 10.1021/acs.chemrev.7b00727

29. Rafiei-Sarmazdeh, Z., Zahedi-Dizaji, S. M., Kang, A. K. (2019). Two-dimensional nanomaterials. In: Ameen, S., Akhtar, M. S., Shin, H., editors. *Nanostructures [Internet]*. London: IntechOpen. Available from: https://www.intechopen.com/chapters/67053 doi: 10.5772/intechopen.85263

30. Maiti, D., Tong, X., Mou, X., Yang, K. (2019 Mar 11). Carbon-based nanomaterials for biomedical applications: a recent study. *Front Pharmacol*, 9, 1401. doi: 10.3389/fphar.2018.01401. PMID: 30914959; PMCID: PMC6421398.

31. Ku, S. H., Lee, M., Park, C. B. (2013). Carbon-based nanomaterials for tissue engineering. *Adv Healthc Mat*, 2(2), 244–260. doi: 10.1002/adhm.201200307

32. Díez-Pascual, A. M. (2021). Carbon-based nanomaterials. *Int J Mol Sci*, 22(14), 7726. 10.3390/ijms22147726

33. Bhattacharya, K., Mukherjee, S. P., Gallud, A., Burkert, S. C., Bistarelli, S., Bellucci, S., Bottini, M., Star, A., Fadeel, B. (2015). Biological interactions of carbon-based nanomaterials: from coronation to degradation. *Nanomed Nanotechnol Biol Med*, S1549963415005845–. doi: 10.1016/j.nano.2015.11.011

34. Xin, Q., Shah, H., Nawaz, A., Xie, W., Akram, M. Z., Batool, A., Tian, L., Jan, S. U., Boddula, R., Guo, B., Liu, Q., Gong, J. R. (2018). Antibacterial carbon-based nanomaterials. *Adv Mater*, 1804838–. doi: 10.1002/adma.201804838

35. Kasas, S., Salicio, V., Pasquier, N., Seo, J. W., Celio, M., Catsicas, S., Schwaller, B., Forró, L., Magrez, A. (2006). Cellular toxicity of carbon-based nanomaterials. *Nano Lett*, 6(6), 1121–1125. doi: 10.1021/nl060162e

36. Cha, C., Shin, S. R., Annabi, N., Dokmeci, M. R., Khademhosseini, A. (2013). Carbon-based nanomaterials: multifunctional materials for biomedical engineering. *ACS Nano*, 7(4), 2891–2897. doi: 10.1021/nn401196a

37. Zhang, B.-T., Zheng, X., Li, H.-F., Lin, J.-M. (2013). Application of carbon-based nanomaterials in sample preparation: a review. *Anal Chim Acta*, 784, 1–17. doi: 10.1016/j.aca.2013.03.054

38. Scida, K., Stege, Patricia W., Haby, G., Messina, Germán A., García, Carlos D. (2011). Recent applications of carbon-based nanomaterials in analytical chemistry: Critical review. *Anal Chim Acta*, 691(1–2), 6–17. doi: 10.1016/j.aca.2011.02.025

39. Siqueira, J. R. (2017). Carbon-based nanomaterials. In: Da Róz, A. L., Ferreira, M., de Lima Leite, F., Oliveira, O. N., editors. *Nanostructures*, 233–249. NY: William Andrew Publishing.

40. Bianco, A., Kostarelos, K., Prato, M. (2008). Opportunities and challenges of carbon-based nanomaterials for cancer therapy. *Expert Opin Drug Deliv*, 5(3), 331–342. doi: 10.1517/17425247.5.3.331

41. Yuan, X., Zhang, X., Sun, L., Wei, Y., Wei, X.. (2019). Cellular toxicity and immunological effects of carbon-based nanomaterials. *Part Fibre Toxicol*, 16, 18. 10.1186/s12989-019-0299-z

42. Patel, K. D., Singh, R. K., Kim, H-W. (2019). Carbon-based nanomaterials as an emerging platform for theranostics. *Mater Horiz*. doi: 10.1039/c8mh00966j

43. Dresselhaus, M. S., Terrones, M. (2013). Carbon-based nanomaterials from a historical perspective. *Proc IEEE*, 101(7), 1522–1535. doi: 10.1109/JPROC.2013.2261271

44. Karimi, M., Zangabad, P. S., Mehdizadeh, F., Malekzad, H., Ghasemi, A., Bahrami, S., Zare, H., Moghoofei, M., Hekmatmanesh, A., Hamblin, M. R. (2017 Jan 26). Nanocaged platforms: modification, drug delivery and nanotoxicity. Opening synthetic cages to release the tiger. *Nanoscale*, 9(4), 1356–1392. doi: 10.1039/c6nr07315h. PMID: 28067384; PMCID: PMC5300024.

45. Kundu, S., Bramhaiah, K., Bhattacharyya, S. (2020). Carbon-based nanomaterials: in the quest of alternative metal-free photocatalysts for solar water splitting. *Nanoscale Adv*, 2(11), 5130–5151.

46. Li, Y. X., Pang, H. B. (2021 Jan 10). Macropinocytosis as a cell entry route for peptide-functionalized and bystander nanoparticles. *J Control Release*, 329, 1222–1230. doi: 10.1016/j.jconrel.2020.10.049. Epub 2020 Oct 24. PMID: 33622520; PMCID: PMC7905157.

47. Zhang, S., Gao, H., Bao, G. (2015 Sep 22). Physical principles of nanoparticle cellular endocytosis. *ACS Nano*, 9(9), 8655–8671. doi: 10.1021/acsnano.5b03184. Epub 2015 Aug 21. PMID: 26256227; PMCID: PMC5681865.

48. Sousa de Almeida, M., Susnik, E., Drasler, B., Taladriz-Blanco, P., Petri-Fink, A., Rothen-Rutishauser, B. (2021 May 7). Understanding nanoparticle endocytosis to improve targeting strategies in nanomedicine. *Chem Soc Rev*, 50(9), 5397–5434. doi: 10.1039/d0cs01127d. Epub 2021 Mar 5. PMID: 33666625; PMCID: PMC8111542.

49. Akinc, A., Battaglia, G. (2013 Nov 1). Exploiting endocytosis for nanomedicines. *Cold Spring Harb Perspect Biol*, 5(11), a016980. doi: 10.1101/cshperspect.a016980. PMID: 24186069; PMCID: PMC3809578.

50. Oh, N., Park, J. H. (2014 May 6). Endocytosis and exocytosis of nanoparticles in mammalian cells. *Int J Nanomed*, 9 (Suppl 1), 51–63. doi: 10.2147/IJN.S26592. PMID: 24872703; PMCID: PMC4024976.

51. Qie, Y., Yuan, H., von Roemeling, C., Chen, Y., Liu, X., Shih, K. D., Knight, J. A., Tun, H. W., Wharen, R. E., Jiang, W., Kim, B. Y. S. (2016). Surface modification of nanoparticles enables selective evasion of phagocytic clearance by distinct macrophage phenotypes. *Sci Rep*. 6, 26269.

52. Foroozandeh, P., Aziz, A. A. (2018). Insight into cellular uptake and intracellular trafficking of nanoparticles. *Nanoscale Res Lett*, 13(339). doi: 10.1186/s11671-018-2728-6

53. Krpetić, Ž., Porta, F., Caneva, E., Dal Santo, V., Scarì, G. (2010). Phagocytosis of biocompatible gold nanoparticles. *Langmuir*, 26(18), 14799–14805. doi: 10.1021/la102758f

54. Gustafson, H. H., Holt-Casper, D., Grainger, D. W., Ghandehari, H. (2015). Nanoparticle uptake: the phagocyte problem. *Nano Today*. doi: 10.1016/j.nantod.2015.06.006

55. Wang, Z., Tiruppathi, C., Minshall, R. D., Malik, A. B. (2009 Dec 22). Size and dynamics of caveolae studied using nanoparticles in living endothelial cells. *ACS Nano*, 3(12), 4110–4116. doi: 10.1021/nn9012274. PMID: 19919048; PMCID: PMC3643811.

56. Dixit, S., Sahu, R., Verma, R., Duncan, S., Giambartolomei, G. H., Singh, S. R., Dennis, V. A. (2018 Mar). Caveolin-mediated endocytosis of the Chlamydia M278 outer membrane peptide encapsulated in poly(lactic acid)-Poly(ethylene glycol) nanoparticles by mouse primary dendritic cells enhances specific immune effectors mediated by MHC class II and CD4$^+$ T cells. *Biomaterials*, 159, 130–145. doi: 10.1016/j.biomaterials.2017.12.019. Epub 2017 Dec 26. PMID: 29324305; PMCID: PMC5801148.

57. Kou, L., Sun, J., Zhai, Y., He, Z. (2013). The endocytosis and intracellular fate of nanomedicines: implication for rational design. *Asian J Pharm Sci*, 8(1), 1–10. doi: 10.1016/j.ajps.2013.07.001

58. Sahay, G., Alakhova, D. Y., Kabanov, A. V. (2010 Aug 3). Endocytosis of nanomedicines. *J Control Release*, 145(3), 182–195. doi: 10.1016/j.jconrel.2010. 01.036. Epub 2010 Mar 10. PMID: 20226220; PMCID: PMC2902597.

59. Hao, X., Wu, J., Shan, Y., Cai, M., Shang, X., Jiang, J., Wang, H. (2012). Caveolaemediated endocytosis of biocompatible gold nanoparticles in living Hela cells. d Matter. *J. Phys.: Condens. Matter*, 24(16), 164207–0. doi: 10.1088/0953-8984/24/16/164207

60. Rennick, J. J., Johnston, A. P. R., Parton, R. G. (2021). Key principles and methods for studying the endocytosis of biological and nanoparticle therapeutics. *Nat Nanotechnol*, 16, 266–276. 10.1038/s41565-021-00858-8

61. Liu, X., Yang, H., Liu, Y., Gong, X., Huang, H. (2019). Numerical study of clathrin-mediated endocytosis of nanoparticles by cells under tension. *Acta Mechanica Sinica*, 35(3), 691–701. doi: 10.1007/s10409-019-00839-0

62. Banerjee, A., Berezhkovskii, A., Nossal, R. (2013). On the size dependence of cellular uptake of nanoparticle via clathrin-mediated endocytosis. *Biophys J*, 104(2), 622a. doi: 10.1016/j.bpj.2012.11.3441

63. Suen, W-L. L., Chau, Y. (April 2014). Size-dependent internalisation of folate-decorated nanoparticles via the pathways of clathrin and caveolae-mediated endocytosis in ARPE-19 cells. *J Pharm Pharmacol*, 66(4), 564–573.

64. Smith, P. J., Giroud, M., Wiggins, H. L., Gower, F., Thorley, J. A., Stolpe, B., Mazzolini, J., Dyson, R. J., Rappoport, J. Z. (2012). Cellular entry of nanoparticles via serum sensitive clathrin-mediated endocytosis, and plasma membrane permeabilization. *Int J Nanomedicine*, 7, 2045–2055. doi: 10.2147/IJN.S29334. PMID: 22619541; PMCID: PMC3356167.

65. Eom, H. J., Choi, J. (2019 Sep 25). Clathrin-mediated endocytosis is involved in uptake and toxicity of silica nanoparticles in *Caenorhabditis elegans*. *Chem Biol Interact*, 311, 108774. doi: 10.1016/j.cbi.2019.108774. PMID: 31369748.

66. Ng, C. T., Tang, F. M., Li, J. J., Ong, C., Yung, L. L., Bay, B. H. (2015 Feb). Clathrin-mediated endocytosis of gold nanoparticles in vitro. *Anat Rec (Hoboken)*, 298(2), 418–427. doi: 10.1002/ar.23051. PMID: 25243822.

67. Deng, H., Dutta, P., Liu, J. (2019 Jun 26). Entry modes of ellipsoidal nanoparticles on a membrane during clathrin-mediated endocytosis. *Soft Matter*, 15(25), 5128–5137. doi: 10.1039/c9sm00751b. PMID: 31190048; PMCID: PMC7570437.

68. Sandvig, K., Kavaliauskiene, S., Skotland, T. (2018). Clathrin-independent endocytosis: an increasing degree of complexity. *Histochem Cell Biol*, 150, 107–118. 10.1 007/s00418-018-1678-5

69. Saha, K., Kim, S. T., Yan, B., Miranda, O. R., Alfonso, F. S., Shlosman, D., Rotello, V. M. (2013 Jan 28). Surface functionality of nanoparticles determines cellular uptake mechanisms in mammalian cells. *Small*, 9(2), 300–305. doi: 10.1002/smll. 201201129. PMID: 22972519; PMCID: PMC4070423.

70. Vanhecke, D., Kuhn, D. A., Jimenez de Aberasturi, D., Balog, S., Milosevic, A., Urban, D., Peckys, D., de Jonge, N., Parak, W. J., Petri-Fink, A., Rothen-Rutishauser, B. (2017). Involvement of two uptake mechanisms of gold and iron oxide nanoparticles in a co-exposure scenario using mouse macrophages. *Beilstein J Nanotechnol*, 8, 2396–2409. doi: 10.3762/bjnano.8.239

71. Wang, C., Chen, S., Bao, L., Liu, X., Hu, F., Yuan, H. (2020 Jun 9). Size-controlled preparation and behavior study of phospholipid-calcium carbonate hybrid nanoparticles. *Int J Nanomed*, 15, 4049–4062. doi: 10.2147/IJN.S237156. PMID: 32606663; PMCID: PMC7293410.

72. Buono, C., Anzinger, J. J., Amar, M., Kruth, H. S. (2009 May). Fluorescent pegylated nanoparticles demonstrate fluid-phase pinocytosis by macrophages in

mouse atherosclerotic lesions. *J Clin Invest*, 119(5), 1373–1381. doi: 10.1172/JCI35548. Epub 2009 Apr 13. PMID: 19363293; PMCID: PMC2673852.

73. Means, N., Elechalawar, C. K., Chen, W. R., Bhattacharya, R., Mukherjee, P. (2021). Revealing macropinocytosis using nanoparticles. *Mol Aspects Med*, 100993. doi: 10.1016/j.mam.2021.100993

74. Li, Yue-Xuan, Pang, Hong-Bo (2020). Macropinocytosis as a cell entry route for peptide-functionalized and bystander nanoparticles. *J Control Release*. doi: 10.1016/j.jconrel.2020.10.049

75. Shang, L., Nienhaus, K., Nienhaus, G. U. (2014). Engineered nanoparticles interacting with cells: size matters. *J Nanobiotechnol*, 12(5). 10.1186/1477-3155-12-5

76. Díaz-Torres, R., López-Arellano, R., Escobar-Chávez, J. J., García-García, E., Domínguez-Delgado, C. L., Ramírez-Noguera, P. (2016). Effect of size and functionalization of pharmaceutical nanoparticles and their interaction with biological systems. *Handbook of Nanoparticles*, 1041–1060. doi: 10.1007/978-3-319-15338-4_46

77. Hoshyar, N., Gray, S., Han, H., Bao, G. (2016 Mar). The effect of nanoparticle size on in vivo pharmacokinetics and cellular interaction. *Nanomedicine (Lond)*, 11(6), 673–692. doi: 10.2217/nnm.16.5. Epub 2016 Mar 22. PMID: 27003448; PMCID: PMC5561790.

78. Gatoo, M. A., Naseem, S., Arfat, M. Y., Dar, A. M., Qasim, K., Zubair, S. (2014). Physicochemical properties of nanomaterials: implication in associated toxic manifestations. *Biomed Res Int*, 2014, 498420. doi: 10.1155/2014/498420. Epub 2014 Aug 6. PMID: 25165707; PMCID: PMC4140132.

79. Fehaid, A., Taniguchi, A. (2019 Feb 27). Size-dependent effect of silver nanoparticles on the tumor necrosis factor α-induced DNA damage response. *Int J Mol Sci*, 20(5), 1038. doi: 10.3390/ijms20051038. PMID: 30818829; PMCID: PMC6429428.

80. Zhu, J., Liao, L., Zhu, L., Zhang, P., Guo, K., Kong, J., Ji, C., Liu, B. (2013). Size-dependent cellular uptake efficiency, mechanism, and cytotoxicity of silica nanoparticles toward HeLa cells. *Talanta*, 107, 408–415. doi: 10.1016/j.talanta.2013.01.037

81. Jin, H., Heller, D. A., Sharma, R., and Strano, M. S. (2009). Size-dependent cellular uptake and expulsion of single-walled carbon nanotubes: single particle tracking and a generic uptake model for nanoparticles. *ACS Nano* 3(1), 149–158. doi: 10.1021/nn800532m

82. Xu, A., Yao, M., Xu, G., Ying, J., Ma, W., Li, B., Jin, Y. (2012). A physical model for the size-dependent cellular uptake of nanoparticles modified with cationic surfactants. *Int J Nanomed*, 7, 3547–3554. doi: 10.2147/IJN.S32188. Epub 2012 Jul 10. PMID: 22848178; PMCID: PMC3405883.

83. Ma, X., Wu, Y., Jin, S., Tian, Y., Zhang, X., Zhao, Y., Yu, Li, Liang, X.-J. (2011). Gold nanoparticles induce autophagosome accumulation through size-dependent nanoparticle uptake and lysosome impairment. *ACS Nano*, 5(11), 8629–8639. doi: 10.1021/nn202155y

84. Mu, Q., Su, G., Li, L., Gilbertson, B. O., Yu, L. H., Zhang, Q., Sun, Y.-P., Yan, B. (2012). Size-dependent cell uptake of protein-coated graphene oxide nanosheets. *ACS Appl Mater Interfaces*, 4(4), 2259–2266. doi: 10.1021/am300253c

85. Chen, L., Xiao, S., Zhu, H., Wang, L., Liang, H. (2016). Shape-dependent internalization kinetics of nanoparticle by membrane. *Soft Matter*, 10.1039.C5SM01869B–. doi: 10.1039/C5SM01869B

86. Vácha, R., Martinez-Veracoechea, F. J., Frenkel, D. (2011). Receptor-mediated endocytosis of nanoparticles of various shapes. *Nano Lett*, 11(12), 5391–5395. doi: 10.1021/nl2030213

87. Xie, X., Liao, J., Shao, X., Li, Q., Lin, Y. (2017). The effect of shape on cellular uptake of gold nanoparticles in the forms of stars, rods, and triangles. *Sci Rep*, 7, 3827. doi: 10.1038/s41598-017-04229-z

88. Kim, S.-N., Park, C. G., Min, C. H., Lee, S. H., Lee, Y. Y., Lee, N. K., Choy, Y. B. (2021). Shape-dependent intracellular uptake of metal–organic framework nanoparticles. *J Ind Eng Chem*. doi: 10.1016/j.jiec.2021.08.042

89. Salatin, S., Maleki Dizaj, S., Yari Khosroushahi, A. (2015). Effect of the surface modification, size, and shape on cellular uptake of nanoparticles. *Cell Biol Int*, 39(8), 881–890. doi: 10.1002/cbin.10459

90. Tang, H., Zhang, H., Ye, H., Zheng, Y. (2017). Receptor-mediated endocytosis of nanoparticles: roles of shapes, orientations, and rotations of nanoparticles. *J Phys Chem B*. doi: 10.1021/acs.jpcb.7b09619

91. Chakraborty, A., Jana, N. R. (2015). Clathrin to lipid raft-endocytosis via controlled surface chemistry and efficient perinuclear targeting of nanoparticle. *J Phys Chem Lett*. doi: 10.1021/acs.jpclett.5b01739

92. Platel, A., Carpentier, R., Becart, E., Mordacq, G., Betbeder, D., Nesslany, F. (2016 Mar). Influence of the surface charge of PLGA nanoparticles on their in vitro genotoxicity, cytotoxicity, ROS production and endocytosis. *J Appl Toxicol*, 36(3), 434–444. doi: 10.1002/jat.3247. Epub 2015 Oct 21. PMID: 26487569.

93. da Rocha, E. L., Caramori, G. F., Rambo, C. R. (2013 Feb 21). Nanoparticle translocation through a lipid bilayer tuned by surface chemistry. *Phys Chem Chem Phys*, 15(7), 2282–2290. doi: 10.1039/c2cp44035k. Epub 2012 Dec 5. PMID: 23223270.

94. Zhao, J., Stenzel, M. H. (2017). Entry of nanoparticles into cells: the importance of nanoparticle properties. *Polymer Chemistry*. doi: 10.1039/C7PY01603D

95. Adler, A. F., Leong, K. W. (2010). Emerging links between surface nanotechnology and endocytosis: impact on nonviral gene delivery. *Nano Today*, 5(6), 553–569. doi: 10.1016/j.nantod.2010.10.007

96. Lee, Y. K., Choi, E. J., Webster, T. J., Kim, S. H., Khang, D. (2014 Dec 18). Effect of the protein corona on nanoparticles for modulating cytotoxicity and immunotoxicity. *Int J Nanomedicine*, 10, 97–113. doi: 10.2147/IJN.S72998. PMID: 25565807; PMCID: PMC4275058.

97. Nguyen, V. H., Lee, B. J. (2017 Apr 18). Protein corona: a new approach for nanomedicine design. *Int J Nanomedicine*, 12, 3137–3151. doi: 10.2147/IJN.S129300. PMID: 28458536; PMCID: PMC5402904.

3 Application of Nanotechnology in Diagnostics of Rheumatoid Arthritis

Devika Tripathi, Krislay Rathour, Jyoti Kumari, Vivek Mishra, and Vikas Shukla

3.1 INTRODUCTION

Rheumatoid arthritis (RA) is characterized by inflammation and other clinical signs that result from immune cells' hyperresponsiveness to self-antigens. It is a long-lasting, systemic autoimmune condition. The various immunologically released enzymes and chemicals in synovial tissues are known causes of RA, which affects all body joints (hand joints, shoulders, knees, hips, cervical spine, ankles, and legs). Commonly, the disease risk increases due to biological and genetic variables. Women above 65 are more affected than men due to hormonal changes. However, the incidence of RA varies in developing nations and is more common in Western nations [1–15]. Severe consequences like joint destruction and remarkable disability in the body were associated with the diagnosis of RA before the 1990s. The pyramid treatment approach was usually followed, nonsteroidal anti-inflammatory drugs (NSAIDs), initiated with rest in bed, and disease-modifying antirheumatic drug therapy that worsened the disease. These methods are neither preventive nor curative yet. The clinical diagnosis of RA is based on two sets of criteria: the 1987 ACR criteria and the 2001 ACR/European League Against Rheumatism (EULAR) criteria. Physical checks and observing characteristic symptoms like pain, stiffness, and multiple joint swelling are considered influential diagnoses. However, early RA diagnosis was made harder by the clinical diagnosis, which was made after a period of six months to a year of RA development. Moreover, the standard approach has not been possible due to RA's non-specificity and unidentified clinical and pathological features. Thus, in 2018, the Chinese Rheumatology Association was responsible for the drafting of the Chinese recommendations for the identification and management of RA. The guidelines have recommended the imaging examinations and laboratory and patient's clinical manifestations for RA. In this regard, serological tests exhibited prospects as biomarkers. Serological tests will detect the antibodies (RF, ACPA), CRP in blood, and erythrocyte sedimentation rate indicative of RA.

DOI: 10.1201/9781003348672-3

Traditional radiography, US, CT, and MRI are all useful for diagnosing RA through imaging. The imaging diagnosis has been selected according to the size, the number of affected joints, and the severity of synovial joints. However, the mandate condition for RA imaging is that patients should have medium, large, or small joints, or the duration of synovitis must be more than six weeks. The structural damage in RA is adequately noticed by X-ray radiography. However, early stages of RA can present with periarticular soft tissue edema as well as periarticular or juxta-articular osteoporosis, which can be shown on X-rays. However, during the course of RA, it has been observed that joint dislocation or fusion, articular surface deterioration, and joint space stenosis cannot be seen. Thus, X-rays are not only inexpensive but also quite efficient. However, their selection in RA has been limited by the risk of radiation exposure as well as their inadequate sensitivity for early detection. The CT scan observed the breakdown of solidified tissue, such as provided a three-dimensional image of the joints and bone erosions in RA [16]. The sensitivity of erosions has increased as a result of this, particularly at complicated places like the wrist, which has aided in the early detection of the condition. Encouraging applications of novel CT techniques (high-resolution CT and dual-energy CT) can detect the appendicular skeleton of RA patients [17,18]. Besides, CT is costly, luminous, and not able to detect dynamic inflammations such as synovitis in RA. The US is suitable and economical for examining the structures of cartilage, bone, and synovial of various joints. The US is more delicate in sensing joint structural deterioration, such as the articular cartilage, shape and thickness of synovium, articular cavity effusion, and synovial sac. Also, able to detect treatment and joint destruction. However, it has been noted that the presence of Doppler signals can cause synovial enlargement with or without effusion. Thus, Doppler ultrasound has been employed. With this, synovitis's presence, monitor disease activity, progression, and inflammation can be assessed. However, mastery is required for US processes. The most sensitive MRI for diagnosing early RA lesions has been recently investigated. The higher expenses are involved in the MRI technique. MRI scans have also revealed bone marrow edema and mild articular surface degradation in addition to synovial thickening. However, after gadolinium injection, studies have shown enhanced MR signal intensity in a synovial compartment. Identifying early inflammation by MRI and US is outstanding for clinical examination. However, several advanced techniques did not solve complications of RA early diagnosis. Surprisingly, nano-based strategies seem advantageous for RA detection and diagnosis. Thus, there has been a brief introduction to the risk factors and pathophysiology of RA, as well as a discussion of various diagnostic techniques and RA therapies.

3.2 PATHOPHYSIOLOGICAL EVENTS OF RHEUMATOID ARTHRITIS

The panoramic view of RA's different stages are pooled results of cell interaction, mediators, auto-antibody, and various innate and adaptive immune system signal transduction pathways. A knowledge of RA pathogenesis insights helps in improving the disease state [19]. Moreover, it contributed to specifying new marks for designing novel disease-modifying treatments. The etiology of RA has been attributed to a complicated network involving several cytokines and cells. Synovial cell proliferation is triggered by cytokines, which also cause damage to cartilage and bone. The cytokines interleukin (IL)-6 and tumor necrosis factor (TNF)-α are critical in RA [20]. The role of other cytokines like IL-7, IL-17, IL-21, IL-23, IL-1β, IL-18, IL-33, IL-2, and factor GM-CSF factors have been researched recently. Multiple roles of autoantibodies have been in the light for the past ten years. Both anti-citrullinated protein antibodies and rheumatoid factor differ significantly from autoantibody-negatives in patients' clinical course of treatment. Activating fibroblasts and macrophages into cells that destroy tissue is the main function of T-cells in RA. Similar to T- and B-cells, activated macrophages release a variety of cytokines and chemokines that promote joint inflammation [16–18].

3.2.1 B-lymphocytes Trigger and Pathogenesis

B-cells have shown an essential role in the pathogenesis of RA. However, autoantibodies and some autoantibody-independent functions (autoreactive T-cells and proinflammatory factors) have promoted autoimmunity. Similarly, B-cells stimulate OC formation by secreting TNF and RANKL and activating other effector molecules. B cells are known to be critical in activating CD4+ T-cells. The interaction between the CD4+ T-cells and I-Ag7 caused T-cell activation and produced autoantibodies that mediated joint damage in the hybrid mouse. Due to the dysfunction of the central and peripheral B-cell tolerance checkpoints in RA, the mature naïve B-cell compartment becomes overpopulated with autoreactive B-cells [21]. Regarding the inhibition of CD4 T-cells, Treg function is compromised in RA. In the pathogenesis of RA, cell-to-cell interaction between B-cells and FLSs may be important [22]. FLSs are effectors that are triggered by B-cells in the immune system. FLSs have the ability to serve as a "nurse-like" cell for mature B-cells. It is possible that this ability is responsible for the sustained survival and homing of B-cells in RA synovium. The introduction of antigens to T-cells has been done by B-cells, which is essential for producing costimulatory signals. These signals help in the initiation of effector function, clonal expansion, and T-cell activation [23].

3.2.2 T-Cells and Pathogenesis

The synovial surroundings in RA have been influenced primarily by T-cells [Figure 3.1]. However, the active role of these cells is yet to be thoroughly comprehended. Despite this, the regulatory T-cells have significantly impacted RA pathogenesis events. These regulatory T-cells suppress T-cell proliferation, cause uncontrolled proinflammatory cytokine production, and support phenotype to CD4+ effector T-cells [24]. The CD4+ T-cell population is represented by the CD4+CD25+ regulatory T-cell subset. This population has been shown to suppress the in vitro proliferation of autologous CD4+ T-cells. In related studies, the differentiation of naïve T-cells into Th 17 cells (cytokine) has been involved in synovitis [25]. **Takemura et al**. have reported that the B-cells are responsible for activating the T-cells and progressing the disease. T-cell activity has been encouraged by B-cell-supported regulatory T-cell homing and survival. However,

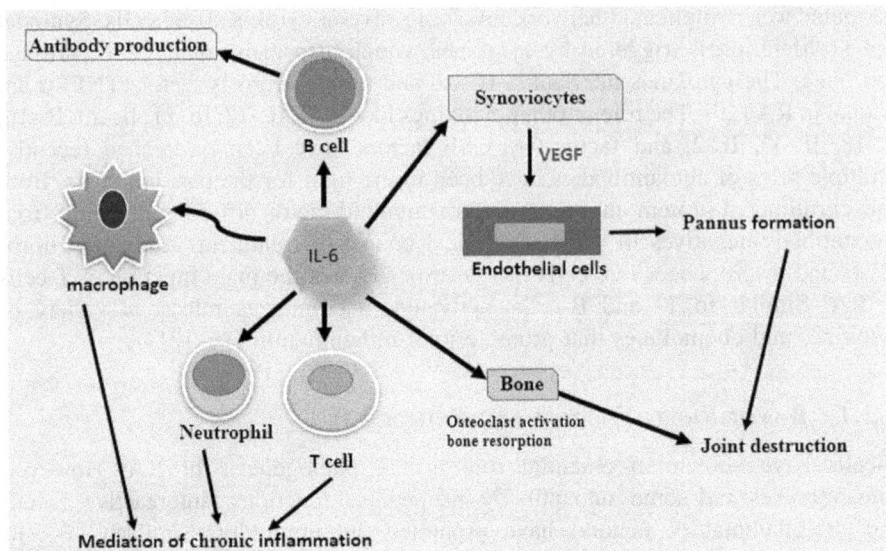

FIGURE 3.1 A schematic presentation of the pathogenesis of rheumatoid arthritis.

T-cell-derived cytokines have activated the synovial fibroblasts and macrophages and formed tissue-invasive pannus [26].

3.2.3 TUMOR NECROSIS FACTOR (TNF-α)

TNF-α is a crucial cytokine that induces inflammations in RA and stimulates numerous inflammatory cytokines. Both TNF-α and IL-7 cytokines can suppress human Tregs' activity [27]. It is reported that TNF-α enables the dysfunctional subset of FoxP3+ Tregs. TNF receptor II (TNFRII) has been expressed by TNF-α, which is directed to arthritis.[28] However, TNF-α has also triggered an NF-κB pathway and has rendered a pro-inflammatory phenotype. As an osteoclast precursor, TNF-α stimulated osteoclast differentiation led to synovitis and initial bone loss [29].

3.2.4 INTERLEUKIN-6 TRIGGER AND PATHOGENESIS

A pleiotropic cytokine, IL-6, is critical in RA pathophysiology. Many systemic manifestations have been included in RA pathophysiology mediated by IL-6. The acute-phase reaction (C-reactive protein (CRP), anemia through hepcidin production, fatigue, and osteoporosis have been considered [30]. Reportedly, IL-6 causes synovitis and destruction mediated by neutrophil migration, osteoclast maturation, and vascular endothelial growth factor (VEGF)-stimulated pannus accumulation. IL-6 exacerbated the local inflammatory reaction. VEGF levels have been involved in disease activity, leading to pannus formation [31]. **Hashizume M et al.** observed that IL-6 provoked tubule formation in human umbilical vein endothelial cells (HUVECs) and fibroblast-like synoviocytes in RA patients. IL-6 has influenced osteoblast differentiation. Illustrative in-vivo and in-vitro stimulation of IL-6 and TNF-α generated osteoclast differentiation from bone marrow-derived macrophages [Figure 3.1] [32].

3.2.5 CYTOKINES IL-1 AND IL-17

Cytokines IL-1 and IL-17 have degraded bone and cartilage and worsened the diseases in RA patients. IL-17 cytokine has evoked several immune and inflammatory responses, resulting in multisystem organ complications [33,34]. The synergistic effects of TNF-α and IL-1, IL-17 have caused joint inflammation, cartilage, and destruction. Recent investigations have revealed that IL-1α and IL-1β increased the glycolysis of rheumatoid synovial cells in RA. It commonly dysregulates the lactate level in rheumatoid joints [35]. Interleukin-17 (IL-17) and the ability of Th17 cells to prevent FLSs from apoptosizing were studied by **Kim E. et al.** Mitochondrial dysfunction was observed in osteoarthritic patients. IL-17 has induced mitochondrial dysfunction and autophagosome formation and progressed the disease (Table 3.1) [36].

TABLE 3.1

Pathogenesis Trigger Factors in Rheumatoid Arthritis and Pathogenesis Effects

Pathogenesis Trigger Factors in Rheumatoid Arthritis	Pathogenesis Effects	References
IL-1	-Implicated in the autoimmune illness rheumatoid arthritis. -Mediates the degradation of cartilage and the resorption of bone	[37]
IL-6	-Prevalent synovium in RA patients, -Advents disease and causes destruction of the joints	[30]
IL-10	-Limiting host immune response to pathogens -Immunoregulator, regulating monocyte and several cytokines including T-cell	[38]
IL-12	-Enhances disease expression and severity in an animal model of RA. -Expressed infiltrating macrophage and synovial lining cells	[39]
IL-15	-Progresses the onset of severe inflammatory arthritis -Physiological triggered cyclosporin A and steroid-sensitive pathways	[40]
IL-18	-Induces leukocyte extravasation -Angiogenic mediator and leukocyte chemoattractant	[41]
IL-22	-Promotes inflammatory responses in RA synovial tissues -induces the proliferation and chemokine production of synovial fibroblasts.	[42]
IL-23	-Stimulates production of IL-17 -Expresses innate-like lymphocytes, such as type 3 innate lymphoid cells.	[43]

(Continued)

TABLE 3.1 *(Continued)*
Pathogenesis Trigger Factors in Rheumatoid Arthritis and Pathogenesis Effects

Pathogenesis Trigger Factors in Rheumatoid Arthritis	Pathogenesis Effects	References
B-cell receptor	-Promotes proliferation and differentiation of T-cells	[44]
	-Activates monocyte osteoclasts in the synovium	
C-receptor protein	-Promotes atherogenic effects	[45]
	-Progress the disease-caused bone destruction	
HLA DRB1 gene	-Increased risk of RA disease	[46]
	-HLA-DRB1 risk alleles induce somatic hypermutation of ACPA	
Epigenetic factor	-Manifested the heritable phenotype changes	[47]

3.3 RISK FACTORS AND THEIR VARIOUS CONSEQUENCES IN RHEUMATOID ARTHRITIS

The risk factors of RA are critically primal to comprehend RA. Various risk factors help identify the exposure consequences of joint and cartilage damage. Regardless, these are virtually important in preventing irreversible synovium damage. Likewise, joint damage has been associated with genetic, sex, and environmental pollutants risk factors, which eventually progressed the RA risk [48].

3.3.1 Host Factors

As with many other immune-mediated illnesses, the host influences the likelihood of RA developing. This mainly includes genetic factors, which account for a sizable portion of disease risk. Recent research has revealed that epigenetic mechanisms directly affect RA's pathogenesis, changing the chance of disease initiation. Notably, the environment links to intrinsic and external components and provides the known prevalence of RA. For instance, in women, hormonal, obstetric, and neuroendocrine factors have long been proposed as the disease's etiology. Lately, it has been suggested that several coexisting conditions may expand the threat of RA [49,50].

3.3.2 Genetic Factor

Numerous autoimmune diseases, including RA, have a genetic basis, which raises the likelihood of developing the illness in people who carry particular genetic traits. Comprehending the disease can be gained by looking into the genetic markers connected to RA. According to studies, four main genetic variables have been associated with RA: The gene most strongly associated with RA is HLA-DR4. People who carry this trait are more likely to get RA than people who do not, and their symptoms may be more severe. Moreover, a specific gene called STAT4 regulates and activates the immune response. Similarly, genes TRAF1 and C5 are vital in the emergence of chronic inflammation [51,52].

3.3.3 EPIGENETIC FACTOR

Epigenetics' role in the onset of RA is only now being comprehended. Epigenetic mechanisms result in heritable gene expression variations, even in the absence of alterations to the DNA sequence. With this strategy, they assist in explaining the disease's small genetic contribution. A significant new epigenome-wide association research demonstrates that monozygotic twin pairs with RA divergence had variable methylation profiles. However, these changes have been linked to the genome and atmosphere interaction with external factors like medications, tobacco, or nutrition [53].

3.3.4 HORMONAL OR REPRODUCTIVE VARIABLES

Female hormonal variables influenced the progression of RA. Early menopause, the postpartum phase, and the use of anti-estrogen medications are all linked to the development of RA. An abrupt reduction in ovarian function and estrogen bioavailability represents all these disorders. Other female hormonal components, on the other hand, are controversial. It is still unknown how systemic hormonal therapies, such as HRT and contraception, affect the development of RA. It is debatable how additional factors (such as PCO, lactation, or parity) connected to various hormonal changes may also have an impact. The duration of estrogen exposure and the effects of female hormonal variables during premenopausal & post-menopause both influenced the onset of RA [54–56].

3.3.5 ALLERGIC AND RESPIRATORY FACTORS

The prevalence of RA was found to be raised by atopy and allergic disorders (such as asthma, nasal congestion, and contact dermatitis). Since then, numerous epidemiological investigations have confirmed an expansion in the incidence of RA in populations with allergies. Despite the disputed nature of the research, the bulk of outstanding population-based cohort studies exhibited a negative connection between atopy and RA. New studies have also associated acute and chronic upper or lower respiratory diseases with a higher risk of seropositive and seronegative RA [57–59].

3.3.6 NEUROLOGICAL AND PSYCHIATRIC FACTORS

People with RA experienced more mental harm than healthy individuals. Moreover, the disease typically advances in a painful, incapacitating manner. The prevalence of comorbid depression and anxiety in RA sufferers was investigated. Approximately 82 RA cases and 41 healthy volunteers of corresponding ages and sexes underwent psychiatric evaluations by DSM-IV guidelines. Patients with anxiety had shorter illness durations than RA patients. Suggestively, patients' ability to adapt to and respond to treatment had encountered specific issues, including anxiety [60,61].

3.3.7 AIRBORNE NOXIOUS CHEMICALS

Investigators initially discussed a meaningful connection between RA and many airborne noxious chemicals. The genomic interplay of smoking with SE alleles and seropositive RA was discussed. However, the key findings have disclosed that multiplier impacted cigarette load and SE danger alleles. According to a proposed hypothesis of RA etiology based on all these epidemiological findings, smoking has caused in situ protein citrullination or transformed the arginine to citrulline in the lungs of SE-positive people, which has produced ACPAs and had advanced RA. This has been supported by the study on smokers' bronchioalveolar compartments, where higher activity and appearance of the citrullination enzyme PAD2 were observed [62–64].

3.3.8 MICROBIAL INFECTION

Numerous studies have shown the clinical connection between microbes and RA. Infection is frequently present in early RA and can manifest before clinical arthritis begins. However, RA-associated infections are solely a reaction to immuno-suppressive medication. Studies using animal models of arthritis have documented the negative influence of infections on RA. The infection occurred before clinical arthritis has repeatedly been found in early RA. P. gingivitis substantially contributes to RA pathogenesis among the microorganisms associated with RA [65]. Figure 3.2 shows various risk factors affecting RA treatment.

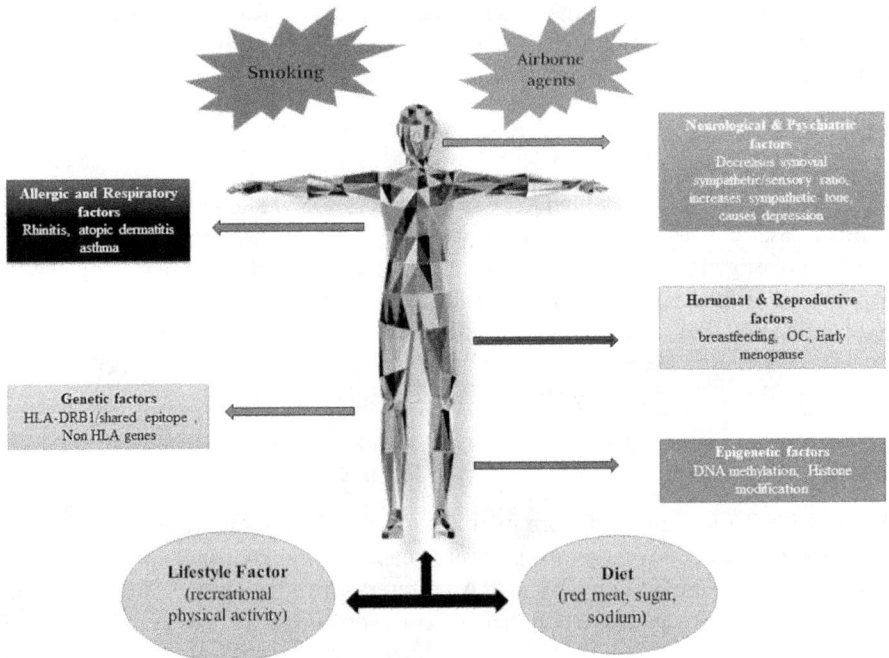

FIGURE 3.2 Risk factors affecting rheumatoid arthritis treatment.

3.4   CONVENTIONAL DIAGNOSTIC METHODS FOR RHEUMATOID ARTHRITIS

The American College of Rheumatology states that early diagnosis can control RA disease progression. At the same time, pain assessment, minor joint stiffness, and symmetrical swelling have been epitomized clinically. However, understanding the levels of anti-citrullinated protein antibody (ACPA), rheumatoid factor (RF), and anti-carbamylated protein depends on the patient's past therapeutic history and diagnosis. Thus, innovative bioimaging techniques have the potential to mark the degeneration, structural changes, and degree of joint destruction in RA. For instance, magnetic resonance imaging, computed tomography, radiography, and ultrasonography efficiently detected joint space narrowing, bone erosion, and destruction of synovial joints. Likewise, biomarkers have opened new gateways in RA diagnosis. Some promising biomarkers genetic markers (HLA-DR) and serological markers have been used. Despite this, about 20% of the patients with RA reported negative ACPA and RF estimation values, necessitating the development of innovative RA diagnostic approaches. For example, RA biomarkers are presently being developed using oral microbiota profiling. Studies have also reported that RA patients have suffered pathogenic complications more from anaerobic bacteria in the oral cavity that induce the production of anti-cyclic citrullinated peptide antibodies and citrullination of self-proteins. Thus, A gram-negative anaerobic bacteria called *Porphyromonas gingivalis* had been identified in the oral cavity of RA patients. In effect, **Bin Chen et al.** presented the utility of oral microbiota in screening RA. However, shotgun and pyrosequencing techniques have relieved the risk of RA development.

3.5   CONVENTIONAL TREATMENT FOR RHEUMATOID ARTHRITIS

Treatment strategies for RA have evolved lately. Indeed, drug therapies are more focused on providing symptomatic relief to delay and control structural joint damage. However, Methotrexate was popular among RA patients without using other drugs. Also, the low tolerance of high doses of Methotrexate was often controversial in achieving maximum effect. Hence, it stayed inadequate responders. Despite this, treatment for RA has grown from salicylates to newer NSAIDs, CSS, DMARDs, and biological response modifiers. Table 3.2 shows conventionally used drugs and their observed side effects while used for RA treatment.

3.6   APPLICATIONS OF NANOTECHNOLOGY IN DIAGNOSTIC OF RHEUMATOID ARTHRITIS

Reportedly, timely and early treatment of RA has improved the treatment outcomes. In this regard, nanomaterials as diagnosis agents have shown inspiring results. The work by **Markides et al.** has shed insight into the usage of superparamagnetic iron oxide nanoparticles to monitor the movement of stem cell populations within rheumatoid mice joints. Advancing SPIONs with MRI was able to track MSCs RA animal models. Similarly, **Chen et al.** used targeted nanoparticles for tracking carboxylated-PEG-SPIONs (IOPC). However, IOPC has been combined with an

TABLE 3.2

Conventionally Used Drugs and Their Observed Side Effects Used during RA Treatment

Conventional Treatment	Drugs Used	Mechanism	Observed Side Effects	References
Non-steroidal anti-inflammatory drugs	Ibuprofen Diclofenac Fenoprofen	-Decreasing the number of prostaglandins in the body -Reduces chemicals that produces pain -Inhibit prostaglandins synthesis by inhibiting COX-1 and COX-2 relative equipotency -Reduction in joint swelling -Increase in grip strength -Reduction in duration of morning sickness	-Ulcers, irritation, burning sensation -Acne, constipation, flatulence -Bloating, impact on decrease hearing, itching	[66–68]
DMARDs	Methotrexate Hydroxychloroquine Leflunomide	-Helps to prevent permanent damage -Reduces the risk of long-term disability -Reduces pain and swelling -Prevent joint damage -Inhibit the mitochondrial enzyme dihydroorotate dehydrogenase	-Nausea, vomiting, mouth sores -Diarrhea, vomiting, nausea -Bloody and cloudy urine, yellow eyes and skin, nausea	[69–71]
Glucocorticoids	Prednisone Betamethasone Dexamethasone	-Stimulate the glucocorticoid receptor in the cells which causes suppression of these harmful cytokines -Rapid, effective and long-lasting inflammatory control -Pain relief -Resulted in a rapid and sustained decrease in RA activity	-Weight gain, increased blood glucose levels, insomnia -Abnormal hair growth, Acne, blindness, weight gain -Leg swelling, insomnia easy bruising	[72–74]
Biologics response modifiers	Abatacept Anakinra Belimumab	-Modulates t-cell costimulation by binding to CD80 and CD86 receptors on antigen-presenting cells thereby inhibiting the t-cell proliferation and B-cell stimulation -Both IL-1alpha and IL-1BETA act through IL-1 receptor 1 to stimulate the production of inflammatory cytokines and TNF alpha that led to the inflammatory cascade -Inhibit the actions of autoreactive, pro-inflammatory B-cells that cause chronic inflammation and tissue damage	-Headache, runny nose, nausea, back pain -Sore throat, vomiting, flu -Depression, anxiety, chest pain, tightness	[75–77]

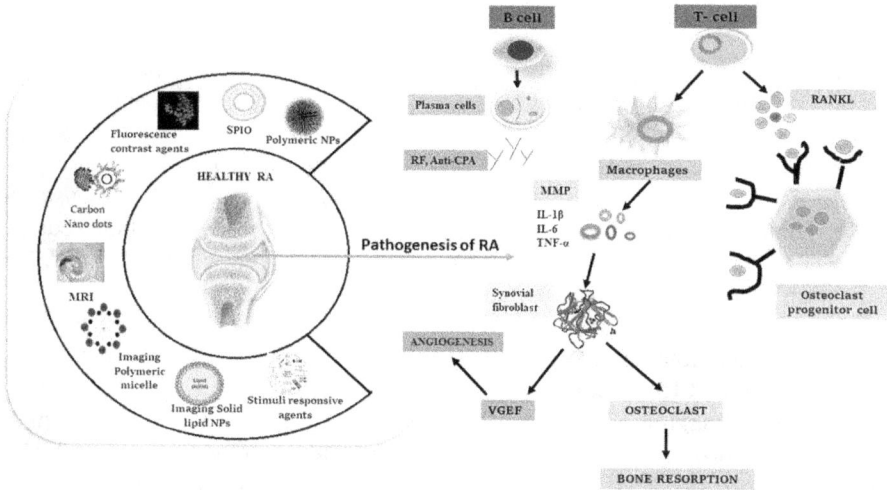

FIGURE 3.3 Nano diagnosis of rheumatoid arthritis.

anti-CD3 monoclonal antibody to target T-cells. Therefore, IOPC-CD3 NPs for bioimaging have been observed *in vitro* cell culture and *in vivo* animal studies. In subsequent studies, the use of magnetic fibrin NPs in the diagnosis of RA has been studied. **Periyathambi et al**. MFNPs were used to target macrophages inside the synovial fluid of rat knee joints. Prepared NPs served as specialized MRI contrast agents that particularly recognized phagocytic macrophages. However, Polymeric NPs were employed by **Vu Quang et al.** to image the inflammatory tissues. By injecting PLGA-PEGFolate NPs with indocyanine green (ICG) and perfluorooctyl bromide, the RA diagnosis has been improved. Comparatively, Rheumatoid factor autoantibodies have been identified and measured using metallic gold nanoparticles. **Veigas et al.** invented an immunosensor using gold nanoprobes and attained early RA diagnosis. Figure 3.3 given below shows nano diagnosis of RA.

3.7 NANOPARTICLE-BASED DIAGNOSTIC OF RHEUMATOID ARTHRITIS

Clinicians can diagnose RA more precisely and swiftly thanks to the constantly evolving molecular imaging technologies. Molecular imaging technology has also made early RA diagnosis possible. Molecule probes provide molecular imaging and non-invasive biological process measurement. Nevertheless, these probes often have short half-lives, nonspecific, simple to release, need high concentrations, and are very lethal. Due to these reasons, molecular imaging applications have been restricted. In this context, a recent study marked the improved execution of imaging probes. Using nanoprobes in early diagnosis has been noted lately. These nanoprobes have reasonable specificity, biocompatibility in vivo, excellent stability, and water solubility. Thus, various nanoscale imaging probes for RA have been included in further discussion of the chapter.

3.7.1 MRI

MR imaging is a form of imaging that does not need any invasive procedures and has good spatial and contrast resolution. In imaging human tissues and organs, it employs both primary and RF magnetic fields. However, imaging effects have been achieved due to hydrogen atoms in the human body. Thus, human organs and tissues may now be seen in sharp, contrasting pictures. MRI was used to collect pictures of soft tissues in various planes, synovial lesions, bone edema, and cartilage degeneration in RA [52–54]. As per the accomplishment belief, MR distinction agents have two longitudinal relaxation contrast agents, and a transverse relaxation contrast has advanced the imaging technique. Typical T1 Gd-based distinction agents, including Gd-DOTA, and Gd-DTPA have been thoroughly studied [55,56]. On the other hand, they have been reported to have tiny molecular imaging methods, a short half-life, and low selectivity. To explicit this, For the purpose of diagnosing RA, **Hou et al.** developed a tailored MRI imaging agent called CB86-DTPA-Gd. TSPO as a suitable candidate biomarker has been included in the preparation. Hence, the ratio of signal to noise at the RA location was 2.49 times higher after it had been raised [57]. The development of Gd_2O_3 nanoparticles and MnOx nanoparticles have been widely studied as T1 contrast agents [58]. They have a greater surface area for high activity. For example, The ultrathin MnO nanoplates with a huge surface area were produced by Park and colleagues. The value of 5.5 L mmol1 for the r1 value indicated high contrast ability [66].

3.7.2 CT Imaging

CT imaging is the benchmark in detecting bone damage and imaging erosion in RA. The different X-ray attenuation abilities are desired for the tissue light and shaded images by CT imaging [71,72]. Despite having a good imaging speed, it is still in its infancy in RA at this point with tissue penetration and spatial resolution [73,74]. Due to its limited ability to contrast soft tissues, CT shares the same limitations as radiography. Consequently, there hasn't been much research on utilizing CT imaging to diagnose RA. Thus, the development of CT contrast agents by researchers has improved imaging, particularly for the early detection of RA. For example, many different contrast agents, including iodine, gold, bismuth, ytterbium, and tungsten, are utilized during CT scans. However, CT contrast agents with tiny molecules require high doses, have low selectivity, and have a short half-life for their effects. Thus, conjugating iodinated compounds has proven to address these issues effectively. Iodine-doped carbon quantum dots (CQDs) were created by Su and colleagues, and they are an effective contrast agent for CT imaging [75]. Iodine, on the other hand, has not been utilized to its full potential as a contrast agent since the K-edge value of the X-ray spectrum is 33 keV [76]. Thus, X-ray attenuation with Au has been used recently [77,78]. For instance, Au nanoparticle (AuNPs) as a contrast agent have proven their versatility in surface chemistry and have developed as multimodal imaging probes.

3.7.3 PHOTOACOUSTIC (PA) IMAGING

Recently, attention has been drawn to a revolutionary non-ionizing and non-invasive PA bioimaging approach. The technique uses pulsed laser energy and ultrasonic wave signals for photothermal effects [79,80]. They have confounded difficulties like tissue blocking by air cavities or bones, as reported in several other imaging techniques. For instance, AuNPs are PA imaging materials with plasmon resonance effects that have improved optical absorption qualities that can be adjusted [81–84]. However, to distinguish the PA signals from blood signals, the optical absorption peak of (AuNS) has been improved [85,86]. Similarly, using ultrasonic diagnostic equipment in RA, PA imaging potentially visualized synovial blood vessels [87,88]. In order to specifically image inflammation in mice with arthritis using PA high-contrast imaging, Jonathan Vonnemann et al. developed polysulfated gold nanorods [89]. According to reports, the QR-PLGA-RES-DS NPs make an effective targeted PA imaging contrast material for examining inflammatory tissues. As a diagnostic tool, these nanoparticles have a core of quadrilateral ruthenium nanoparticles surrounded by a shell of dextran sulfate (DS) modified poly (PLGA) [90–92].

3.7.4 FLUORESCENCE (FL) IMAGING

The efficacy of FL imaging in RA has been limited due to in-vivo weak penetration ability. However, the practical prognostic evaluation and diagnostic of altered molecular distortion of RA by FL imaging can be accessed. Fortunately, using contrast agents (organic dyes, carbon nanodots, quantum dots) in FL imaging has disclosed promising performance. Specifically, contrasting FL agents (organic dyes such as fluorescein, cyanines, and BODIPYs) have been prevalent in RA diagnosis [93,94]. For example, indocyanine green has been approved by the FDA for clinical use. It is utilized in angiography with an emission peak of 835 nm and 13% quantum field. Similarly, semiconductor QDs of elemental 2–6, 2–5, 3–5, 4–6, 1–6, 1–3–6, and four groups exhibited excellent FL contrast ability for deeper imaging [95,96]. However, the emission wavelength of QDs can be improved significantly by controlling the varied synthesis temperature and core precursor ratios [8,97–108].

3.7.5 MULTIMODAL IMAGING

Molecular imaging technology in the clinical diagnosis of RA has been exceptionally reported, but their applications are restricted due to their respective imaging code defects. For illustration, FL imaging offers excellent sensitivity for superior compatibility, real-time diagnosis, and less tissue penetration [109]. Whereas low sensitivity of MRI has been observed in osteosclerosis and bone erosion detection [110,111]. Thus, this single imaging technology has not yet achieved comprehensive imaging for RA diagnosis. In this case, multimodality imaging has shown a remarkable way of improving diagnostic outcome accuracy in RA. Multimodality imaging is a technique of combining more than two imaging methods to have multiple imaging functions. In this context, a nanocomposite for focused T2-MR and NIR optical imaging has been created by Kim et al. [112]. Nanocomposites had

RGD active target molecule for RA site with contrast agents Fe and Au for imaging. Indeed, this unique combination of MRI and optical imaging (T2-MR) has increased the absorbance intensity in inflamed paws of CIA mice and attained the targeted effects. Moreover, several multimodal imaging such as US/PA, FL/PA, and FL/MR have been discovered for the diagnosis of RA.

3.7.6 STIMULI-RESPONSIVE IMAGING

While viewing imaging sensitivity, numerous contrast agents have shown robust applications effectively in improving imaging quality. The excellent retention time due to accumulation in RA sites and other body parts has been reported. Eventually, signals from lesion sites and healthy sites have been enhanced. Lately, stimuli-responsive imaging (always on probe) has become the central research topic. For example, HOCl has been noted as a significant biomarker for inflammatory-related responses in RA. Improvements in in-vivo sensitivity have been made to two FL turn-on probe designs [113]. For instance, ROS as RA biomarker has been utilized in stimuli-responsive UCNPs probe preparation. Further, HAR-UCNPs were prepared by conjugation with rhodamine-B-labeled HA where UCNPs acted as energy donors for luminescence excitation [114]. Similarly, **Xiao D et al.,** [115] reported the trypsin-responsive NIR FL/MR nanoparticle coacervate nanoprobes for dual-imaging in RA. Nanoprobes were created using self-assembling Cy5.5-modified poly-L-lysine and polyacrylate-modified Fe3O4 magnetic nanoparticles. The pancreatin-responsive FL/MR imaging has been remarkably achieved by using probes. However, the MR signal was improved due to enhanced cellular uptake aided by smaller particle sizes. Moreover, in-vivo tumor-bearing mice showed an increased FL/MR signal of trypsin overexpression. Consequently, the non-trypsin expression tumor group has not shown any discernible differences (Table 3.3).

TABLE 3.3
Showing Some Recent Development of Diagnostic Methods for Rheumatoid Arthritis

Recent Diagnostic Technology	Purpose	Diagnostic Interventions	References
Non-specific fluorescence imaging	*Fluorescence imaging of finger joints*	-NIR dyes showed different kinetic behavior inflammatory joints than normal joints. -Enhanced fluorescence imaging in early changes in finger joints by RA	[116]
Microchip diagnostic biomarker	*-In vitro diagnostic and profiling of cytokines in RA* *-To detect TNF-α expression in RA*	- On/ off cytokine detection in human -High-density one-step immobilization of anti-TNF-α antibody on nanobead-coated glass slide chip achieved	[117]

TABLE 3.3 *(Continued)*

Showing Some Recent Development of Diagnostic Methods for Rheumatoid Arthritis

Recent Diagnostic Technology	Purpose	Diagnostic Interventions	References
Self-assembled immunosensor	*IgM-RF detection in RA*	-IgG-Fc fragments on a gold surface covalent coupling showed significant biocompatibility to the bioelectrode - Used as an impedimetric biosensor.	[118]
A PVA-Polymer-coated SPION	*Detection of specific immune cell viability and cytokine secretion as an immune cell indicator for early diagnosis*	-Promoted differentiation to and increased survival of MDMs -Favored the expression of immunity -Taken up by human macrophages and migrated into inflamed tissue and facilitated the early tissue visualization by MRI.	[119]
Wearable Sensor Gloves	*Morning stiffness and the assessment of hand function*	-Assisted with the diagnosis and rehabilitation activities	[120]
Rapid response fluorescence probe	*Visualization of inflammatory response–related HOCl levels in vitro and in vivo*	Showed high effectiveness for early assessment of the treatment response of HOCl-mediated RA in mice with a Methotrexate.	[121]

3.8 CONCLUSION

RA is an inflammatory arthritis condition that leaves people severely disabled. However, it significantly affects people's lives all over the world. As a result, RA may be effectively diagnosed and treated to help people feel better and heal faster. Hence The prime objective of this chapter is to present current diagnostic treatment and novel imaging technologies and their explored possibilities in RA. The chapter has summarized the robust applications of nanotechnological medical imaging techniques. Illustrative diagnostic techniques like FL, MR, PA, and CT imaging that precisely interpret RA have been discussed. However, research has been expanded by describing the typical worth agents with unique contrast features in the RA diagnosis overview. Then, the novel multimodal imaging has also been explored in obtaining high-quality imaging. Similarly, high background signals are feasible with "always on" digital probes. Hence, stimuli-responsive imaging in RA has been proposed.

REFERENCES

1. Bullock J, Rizvi SA, Saleh AM, Ahmed SS, Do DP, Ansari RA, Ahmed J. Rheumatoid arthritis: a brief overview of the treatment. Medical Principles and Practice. 2018;27(6):501–507.

2. Abbasi M, Mousavi MJ, Jamalzehi S, Alimohammadi R, Bezvan MH, Mohammadi H, Aslani S. Strategies toward rheumatoid arthritis therapy; the old and the new. Journal of Cellular Physiology. 2019 Jul;234(7):10018–10031.

3. Zhao J, Chen X, Ho KH, Cai C, Li CW, Yang M, Yi C. Nanotechnology for diagnosis and therapy of rheumatoid arthritis: evolution towards theranostic approaches. Chinese Chemical Letters. 2021 Jan 1;32(1):66–86.

4. Wang Y, Jia M, Zheng X, Wang C, Zhou Y, Pan H, Liu Y, Lu J, Mei Z, Li C. Macrovesicle-camouflaged biomimetic nanoparticles encapsulating a metal-organic framework for targeted rheumatoid arthritis therapy. Journal of Nanobiotechnology. 2022 Dec;20(1):1–8.

5. Prasad LK, O'Mary H, Cui Z. Nanomedicine delivers promising treatments for rheumatoid arthritis. Nanomedicine. 2015 Jul;10(13):2063–2074.

6. Li C, Zheng X, Hu M, Jia M, Jin R, Nie Y. Recent progress in therapeutic strategies and biomimetic nanomedicines for rheumatoid arthritis treatment. Expert Opinion on Drug Delivery. 2022 Jul 7;19(8):883–898.

7. Kumar S, Ali J, Baboota S. Polysaccharide nanoconjugates for drug solubilization and targeted delivery. Polysaccharide Carriers for Drug Delivery. 2019 Jan 1;Ch 16:443–475.

8. Gadeval A, Chaudhari S, Bollampally SP, Polaka S, Kalyane D, Sengupta P, Kalia K, Tekade RK. Integrated nanomaterials for non-invasive photothermal therapy of rheumatoid arthritis. Drug Discovery Today. 2021 Oct 1;26(10):2315–2328. ISSN 1359-6446

9. Fang G, Zhang Q, Pang Y, Thu HE, Hussain Z. Nanomedicines for improved targetability to inflamed synovium for treatment of rheumatoid arthritis: multi-functionalization as an emerging strategy to optimize therapeutic efficacy. Journal of Controlled Release. 2019 Jun 10;303:181–208.

10. Pham CT. Nanotherapeutic approaches for the treatment of rheumatoid arthritis. Wiley Interdisciplinary Reviews: Nanomedicine and Nanobiotechnology. 2011 Nov;3(6):607–619.

11. American College of Rheumatology Subcommittee on Rheumatoid Arthritis Guidelines. Guidelines for the management of rheumatoid arthritis: 2002 update. Arthritis & Rheumatism. 2002 Feb;46(2):328–346.

12. Firestein GS. Evolving concepts of rheumatoid arthritis. Nature. 2003 May; 423(6937): 356–361.

13. Smolen JS, Aletaha D. Rheumatoid arthritis therapy reappraisal: strategies, opportunities and challenges. Nature Reviews Rheumatology. 2015 May;11(5):276–289.

14. Koenders MI, van den Berg WB. Novel therapeutic targets in rheumatoid arthritis. Trends in Pharmacological Sciences. 2015 Apr 1;36(4):189–195.

15. Singh JA, Cameron C, Noorbaloochi S, Cullis T, Tucker M, Christensen R, Ghogomu ET, Coyle D, Clifford T, Tugwell P, Wells GA. Risk of serious infection in biological treatment of patients with rheumatoid arthritis: a systematic review and meta-analysis. The Lancet. 2015 Jul 18;386(9990):258–265.

16. Stoffer MA, Schoels MM, Smolen JS, Aletaha D, Breedveld FC, Burmester G, Bykerk V, Dougados M, Emery P, Haraoui B, Gomez-Reino J. Evidence for treating rheumatoid arthritis to target: results of a systematic literature search update. Annals of the Rheumatic Diseases. 2016 Jan 1;75(1):16–22.

17. Bijlsma JW, Welsing PM, Woodworth TG, Middelink LM, Pethö-Schramm A, Bernasconi C, Borm ME, Wortel CH, Ter Borg EJ, Jahangier ZN, van der Laan WH. Early rheumatoid arthritis treated with tocilizumab, methotrexate, or their combination (U-Act-Early): a multicentre, randomised, double-blind, double-dummy, strategy trial. The Lancet. 2016 Jul 23;388(10042):343–355.

18. Firestein GS, McInnes IB. Immunopathogenesis of rheumatoid arthritis. Immunity. 2017 Feb 21;46(2):183–196.

19. Chen J, Wright K, Davis JM, Jeraldo P, Marietta EV, Murray J, Nelson H, Matteson EL, Taneja V. An expansion of rare lineage intestinal microbes characterizes rheumatoid arthritis. Genome Medicine. 2016 Dec;8(1):1–4.

20. McInnes IB, Buckley CD, Isaacs JD. Cytokines in rheumatoid arthritis—shaping the immunological landscape. Nature Reviews Rheumatology. 2016 Jan;12(1):63–68.

21. Sun W, Meednu N, Rosenberg A, Rangel-Moreno J, Wang V, Glanzman J, Owen T, Zhou X, Zhang H, Boyce BF, Anolik JH. B cells inhibit bone formation in rheumatoid arthritis by suppressing osteoblast differentiation. Nature Communications. 2018 Dec 3;9(1):1–4.

22. Bugatti S, Vitolo B, Caporali R, Montecucco C, Manzo A. B cells in rheumatoid arthritis: from pathogenic players to disease biomarkers. BioMed Research International. 2014 Oct;2014.

23. Wang Q, Ma Y, Liu D, Zhang L, Wei W. The roles of B cells and their interactions with fibroblast-like synoviocytes in the pathogenesis of rheumatoid arthritis. International Archives of Allergy and Immunology. 2011;155(3):205–211.

24. Ehrenstein MR, Evans JG, Singh A, Moore S, Warnes G, Isenberg DA, Mauri C. Compromised function of regulatory T cells in rheumatoid arthritis and reversal by anti-TNFα therapy. The Journal of Experimental Medicine. 2004 Aug 2;200(3):277–285.

25. Paliard X, West SG, Lafferty JA, Clements JR, Kappler JW, Marrack P, Kotzin BL. Evidence for the effects of a superantigen in rheumatoid arthritis. Science. 1991 Jul 19;253(5017):325–329.

26. Takemura S, Klimiuk PA, Braun A, Goronzy JJ, Weyand CM. T cell activation in rheumatoid synovium is B cell dependent. Journal of Immunology. 2001 Oct 15; 167(8):4710–4718.

27. Farrugia M, Baron B. The role of TNF-α in rheumatoid arthritis: a focus on regulatory T cells. Journal of Clinical and Translational Research. 2016 Nov 10;2(3):84.

28. Vasanthi P, Nalini G, Rajasekhar G. Role of tumor necrosis factor-alpha in rheumatoid arthritis: a review. APLAR Journal of Rheumatology. 2007 Dec;10(4):270–274.

29. Moelants EA, Mortier A, Van Damme J, Proost P. Regulation of TNF-α with a focus on rheumatoid arthritis. Immunology and Cell Biology. 2013 Jul;91(6):393–401.

30. Srirangan S, Choy EH. The role of interleukin 6 in the pathophysiology of rheumatoid arthritis. Therapeutic Advances in Musculoskeletal Disease. 2010 Oct;2(5):247–256.

31. Takeuchi T, Yoshida H, Tanaka S. Role of interleukin-6 in bone destruction and bone repair in rheumatoid arthritis. Autoimmunity Reviews. 2021 Sep 1;20(9): 102884.

32. Hashizume M, Mihara M. The roles of interleukin-6 in the pathogenesis of rheumatoid arthritis. Arthritis. 2011 Oct;2011: 765624.

33. Tan Q, Huang Q, Ma YL, Mao K, Yang G, Luo P, Ma G, Mei P, Jin Y. Potential roles of IL-1 subfamily members in glycolysis in disease. Cytokine & Growth Factor Reviews. 2018 Dec 1;44:18–27.

34. Sarafan N, Fakoor M, Mehdinasab A, Bahadoram M, Ashtary-Larky D, Mahdavi H, Javanmardi F. Post-traumatic arthritis: the role of cytokine levels in serum and synovial fluid. Global Journal of Health Science. 2018;10(1):166–174.

35. Vickers NJ. Animal communication: when I'm calling you, will you answer too? Current Biology. 2017 Jul 24;27(14):R713–R715.

36. Kim EK, Kwon JE, Lee SY, Lee EJ, Kim DS, Moon SJ, Lee J, Kwok SK, Park SH, Cho ML. IL-17-mediated mitochondrial dysfunction impairs apoptosis in rheumatoid arthritis synovial fibroblasts through activation of autophagy. Cell Death & Disease. 2018 Jan;8(1):e2565.

37. Schiff MH. Role of interleukin 1 and interleukin 1 receptor antagonist in the mediation of rheumatoid arthritis. Annals of the Rheumatic Diseases. 2000 Nov 1;59(suppl 1):i103–i108.
38. Iyer SS, Cheng G. Role of interleukin 10 transcriptional regulation in inflammation and autoimmune disease. Critical Reviews™ in Immunology. 2012;32(1):23–63.
39. Yang X, Chang Y, Wei W. Emerging role of targeting macrophages in rheumatoid arthritis: focus on polarization, metabolism and apoptosis. Cell Proliferation. 2020 Jul;53(7):e12854.
40. Yang XK, Xu WD, Leng RX, Liang Y, Liu YY, Fang XY, Feng CC, Li R, Cen H, Pan HF, Ye DQ. Therapeutic potential of IL-15 in rheumatoid arthritis. Human Immunology. 2015 Nov 1;76(11):812–818.
41. Volin MV, Koch AE. Interleukin-18: a mediator of inflammation and angiogenesis in rheumatoid arthritis. Journal of Interferon & Cytokine Research. 2011 Oct 1;31(10):745–751.
42. Ikeuchi H, Kuroiwa T, Hiramatsu N, Kaneko Y, Hiromura K, Ueki K, Nojima Y. Expression of interleukin-22 in rheumatoid arthritis: potential role as a proinflammatory cytokine. Arthritis & Rheumatism. 2005 Apr;52(4):1037–1046.
43. Yuan N, Yu G, Liu D, Wang X, Zhao L. An emerging role of interleukin-23 in rheumatoid arthritis. Immunopharmacology and Immunotoxicology. 2019 Mar 4;41(2):185–191.
44. Wu F, Gao J, Kang J, Wang X, Niu Q, Liu J, Zhang L. B cells in rheumatoid arthritis: pathogenic mechanisms and treatment prospects. Frontiers in Immunology. 2021;12:750753.
45. Pope JE, Choy EH. C-reactive protein and implications in rheumatoid arthritis and associated comorbidities. In Seminars in Arthritis and Rheumatism 2021 Feb 1 (Vol. 51, No. 1, pp. 219–229). WB Saunders.
46. Fugger L, Svejgaard A. Association of MHC and rheumatoid arthritis: HLA-DR4 and rheumatoid arthritis-studies in mice and men. Arthritis Research & Therapy. 2000 Apr;2(3):1–5.s
47. Shaker O, Ayeldeen G, Abdelhamid A. The impact of single nucleotide polymorphism in the long non-coding MEG3 gene on microRNA-182 and microRNA-29 expression levels in the development of breast cancer in Egyptian women. Frontiers in Genetics. 2021;12:683809.
48. Pradeepkiran JA. Insights of rheumatoid arthritis risk factors and associations. Journal of Translational Autoimmunity. 2019 Dec 1;2:100012.
49. Wang D, Zhang J, Lau J, Wang S, Taneja V, Matteson EL, Vassallo R. Mechanisms of lung disease development in rheumatoid arthritis. Nature Reviews Rheumatology. 2019 Oct;15(10):581–596.
50. Maeda Y, Takeda K. Host–microbiota interactions in rheumatoid arthritis. Experimental & Molecular Medicine. 2019 Dec;51(12):1–6.
51. Van Drongelen V, Holoshitz J. HLA disease associations in rheumatoid arthritis. Rheumatic Disease Clinics. 2017 Aug;43(3):363–376.
52. Deane KD, Demoruelle MK, Kelmenson LB, Kuhn KA, Norris JM, Holers VM. Genetic and environmental risk factors for rheumatoid arthritis. Best Practice & Research Clinical Rheumatology. 2017 Feb 1;31(1):3–18.
53. Svendsen AJ, Kyvik KO, Houen G, et al. On the origin of rheumatoid arthritis: the impact of environment and genes—a population based twin study. PLoS ONE. 2013;8:e57304. doi: 10.1371/journal.pone.0057304
54. Smith-Bouvier DL, Divekar AA, Sasidhar M et al. A role for sex chromosome complement in the female bias in autoimmune disease. Journal of Experimental Medicine. 2008;205:1099–1108.

55. Rak JM, Maestroni L, Balandraud N et al. Transfer of the shared epitope through microchimerism in women with rheumatoid arthritis. Arthritis & Rheumatology. 2009;60:73–80.
56. Wolfberg AJ, Lee-Parritz A, Peller AJ, Lieberman ES. Association of rheumatologic disease with preeclampsia. Obstetrics & Gynecology. 2004;103:1190–1193.
57. Gomez A, Luckey D, Taneja V. The gut microbiome in autoimmunity: sex matters. Clinical Immunology. 2015;159:154–162
58. Rolfes MC, Juhn YJ, Wi C-I, Sheen YH. Asthma and the risk of rheumatoid arthritis: an insight into the heterogeneity and phenotypes of asthma. Tuberculosis and Respiratory Diseases. 2017;80:113. doi: 10.4046/trd.2017.80.2.113
59. Hou Y-C, Hu H-Y, Liu I-L, Chang Y-T, Wu C-Y. The risk of autoimmune connective tissue diseases in patients with atopy: a nationwide population-based cohort study. Allergy and Asthma Proceedings. 2017;38:383–389. doi: 10.2500/aap.2017.38.4071
60. Sheen YH, Rolfes MC, Wi C, et al. Association of asthma with rheumatoid arthritis: a population-based case-control study. Journal of Allergy and Clinical Immunology. 2018;6:219–226. doi: 10.1016/j.jaip.2017.06.022.
61. Horta-Baas G, Romero-Figueroa MD, Montiel-Jarquín AJ, Pizano-Zárate ML, García-Mena J, Ramírez-Durán N. Intestinal dysbiosis and rheumatoid arthritis: a link between gut microbiota and the pathogenesis of rheumatoid arthritis. Journal of Immunology Research. 2017 Oct;2017: Article ID 4835189.
62. Malmström V, Catrina AI, Klareskog L. The immunopathogenesis of seropositive rheumatoid arthritis: from triggering to targeting. Nature Reviews Immunology. 2017;17:60–75. doi: 10.1038/nri.2016.124
63. Makrygiannakis D, Hermansson M, Ulfgren AK, et al. Smoking increases peptidylarginine deiminase 2 enzyme expression in human lungs and increases citrullination in BAL cells. Annals of the Rheumatic Diseases. 2008;67:1488–1492. doi: 10.1136/ard.2007.075192.
64. Jiang X, Alfredsson L, Klareskog L, Bengtsson C. Smokeless tobacco (Moist Snuff) use and the risk of developing rheumatoid arthritis: results from a case-control study. Arthritis Care & Research. 2014;66:1582–1586. doi: 10.1002/acr.22325
65. Holers VM, Demoruelle MK, Kuhn KA, Buckner JH, Robinson WH, Okamoto Y, Norris JM, Deane KD. Rheumatoid arthritis and the mucosal origins hypothesis: protection turns to destruction. Nature Reviews Rheumatology. 2018 Sep;14(9): 542–557.
66. Derry CJ, Derry S, Moore RA. Single dose oral ibuprofen plus paracetamol (acetaminophen) for acute postoperative pain. Cochrane Database of Systematic Reviews. 2013(6): Art. ID CD010210.
67. Gan TJ. Diclofenac: an update on its mechanism of action and safety profile. Current Medical Research and Opinion. 2010 Jul 1;26(7):1715–1731.
68. Agotegaray M, Gumilar F, Boeris M, Toso R, Minetti A. Enhanced analgesic properties and reduced ulcerogenic effect of a mononuclear copper (II) complex with fenoprofen in comparison to the parent drug: promising insights in the treatment of chronic inflammatory diseases. BioMed Research International. 2014 Jun 19;2014.
69. Wenham CY, Grainger AJ, Hensor EM, Caperon AR, Ash ZR, Conaghan PG. Methotrexate for pain relief in knee osteoarthritis: an open-label study. Rheumatology. 2013 May 1;52(5):888–892.
70. Han J, Li X, Luo X, He J, Huang X, Zhou Q, Han Y, Jie H, Zhuang J, Li Y, Yang F. The mechanisms of hydroxychloroquine in rheumatoid arthritis treatment: inhibition of dendritic cell functions via Toll like receptor 9 signaling. Biomedicine & Pharmacotherapy. 2020 Dec 1; 132:110848.

71. Fox RI. Mechanism of action of leflunomide in rheumatoid arthritis. The Journal of Rheumatology. Supplement. 1998 Jul 1; 53:20–26.

72. Townsend HB, Saag KG. Glucocorticoid use in rheumatoid arthritis: benefits, mechanisms, and risks. Clinical and Experimental Rheumatology. 2004 Sep 1;22: S77–S82.

73. Oliveira IM, Gonçalves C, Shin ME, Lee S, Reis RL, Khang G, Oliveira JM. Anti-inflammatory properties of injectable betamethasone-loaded tyramine-modified gellan gum/silk fibroin hydrogels. Biomolecules. 2020;10(10):1456.

74. De A, Blotta HM, Mamoni RL, Louzada P, Bertolo MB, Foss NT, Moreira AC, Castro M. Effects of dexamethasone on lymphocyte proliferation and cytokine production in rheumatoid arthritis. The Journal of Rheumatology. 2002 Jan 1;29(1): 46–51.Oct 17;10(10):1456.

75. Vital EM, Emery P. Abatacept in the treatment of rheumatoid arthritis. Therapeutics and Clinical Risk Management. 2006 Dec;2(4):365.

76. Clark W, Jobanputra P, Barton P, Burls A. The clinical and cost-effectiveness of anakinra for the treatment of rheumatoid arthritis in adults: a systematic review and economic analysis. Health Technology Assessment (Winchester, England). 2004 Jan 1;8(18):iii–v.

77. Ding C. Belimumab, an anti-BLyS human monoclonal antibody for potential treatment of inflammatory autoimmune diseases. Expert Opinion on Biological Therapy. 2008 Nov 1;8(11):1805–1814.

78. Chando A, Momin M, Quadros M, Lalka S. Topical nanocarriers for management of rheumatoid arthritis: a review. Biomedicine & Pharmacotherapy. 2021;141: 111880, ISSN 0753-3322.

79. Oliveira IM, Gonçalves C, Reis RL, et al. Engineering nanoparticles for targeting rheumatoid arthritis: past, present, and future trends. Nano Research. 2018;11: 4489–4506.

80. Prasad LK, O'Mary H, Cui Z. Nanomedicine delivers promising treatments for rheumatoid arthritis. Nanomedicine. 2015;10(13):2063–2074. doi:10.2217/nnm.15.45

81. Li Y, Wei S, Sun Y, et al. Nanomedicine-based combination of dexamethasone palmitate and MCL-1 siRNA for synergistic therapeutic efficacy against rheumatoid arthritis. Drug Delivery and Translational Research. 2021;11:2520–2529.

82. Wang Q, Li Y, Chen X, et al. Optimized in vivo performance of acid-liable micelles for the treatment of rheumatoid arthritis by one single injection. Nano Research. 2019;12:421–428.

83. Yu Z, Reynaud F, Lorscheider M, Tsapis N, Fattal E. Nanomedicines for the delivery of glucocorticoids and nucleic acids as potential alternatives in the treatment of rheumatoid arthritis. WIREs Nanomedicine and Nanobiotechnology. 2020;12:e1630

84. van Vollenhoven R. (2019). Treat-to-target in rheumatoid arthritis—are we there yet? Nature Reviews Rheumatology. doi:10.1038/s41584-019-0170-5

85. Holten K, Sundlisater NP, Lille Graven S, Sexton J, Nordberg LB, Moholt E, Hammer HB, Uhlig T, Kvien TK, Haavardsholm EA, Aga AB. Fatigue in patients with early rheumatoid arthritis undergoing treat-to-target therapy: predictors and response to treatment. Annals of the Rheumatic Diseases. 2022 Mar 1;81(3): 344–350.

86. Kumar V, Leekha A, Tyagi A, Kaul A, Mishra AK, Verma AK. Preparation and evaluation of biopolymeric nanoparticles as drug delivery system in effective treatment of rheumatoid arthritis. Pharmaceutical Research. 2017 Mar;34(3): 654–667.

87. Yang M, Feng X, Ding J, Chang F, Chen X. Nanotherapeutics relieve rheumatoid arthritis. Journal of Controlled Release. 2017 Apr 28;252:108–124.

88. Shen Q, Shu H, Xu X, Shu G, Du Y, Ying X. Tofacitinib citrate-based liposomes for effective treatment of rheumatoid arthritis. Die Pharmazie-An International Journal of Pharmaceutical Sciences. 2020 Apr 6;75(4):131–135.

89. Siddique R, Mehmood MH, Haris M, et al. Promising role of polymeric nanoparticles in the treatment of rheumatoid arthritis. Inflammopharmacology. 2022; 30:1207–1218.

90. Ishihara T, Kubota T, Choi T, Higaki M. Treatment of experimental arthritis with stealth-type polymeric nanoparticles encapsulating betamethasone phosphate. Journal of Pharmacology and Experimental Therapeutics. 2009 May 1;329(2):412–417.

91. Bashir S, Aamir M, Sarfaraz RM, Hussain Z, Sarwer MU, Mahmood A, Akram MR, & Qaisar MN. Fabrication, characterization and in vitro release kinetics of tofacitinib-encapsulated polymeric nanoparticles: a promising implication in the treatment of rheumatoid arthritis. International Journal of Polymeric Materials and Polymeric Biomaterials. 2021;70(7):449–458.

92. Li Y, Liang Q, Zhou L, et al. Metal nanoparticles: a platform integrating diagnosis and therapy for rheumatoid arthritis. Journal of Nanoparticle Research. 2022;24:84.

93. An H, Song Z, Li P, et al. Development of biofabricated gold nanoparticles for the treatment of alleviated arthritis pain. Applied Nanoscience. 2020;10: 617–622.

94. Alam MM, Han HS, Sung S, Kang JH, Sa KH, Al Faruque H, Hong J, Nam EJ, San Kim I, Park JH, Kang YM. Endogenous inspired biomineral-installed hyaluronan nanoparticles as pH-responsive carrier of methotrexate for rheumatoid arthritis. Journal of Controlled Release. 2017 Apr 28;252:62–72.

95. Wu H, Wang K, Wang H, Chen F, Huang W, Chen Y, Chen J, Tao J, Wen X, Xiong S. Novel self-assembled tacrolimus nanoparticles cross-linking thermosensitive hydrogels for local rheumatoid arthritis therapy. Colloids and Surfaces B: Biointerfaces. 2017 Jan 1;149:97–104.

96. Prasad SR, Elango K, Damayanthi D, Saranya JS. Formulation and evaluation of azathioprine loaded silver nanoparticles for the treatment of rheumatoid arthritis. AJBPS. 2013 Sep 15;3(23):28–32.

97. Yang Y, Guo L, Wang Z, Liu P, Liu X, Ding J, Zhou W. Targeted silver nanoparticles for rheumatoid arthritis therapy via macrophage apoptosis and re-polarization. Biomaterials. 2021;264:120390, ISSN 0142-9612.

98. Rao K, Roome T, Aziz S, Razzak A, Abbas G, Imran M, Jabri T, Gul J, Hussain M, Sikandar B, Sharafat S. Bergenin loaded gum xanthan stabilized silver nanoparticles suppress synovial inflammation through modulation of the immune response and oxidative stress in adjuvant induced arthritic rats. Journal of Materials Chemistry B. 2018;6(27):4486–4501.

99. Lorscheider M, Tsapis N, ur-Rehman M, Gaudin F, Stolfa I, Abreu S, Mura S, Chaminade P, Espeli M, Fattal E. Dexamethasone palmitate nanoparticles: an efficient treatment for rheumatoid arthritis. Journal of Controlled Release. 2019;296: 179–189, ISSN 0168-3659.

100. Zhu Y, Zhao T, Liu M, Wang S, Liu S, Yang Y, Nan Y, Huang Q, Ai K, Rheumatoid arthritis microenvironment insights into treatment effect of nanomaterials. Nano Today. 2022 Feb 1;42:101358.

101. Zheng M, Jia H, Wang H, Liu L, He Z, Zhang Z, Yang W, Gao L, Gao X, Gao F. Application of nanomaterials in the treatment of rheumatoid arthritis. RSC Advances. 2021;11(13):7129–7137.

102. Hosseinikhah SM, Barani M, Rahdar A, Madry H, Arshad R, Mohammadzadeh V, Cucchiarini M. Nanomaterials for the diagnosis and treatment of inflammatory arthritis. International Journal of Molecular Sciences. 2021 Mar 18;22(6):3092.

103. Zhao Y, Liu Y, Li X, Wang H, Zhang Y, Ma H, Wei Q. Label-free ECL immunosensor for the early diagnosis of rheumatoid arthritis based on asymmetric heterogeneous polyaniline-gold nanomaterial, Sensors and Actuators B: Chemical. 2018;257:354–361, ISSN 0925-4005,

104. Zhou B, Yan Y, Xie J, Huang H, Wang H, Gopinath SC, Anbu P, He S, Zhang L. Immunosensing the rheumatoid arthritis biomarker through bifunctional aldehyde-amine linkers on an iron oxide nanoparticle seeded voltammetry sensor. Nanomaterials and Nanotechnology. 2022 Mar 7;12:18479804221085103.

105. Li X, Hou Y, Meng X, Li G, Xu F, Teng L, Sun F, Li Y. Folate receptor-targeting mesoporous silica-coated gold nanorod nanoparticles for the synergistic photothermal therapy and chemotherapy of rheumatoid arthritis. RSC Advances. 2021; 11(6):3567–3574.

106. Vonnemann J, Beziere N, Böttcher C, Riese SB, Kuehne C, Dernedde J, Licha K, von Schacky C, Kosanke Y, Kimm M, Meier R, Ntziachristos V, Haag R. Polyglycerolsulfate functionalized gold nanorods as optoacoustic signal nanoamplifiers for in vivo bioimaging of rheumatoid arthritis. Theranostics. 2014 Mar 20;4(6):629–641. doi: 10.7150/thno.8518.

107. Li C, Liu R, Song Y, Zhu D, Yu L, Huang Q, Zhang Z, Xue Z, Hua Z, Lu C, Liu Y. Intra-articular administrated hydrogels of hyaluronic acid hybridized with triptolide/gold nanoparticles for targeted delivery to rheumatoid arthritis combined with photothermal-chemo therapy Res. Sq. 2021, 1–22.

108. Lee SM, Kim HJ, Ha YJ, Park YN, Lee SK, Park YB, Yoo KH. Materials chemistry B accepted manuscript chemistry B accepted manuscript. ACS Nano. 2013;7:50–57.

109. Zhang Y, Li Y, Zhang J, Chen X, Zhang R, Sun G, Jiang B, Fan K, Li Z, Yan X. Nanocage-based capture-detection system for the clinical diagnosis of autoimmune disease. Small. 2021 Jun;17(25):2101655.

110. Zhao J. Hyaluronic acid-modified and TPCA-1-loaded gold nanocages alleviate inflammation. Pharmaceutics. 2019 Mar 25;11(3):143.

111. Zhang N, Li M, Hou Z, Ma L, Younas A, Wang Z, Jiang X, Gao J. From vaccines to nanovaccines: a promising strategy to revolutionize rheumatoid arthritis treatment. Journal of Controlled Release. 2022 Oct 1; 350:107–121.

112. Gheibi Hayat SM, Darroudi M. Nanovaccine: a novel approach in immunization. Journal of Cellular Physiology. 2019 Aug;234(8):12530–12536.

113. Wells C.M, Harris M, Choi L, Murali V.P, Guerra F.D, Jennings J.A. Stimuli-responsive drug release from smart polymers. Journal of Functional Biomaterials 2019;10:34.

114. Zhang M, Hu W, Cai C, Wu Y, Li J, Dong S. Advanced application of stimuli-responsive drug delivery system for inflammatory arthritis treatment. Materials Today Bio. 2022 Feb 21:100223.

115. Xiao D, Lu T, Zeng R, Bi Y. Preparation and highlighted applications of magnetic microparticles and nanoparticles: a review on recent advances. Microchimica Acta. 2016 Oct;183(10):2655–2675.

116. Fischer T, Ebert B, Voigt J, Macdonald R, Schneider U, Thomas A, Hamm B, Hermann KG. Detection of rheumatoid arthritis using non-specific contrast enhanced fluorescence imaging. Academic Radiology. 2010 Mar 1;17(3):375–381.

117. Marulli E, Aloisi A, Di Giuseppe P, Rinaldi R. Micro and nanotechnology for early diagnosis and detection of rheumatic diseases-molecular markers. BioChip Journal. 2016 Sep;10(3):189–197.

118. Chinnadayyala SR, Park J, Abbasi MA, Cho S. Label-free electrochemical impedimetric immunosensor for sensitive detection of IgM rheumatoid factor in human serum. Biosensors and Bioelectronics. 2019 Oct 15;143:111642.

119. Strehl C, Gaber T, Maurizi L, Hahne M, Rauch R, Hoff P, Häupl T, Hofmann-Amtenbrink M, Poole AR, Hofmann H, Butteries F. Effects of PVA coated nanoparticles on human immune cells. International Journal of Nanomedicine. 2015;10:3429.

120. Henderson J, Condell J, Connolly J, Kelly D, Curran K. Review of wearable sensor-based health monitoring glove devices for rheumatoid arthritis. Sensors. 2021 Feb 24;21(5):1576.

121. Feng H, Zhang Z, Meng Q, Jia H, Wang Y, Zhang R. Rapid response fluorescence probe enabled in vivo diagnosis and assessing treatment response of hypochlorous acid-mediated rheumatoid arthritis. Advanced Science. 2018 Aug;5(8):1800397.

4 Classification of Nanomedicines

Mamata Singh, Keshva Sai Pentapati, and
N.P. Singh

4.1 INTRODUCTION

The phrase "nanomedicine" first arose around the turn of the century, and less than 30 papers using this word had been published by 2005. References to nano-particles in connection to bio-medicine began at the end of the 1970s and are currently the topics of over 10,000 publications annually [1]. Science Web reports that more than ten times as many publications concerning nanoparticles for biomedical use—more than 1000 articles—were published nearly a decade later in 2015. **Nanomedicines** can be defined as the European Science Foundation's forward reads: "To diagnose, prevent, and cure disease as well as to better understand the intricate pathophysiology of the illness, nanomedicine employs tiny instruments. The ultimate objective is to raise the standard of living" [2].

Metchnikoff and Ehrlich, who in 1908 were jointly awarded the medical Nobel Prize for their research on phagocytosis, are, respectively, the modern ancestors of nanomedicine. Nanomedicine has a connection to the ancient practice of using solid colloidal gold, cell-specific diagnostics, and therapy [2–4]. Liposomes, DNA-drug conjugates, polymer-drugs, antibody-drugs, polymer nanoparticles, polymer-protein conjugates, albumin-drugs, gold nanoparticles that fight arthritis and block-copolymer micelles, and anti-microbial silver nanoparticles are a few of the groundbreaking discoveries. Over the last 30 years of the 20th century, more and more nanoparticles for nanomedicine have been produced [5–7].

Nanotechnology has entered our daily lives over the past few years [8]. Through an integrated approach, this ground-breaking technology has been used in several sectors. There are now more and more goods and applications that either claim to use nanoparticles or incorporate them. The same thing takes place in pharmaceutical research. Our research currently includes the use of nanotechnology for creating new medications [9,10].

The usage of nanoparticles for illness monitoring, regulating, prevention, and therapy is known as nanomedicine, or the application of nanotech for medical reasons. Nevertheless, major scientific and international regulatory bodies disagree on what constitutes a nanomaterial [8,10,11]. Because nanomaterials have new physicochemical features that are distinct from their traditional bulky chemical counterparts because of their tiny size, several efforts have been made to come up

DOI: 10.1201/9781003348672-4

with a consensus definition. These characteristics considerably expand the number of potential therapeutic development prospects, but certain safety concerns have also surfaced. Concerns about the use of nanomaterials include their potential to easily cross biological barriers, toxic properties, and persistence in the environment and the human body, as well as their physicochemical characteristics that can result in changes to **pharmacokinetics**, or the body's absorption, distribution, elimination, and metabolism [12].

4.1.1 NANOMEDICINE

The use of nanotechnology in medicine is known as nanomedicine. Nanomaterials, biological devices, nanoelectronic biosensors [13], and even potential future uses of molecular nanotechnology, including biological machines, are all included in the field of nanomedicine. Three main fields of medicine can use **nanomaterials** in **nanomedicine**: regenerative medicine, controlled medication delivery (mono-therapy), and diagnostics (nano diagnosis) [8–10,14,15].

The Food and Drug Administration (FDA) has adopted the definitions commonly used for the creation of materials with at least one dimension in the 1 to 100 nm (nanometers) range in size [16], rather than developing "nanotechnology," "nanomaterial," "nanoscale," or other terminology related to it are defined here [8,10]. The FDA also advised that assessments of the security, effects, impact on public health, and the legal position of nanotechnology goods should be considered with any distinctive characteristics and actions that the use of nanotechnology may produce [8,10,16]. This depends on the current state of science and knowledge of nanoparticles and their properties as it relates to technology [9,17,18].

4.2 PRINCIPLES OF NANOMEDICINES

Three main fields of medicine can use nanomaterials in nanomedicine: regenerative medicine, controlled medication delivery (monotherapy), and diagnostics (nano diagnosis) [15,19]. Theranostics, a developing field that combines diagnosis and therapy, is a promising strategy that holds both the imaging/diagnosis tool and the medication in the same system [19,20].

The evolution of creative drugs for both diagnosis and therapy through the use of nanomedicine holds the potential to significantly alter clinical practice efficient molecules that would not otherwise be usable due to their high toxic level (like Impact), also by enhancing effectiveness (e.g., by improving bioavailability and decreasing the dosage), by utilizing several modes of action (like Nanomag, multifunctional gels), and to address [19].

This is a result of the inherent qualities of nanomaterials, which have greatly aided the creation of pharmaceuticals. Nano molecules have the highest certain surface area in comparison to volume because of their tiny size. The result is an increase in particle surface energy, which greatly increases the reactivity of the nanomaterials. The effects of nanoparticles on biological fluids are a propensity to adsorb the biomolecules, including lipids and proteins, among other things [19,21].

The plasma/serum biomolecule-adsorption layer, or "corona," that develops on colloidal nanoparticles' exterior is responsible for one of the most significant interactions with living things. Its composition depends on the body's entrance point and the specific fluid from which the nanoparticles originate in contact (such as blood serum, lung fluid, digestive fluid, etc.) [22]. The "corona" composition may undergo additional dynamic alterations as the nanoparticle switches between several biological compartments [19,20].

Additionally, electron confinement in nanomaterials allows for the modification and tuning of optical, electrical, and magnetic characteristics [13]. Furthermore, nanomaterials may be created with a variety of sizes, shapes, chemical compositions, and surfaces to enable them to interact with a variety of biological targets [19]. Only precise particle design will result in a successful biological consequence [21]. For two key reasons, it is therefore essential to have a thorough understanding of how nanomaterials and biological systems interact. Critical guidelines for the design of nanomaterials will thus be provided by a clearer understanding of how the physical and chemical characteristics of the bio-interface affect cellular dynamics, transport, and the signaling pathway [23].

4.3 PROPERTIES OF NANOMEDICINES

There are different types of principle methods for the characterization, and also to define the usage and application of nanomedicine to the targeted location inside the human body [19,21].

4.3.1 SIZE DISTRIBUTION OF PARTICLES

The PSD, which reflects the range of size fluctuation, is a measure that is frequently used in the identification of nanomaterials [24]. Because a nanomaterial is often polydisperse or made up of particles of various sizes, it is crucial to establish the PSD [21,25].

4.3.2 AREA OF SURFACE

When extra regulation requires it, it calculates the ratio of surface to volume, which is a parameter in a relation [26]. If the material's surface area to volume ratio exceeds 60 m^2/cm^3, as previously stated, it falls within the definition. Even if a material's surface area to volume ratio is less than the required 60 m^2/cm^3, the PSD will still be used to determine the material's classification as a nanomaterial [20].

4.3.3 SIZE

Size is the most crucial consideration since it applies to a wide variety of materials. One to one hundred nanometers is the usual range [19]. The limit is not, however, clearly defined. Since the materials' physiochemical and biological characteristics do not suddenly change at 100 nm, the greatest size that a substance may have before being designated a nanomaterial is an arbitrary value. To this degree, it is presumed that other qualities should be considered [20,21,25].

The methods are mentioned below along with their principle and limitations:

- **Transmission Electron Microscopy**
  Principle: The sample is traversed by an electron beam, and the dispersed electrons are concentrated to produce a picture [13].

  Limitations: High-vacuum operation, only used for solid samples, time-consuming, costly, and complex sample preparation.

- **Scanning Electron Microscopy**
  Principle: While interacting with the material, an electron beam passes across the surface where secondary electrons are expelled by inelastic scattering, leading to the formation of the picture [13,21].

  Limitations: Operate in a high vacuum; take a long time and cost money; use solid and conductive materials; take a complex sample.

- **Atomic Force Microscopy**
  Principle: By measuring the forces created by the contact of the two surfaces, a scanning probe glides across the sample's surface and identifies the surface topography [21].

  Limitations: It takes time to spread samples on a substrate or have them adhere to it [19].

- **Particle Tracking Analysis**
  Principle: The sample is positioned against a black backdrop and illuminated by a powerful laser beam. A sensitive camera on the optical microscope is used to measure the scattered light and the Brownian motion of the particles [27].

  Limitations: The sample must be in suspension; short particle distances make the sample less sensitive.

- **X-ray Diffraction (XRD)**
  Principle: The sample is penetrated by an X-ray beam, which interacts with the repeating atomic planes. The atoms in a crystalline structure will cause the beam to diffract. The spacing between the atoms' planes is determined by Bragg's law [21].

  Limitations: Can only be applied to crystalline particles.

- **Dynamic Light Scattering**
  Principle: The Stokes-Einstein equation's assessment of the variations in scattered light brought on by the motion of the particles in suspension yields information on the hydrodynamic diameter.

  Limitations: Only used for suspensions; polydisperse sample resolution is poor.

4.4 NECESSITY AND BENEFITS OF NANOMEDICINE

Although nanomedicine, nanotechnology is only recently being used in medicine, in health care, it is expected to have a revolutionary impact [18,21]. Public funding and legislation have greatly aided the advancement of nanomedical research. The potential benefits of ongoing nanomedicine development offer several advantages over traditional medications, including increased targeting, efficiency, bio-availability, dosage response capability, personalization, and safety.

The development of multipurpose nanoparticle (NP) complexes that may transport substances for both diagnosis and treatment desired at the same time may be the most intriguing idea in the nanomedical investigation. These skills include completely new and marked improvements in patient diagnosis, treatment, and follow-up that are noteworthy [28]. However, there is currently a lack of information on the pharmacokinetics, pharmacodynamics, and toxicity of many nanomaterials, despite these potential advantages [12,24,28].

Drug delivery systems using nanoparticles can function in a variety of ways. Nanoparticles can be designed to carry particular chemicals that will enable them to bind to molecules on tumor cells [29], in addition to the medicine for delivery [4,15,30]. They can safely transport the medicine to the particular tumor spot once connected [31,32].

Drug solubility can also be improved by nanoparticles. Medicine must be soluble to be able to reach the bloodstream, which is needed for it to function. For instance, paclitaxel (Taxol), a cancer medication [33–35], is insoluble and needs to be dissolved in a delivery agent to enter the bloodstream. But people who are exposed to this substance may develop allergies [36,37].

Scientists have created a nanoparticle out of the naturally occurring protein albumin to solve these problems. It renders paclitaxel soluble and transports it while preventing allergic responses. Blood arteries that are disorganized and leaky frequently develop through and off of tumors [30,32]. Because chemotherapy molecules are so tiny, they easily diffuse through the capillaries and leave the tumor, affecting the tissues around it. These vessels make it easy for chemotherapy medications to penetrate the tumor [30]. Larger molecules known as nanoparticles become stuck inside the tumor, where they cause all of the harm [4,31,32].

Nanoparticles can be made to degrade into harmless metabolites after delivering their pharmacological payload to cells [23]. For young children who are still growing, this is especially crucial.

4.5 CLASSIFICATION OF NANOMEDICINES

The two primary categories of nanomedicines are organic nanoparticles like polymers, liposomes [6], and micelles or inorganic nanoparticles like gold, silica, and iron oxide [5,38,39]. The majority of the time, these nanoparticles are utilized for therapies and diagnosis purposes. Applications for inorganic nanoparticles include the treatment of anemia, lymph node imaging, and hyperthermia. Some of them have completed preclinical research and clinical testing [28]. Organic nanoparticles have similar properties to inorganic nanoparticles, however, also successfully entered the clinical stage and are now available on the market for a variety of uses, including cancer, microbial infection, and immunization [11,40,41].

4.5.1 NANOMEDICINES BASED ON ALBUMIN

Another type of nanosystem is albumin-based nanomedicine, which uses albumin, particularly a carrier protein called human serum albumin [42]. Through a straightforward self-assembly process, Albumin nanosystems may carry a variety of cargos thanks to a simple crosslinking procedure in an aqueous medium solution of albumin [42]. Biocompatibility is albumin's key benefit. Although this is the case, only 2 of the 29, and 2 of the 65 authorized nanomedicines were also listed, and now undergoing clinical tests are albumin-based [42]. Currently, it is utilized for imaging and medicine delivery to combat cancer [15,33,34,43].

4.5.2 LIPID-BASED NANOMEDICINES

Another kind of nanomedicine is lipid nanosystems, which are often employed to encapsulate hydrophobic cargos to enhance penetration and manage release profiles. Lipid nanosystems include solid lipid-based nanoparticles and nanoemulsions [44]. A surfactant is frequently used to offer a stable dispersion. Lipid nanomedicine can also contain gene therapies like siRNA or contrast agents used in imaging, including F-butane. Lipid using nanomedicine often increases the drug's bio-compatibility as well as its ability to accumulate in the target tissues, which can enhance the pharmacological impact. But there are several disadvantages, including quick clearance brought on by reticuloendothelial system (RES) absorption, certain restrictions on administration routes, and difficulties with system stability. Lipid-based nanomedicines are not restricted to treating cancer-related disorders, in contrast to liposomal-based nanomedicines [5,33,34,45]. Hepatitis B, hepatic fibrosis, and amyloidosis are a few of the disorders that are being treated using lipid-based nano-medicines. Coenzyme Q10, cyclosporine, simvastatin, and cinnarizine, which are utilized as antihyperlipidemic, antihistamines, antioxidants, respectively, and im-munosuppressants, were also added to various types of nanoemulsion [40,46].

4.5.3 LIPOSOME-BASED NANOMEDICINES

A kind of medication formulation called liposome-based nanomedicine encapsu-lates a drug inside a bilayer structure of phospholipids to increase its therapeutic efficacy and bioavailability action. One of the earliest nanomedicines with a proven method is liposome formulations. The use of liposomes to encapsulate various cargos, including small molecules like RNAs, biological compounds like hepatitis A virus vaccinations, nucleic acids like doxorubicin, and, was the focus of a lot of research [6,40,47]. Furthermore, if the liposome components, such as sphingo-myelin and cholesterol, have a specific therapeutic effect, delivery of the liposomes without an encapsulating medication is also an option. Due to the significance of PEGylation in enhancing the delivery system's stealth, PEGylation should be taken into consideration while using liposomes. Licensing liposome-based nanomedicines are frequently utilized to treat cancer-related diseases [35,43,48,49]. Since 10 of the 29 authorized nanomedicines are based on liposomes, they play a significant role in research [6,45].

4.5.4 MICELLE-BASED NANOMEDICINES

Amphiphilic molecules with a hydrophilic and a hydrophobic portion create micelles, which are self-assembling nanosystems. Their high permeability and solubility, among other benefits, increase the bioavailability of drugs. They nevertheless suffer from issues including inadequate drug release control and cytotoxicity brought on by the use of amphiphilic molecules that interact with cell membranes [23,40,47]. There are no licensed micelle-based nanomedicines, although multiple papers have employed micelles made of block copolymers to decrease the consent and boost the chemotherapeutic drug bioavailability and other forms of medications. However, nine nanomedicines based on micelles are now being tested in humans. The majority of them are used to treat cancer [37].

4.5.5 POLYMERIC-BASED NANOMEDICINES

One of the most often utilized nanosystems for drug delivery is polymeric nanoparticles [44]. Ethylcellulose, alginate, cyclodextrin, chitosan, poly(lactic-co-glycolic acid), and polylactic acid are just a few of the polymers that have been employed [22]. Many methods have been utilized to create polymeric nanoparticles, depending on whether the polymer is hydrophilic or hydrophobic [50]. Polymeric nanoparticles are a market-promising technology because of several benefits like relative stability and longer duration of action [22]. However, there are no commercially available goods made with polymeric nanoparticles [44]. There are presently just three products in cancer clinical trials [33,34].

4.5.6 NANOMEDICINES BASED ON INORGANIC COMPOUNDS

Several subtypes of inorganic-based nanomedicines exist. A few types have been employed for therapeutic purposes because of concerns with degradability and biocompatibility, whereas other types, including imaging agents, have been utilized for diagnostic purposes. Metal oxide nanoparticles are one of these classes; examples include nanoparticles of hafnium oxide, which promote tumor cell death by electron generation when stimulated with external radiation [13,23,30,32]. Unusually used to treat iron-deficiency anemia, containing iron gluconate and iron dextran colloids, for example, colloids, and other comparable derivatives constitute another kind [39]. The final subtype is described as nanomedicines based on iron, silica, and gold, either in the form of nanoparticles for the treatment of cancer with medications arrayed on the surface or as nano-shells or the use of nanoparticles in thermal ablation of malignancies [33,34,50]. There are 12 items of this sort on the market [39,44]. Therapy for iron replacement was utilized in eight products. Four products, however, are now undergoing clinical testing to treat cancer [35,37,51].

4.6 DRUG DELIVERY MECHANISM

Nanotechnology is a young field that has opened up several possibilities for medicine delivery and targeting [16–18]. Simply put, it is obtaining enormous things from a little planet. Research is currently being conducted in all fields, including engineering, medicine, and pharmacy, to maximize the advantages of cutting-edge technology while minimizing costs. However, moving drugs and goods based on nanotechnology from the lab to the clinic requires a multi-disciplinary approach [8]. Numerous nanomaterials and nanodevices are used in nanotechnology, including carbon nanotubes, gold nanoparticles, magnetic nano-particles, dendrimers, lipoidal nanoparticles, quantum dots, polymeric nanoparti-cles, and many others [10,22,24,44].

The sizes of these 1 to 100 nm-sized solid colloidal particles. Vaccine adjuvants or drug carriers that carry the active pharmacological ingredient are adsorbed, dissolved, imprisoned, enclosed, encased, or chemically bound, they are composed of macro-molecular materials and can be utilized therapeutically [25,52,53]. In addition to being effective drug delivery vehicles, because they provide non-invasive adminis-tration methods for oral, nasal, and ocular channels, nanoparticles also function well as vaccine adjuvants. When it comes to early detection, medication administration, and noninvasive imaging, nanoparticles exhibit extraordinary certainty. The term "nanomedicine" is frequently used to describe nanoparticles used in medication delivery [44].

The field of nanoengineered devices has some of the most cutting-edge and original applications of nanotechnology in medication delivery [17,18]. The number of drugs that can be loaded onto a single nanoparticle limits the drug delivery capabilities of these systems, and they are only capable of controlling drug release in response to one trigger, such as the particle's disintegration [52,54]. Additionally, there is a growing need for more sophisticated systems that can hold a lot of active molecules and release them in controlled amounts gradually in response to pulsatile inputs. As a result, nanoscale manufacturing methods are being researched more and more for the construction of devices with controllable surface characteristics as well as for devices that may serve as stimuli-sensitive delivery systems and biosensors [55,56].

The debate concludes that simple polymer and lipid-based particles may be used for medication administration, but diagnostic devices also seem to be moving quickly toward development. Despite the enormous advancements and revolution in drug delivery, one must concentrate on recent advances in nanomedicine from the standpoint of physical fundamentals, biological considerations, medical applica-tions, and worries about the production, dependability, and safety of nano-scale medicines [46,52,57].

The mechanism of **nanomedicines** is mainly done by the interactions of these nanoparticles with the targeted cells. Participants engaged in lengthy debates about how nanocarriers affect the immune system [3,58,59]. Nanoparticles mostly activate/affect innate immune responses, even while some forms of adaptive immunity such as the production of anti-poly(ethylene glycol), PEG, and antibodies may contribute to toxicities associated with the use of nanomedicine [26,50,59,60]. Utilizing associations with circulating and organ-dwelling mononuclear phagocyte system (MPS) cells, complement activation, interactions with immune cells in the tumor microenvironment [61–63], and more, and more are a few of the factors that have been discussed regarding the relationship between nanoparticles and the immune system [15,53,59].

An essential component of innate immunity is the complement system, which is made up of more than 30 soluble and membrane-bound proteins that work to destroy invasive pathogens [59]. Complement activation by nanosurfaces has a dual effect: While opsonization of nanoparticles with the help of C3b/iC3b may cause phagocytic cells to absorb them; however, uncontrolled production of anaphylatoxins, also known as C3a, C4a, and C5a, may result in unpleasant responses in susceptible people. Even Concerning the complement activation-related pseudoallergy (CARPA) brought on by nanocarriers [3], there was disagreement at the conference about the necessity of taking precautions to prevent complement activation by nanomedicines.

Although the first anticancer nano-drug [64,65], PEGylated Liposomal Doxorubicin (Doxil), causes considerable complement activation in vitro, initial infusion responses in humans are generally less than 10% and may be prevented by premedication and reducing the pace of infusion [5,45,47,66]. This distinction suggests that complement activation may only be incidentally involved in the regulation of unfavorable reactions through other integrative immune mechanisms [26,59]. Others emphasized that complement activation induced significant pro-inflammatory reactions and might perhaps be harmful to the payload's ability to treat patients [61]. There is evidence that some nanocarriers do promote the growth of malignancies, perhaps as a result of the release of C5a and the subsequent draw of regulatory T-cells and inflammatory macrophages [3,26,51,67].

While some of the symptoms could be brought on by anti-PEG antibodies, which in certain people cause complement activation, there may be more processes that are still unknown. Collectively, these observations imply that the carrier's ability to promote tumor growth may reduce the benefits of carrier-mediated medication delivery and may provide insight into why the clinical performance of liposomal medicines has not significantly outperformed free pharmaceuticals [4,53]. It is debatable whether further preclinical understanding of the impact of complement activation on the functioning of nanocarriers requires clinical investigations [32,45].

Nanomedicine is the term for the application of nanotechnology in medicine. Working with materials at the nano level, which is too tiny to be seen with a standard lab microscope, is known as nanotechnology [8,9,18]. One-millionth of a millimeter is a nanometer. The diameter of human hair is hundreds of times larger than that. Nanoscale particles are abundant in nature. They may also be produced by humans using materials like silver or carbon. Human-made compounds with a nanometer scale are called nanomaterials [24]. Scientists are developing materials and tools for nanomedicine that interact with your body at the atomic or molecular level. This enables extremely focused, targeted outcomes and may reduce adverse effects.

4.7   FIELD OF DIAGNOSIS

Think of nanomedicine as small, incredibly accurate instruments that scientists design and manipulate within your body. For instance, nanomedicine may deliver medications to your body extremely precisely since it works on such a small scale. Depending on the location of the targeted cells, the nanomedicines are applied and the field of diagnosis is divided into three types, and they are as follows:

4.7.1 DIAGNOSIS (NANO-DIAGNOSIS)

The phrase "nanodiagnostics" refers to the use of nano-biotechnology in molecular diagnosis, which is crucial for creating customized cancer treatments [37,51,52]. It often relies on data from pharmacogenetics, pharmacogenomics, and pharmaco-proteomics but also takes into account environmental variables that affect treatment response [62,68]. Applications of presently developed nanoparticles, as well as longer-range research including the employment of created nano-robots to perform cellular repairs, are both possible with the help of nanotechnology in medicine [8,17,18].

Since nanoparticles have benefits such as a high volume-to-surface ratio and multifunctionality, nano-diagnostic technologies are also being applied to improve the identification of biomarkers [69]. The use of biomarkers in cancer treatment is also possible and is one of the fundamental elements of personalized medicine [37,50,65,70]. There are several moral questions raised by the science of nanodiagnostics about blood testing [62,68]. Medical professionals will be able to do thorough health checks on patients swiftly and frequently because of advancements in diagnostic technologies. If the medicine is necessary, it will be uniquely formulated for each person based on their genetic profile, minimizing unintended adverse effects.

4.7.2 CONTROL DRUG DELIVERY (NANOTHERAPY)

Despite improvements in the understanding of tumor biology and the creation of chemotherapy, cancer continues to be a common and deadly illness [32,63,71]. Tumor heterogeneity, medication resistance, and systemic toxicity are the three main challenges in the treatment of cancer [4,52,72]. Because of their potential for targeting and versatility, nanoscale delivery systems, or nano therapies, are becoming increasingly important as carriers for anti-cancer drugs [37,73]. We talk about the state of cancer therapy today and potential approaches to overcome barriers to cancer treatment with nano therapies [51,63,74,75]. In particular, we discuss the methods for logically designing nanoparticles for focused, multimodal therapeutic drug delivery [17,55,76].

In addition to the difficulties provided by tumor cell biology, host variables, and the tumor microenvironment can affect how effectively the current chemotherapy regimens work [74,76]. The aberrant vasculature and nearby stromal cells that make up the tumor microenvironment can both hinder medication delivery and speed up drug clearance [32,71,77]. Delivery to big, necrotic tumors may be compromised [57,58,62]. Lowered absorption, quick metabolism, and accelerated clearance of drugs are examples of host variables that can lower blood medication concentrations. Additionally, medication size and solubility might obstruct tumor penetration and delivery. Additionally, a patient's ability to take chemotherapy drugs varies, and the emergence of side effects can seriously impede the dose and treatment length [54,74,78].

Future therapy regimens will probably include combination multimodal medicines due to the heterogeneity of tumors and the emergence of medication resistance. The effectiveness of targeted monotherapy and combination medicines on tumor growth may be assessed using mathematical models [32,39,71]. According to these models, triple therapy may be necessary for individuals with more severe initial disease burdens even if dual therapy is frequently sufficient for long-term illness management [48]. Additionally, the models imply that simultaneous therapy is superior to sequential therapy in terms of efficacy [76].

4.7.3 REGENERATIVE MEDICINES

The need for treatments that can regenerate tissues and lessen the need for transplants is driven by the disease- and damage-related loss of organs and tissues [79]. Regenerative medicines are an interdisciplinary subject that combines principles from engineering and biology to encourage regeneration and may be able to repair damaged and diseased tissues as well as whole organs [11,48,79]. Ever since the industry began a few decades ago, several regenerative medicine therapies, such as those created for orthopedic and wound healing, have obtained Food and Drug Administration (FDA) approval and are currently marketed [16,78,80].

This chapter also addresses the treatments to other forms of regenerative medicine strategies that are being currently investigated in contexts both preclinical and clinical [52,79]. Particularly, innovations for integrating grafts with host vasculature and advancements in producing complex grafts and tissue mimics will be covered. Methods for utilizing recently developed cell sources as well as ways to change the host's environment to increase its inherent ability for regeneration will be covered [62]. Finally, we suggest potential avenues for therapeutics utilizing regenerative medicine [74,81].

In addition to normalizing congenital anomalies, regenerative medicine can repair or replace damaged tissues and organs harmed by illness, trauma, aging, or other factors [9,24,28,52,79]. The potential for both chronic disorders will be treated using regenerative medicine and acute injuries, as diseases impacting many different organ systems and situations, such as dermal wounds, trauma, some cancer therapies [35,51,65], cardiovascular disorders, and more, are supported by promising preclinical and clinical data to date [70]. Due to a lack of available donors and frequently serious immunological problems, the current therapy method of treating organ and tissue failures and loss by transplanting healthy organs and tissues faces challenges [59,74]. However, these challenges may be overcome by using regenerative medicine techniques [80,82].

The field of regenerative medicine includes many various types of techniques, such as the usage of materials and newly created cells, and also other combinations, to replace the lost tissue and do so in a way that is both structurally and functionally equivalent, or to help in tissue recovery [81]. Though adult humans have a restricted potential for regeneration when compared to smaller vertebrates, the body's natural response to healing can nevertheless be used to support it. The market-available regenerative medicine treatments will be covered first in this study [81,82]. The study will then focus on early clinical stages and preclinical research that aims to impact the patient's physiological surroundings through the administration of components, living cells, or growth elements, either to replace the lost tissue or to improve the human body's natural healing capacity and repair systems [78].

The use of recently developed cell sources and methods for enhancing the structural complexity of implantable grafts will also be covered. Finally, prospective avenues for the field's future research will be suggested. We grouped these efforts in this study under the topic of regenerative medicine because of the significant overlap in the terminology used by scholars in tissue engineering and regenerative medicine [24,81,82].

4.8 APPLICATIONS OF NANOMEDICINES

More and more research is being done on the creation and application of the use of materials with properties at the nanoscale to address medical and health-related issues. Research in nanomedicine examines a variety of subjects, such as employing biotic, abiotic, fingerprints, or hybrid materials, for example, medication delivery, creation of vaccines, antimicrobial, diagnostic, and also imaging tools, wearable technologies, implants, high-tech screening platforms, etc. Many of these innovations are now starting to be developed into therapeutically helpful products [74]. Here is a summary of recent advances in the nanomedicine field and emphasizes the problems the field is now facing as well as potential prospects for research and clinical application.

Disease detection, monitoring, treatment, prevention, and cure are the science, engineering, and practice of medicine [49]. Most people think about nanomedicine in terms of pharmacological formulations, which involve injecting soft or hard particles with diameters of a few nanometers into patients to diagnose and cure them. However, there are many types of research and development included in this topic. The discovery and use of distribution of medication, development of vaccinations, and antimicrobial uses materials and technology with nanoscale length scales to function in all ways.

The characteristics of nanoscale objects are transformed from the molecular and bulk regimes. All materials, whether made of natural or synthetic materials, exhibit nanoscale properties. But typically, the characterization of biological nanoscale structures is done without considering biological characteristics, whereas only synthetic items are generally considered to be a part of "nanoscience and engineering." Because "nanoscale" materials are transitional, it is challenging to identify a material's boundaries and set rigid boundaries for it (less than 100 nm yet bigger than atoms or tiny molecules, for example). More importantly, nanoscale particles can display unique properties that can be applied in the creation of innovative therapeutic and diagnostic modalities [74].

Chemotherapy medications are frequently recommended in the greatest dose that may be tolerated for a kid of the child's age or size, based on adult doses, as routine treatment for childhood cancer [52,63,65,73]. Children, however, are not little grown-ups. Children's growth and development processes may cause a chemotherapeutic treatment to have effects and responses that are different from those found in adults [51].

Additionally, if a child develops resistance to medication and is already taking the maximum dosage, there is no way to raise it without having severe adverse effects. Theoretically, nanomedicine enables the use of bigger quantities of medications by encapsulating them and delivering them through the body directly to sick cells to minimize collateral harm.

Cancer in youngsters has a strong chance of being safely treated using nanomedicine. But there is presently insufficient research to advance it [51,73]. Out of more than 250 nanomedicine items, cancer research receives around two-thirds of the attention [81–83]. However, this hasn't resulted in any novel pediatric cancer medicines entering the market [37,55,65,73].

However, we are moving forward. Our research focuses on developing nanoparticles that can carry medications that silence genes to treat medulloblastoma, the most prevalent brain tumor in children [50,71].

Additionally, we are developing nanomedicines to treat important pediatric tumors [71]. These include neuroblastoma, the disease that kills more children under five than any other, and drug-refractory acute lymphoblastic leukemia, the most prevalent childhood cancer [37,49,83].

Here are some specific applications of nanomedicine that are being researched or used:

4.8.1 VACCINES FOR COVID-19

The two COVID vaccines produced by Pfizer and Moderna heavily rely on nanoparticles [50,84]. These vaccines work by using messenger RNA (mRNA) to aid in the development of COVID viral immunity [79]. However, mRNA degrades fast. Before it disintegrates, it requires something to transport it through your body. Therefore, scientists enclosed it in nanoparticles, which then transported it to your immune cells. It can complete its work there [28,85].

4.8.2 CANCER THERAPY

Your entire body receives cancer-fighting medications from chemotherapy. Because of this, you can have adverse effects like nausea and hair loss [23,73,79,85]. With the use of nanomedicine, doctors can only harm the cancer cells in your body while limiting harm to healthy cells [37,52,65,83].

4.8.3 MRIs

Radio waves and magnetic fields are used in magnetic resonance imaging (MRI) to produce precise images of your organs and tissue. Through an IV, some patients receive what is referred to as a contrast substance [84]. It improves the clarity of details in the photographs [84]. But compared to conventional contrast agents, luminous nanoparticles provide crisper images [18]. They may eventually reduce the cost of MRIs by making the imaging techniques that utilize them more straightforward and economical [86].

4.8.4 MEDICAL EQUIPMENT

Scientists anticipate using nanotechnology to create more advanced versions of implantable devices including pacemakers, defibrillators, and stents. These gadgets' small chips and sensors might communicate data and alerts, release medications, or let your doctor keep an eye on you from a distance [18].

4.8.5 DETECTION OF BIOMARKERS

Biomarkers provide information about the current state of a cell in your body. They could serve as illness indicators [69,84]. For instance, a biomarker for heart disease is elevated cholesterol [48]. Doctors use tests on your tissue, blood, and urine to seek biomarkers [69]. Your body also contains biomarkers in the form of individual cells and proteins [87]. Since nanoparticles are more responsive to biomarkers, doctors may be able to take more accurate readings. As a consequence, they might be able to identify infections early [41,69,88].

4.9 EFFECTS OF NANOMEDICINES

Nanomedicine has the potential to cure the following illnesses in addition to cancer:

A **neurological** condition where larger chemicals are blocked from entering your brain by a layer of guarding cells. When medications need to reach your brain, the blood-brain barrier (BBB), often known as the BBB, causes issues. Due to their small size, nanoparticles can pass through the BBB. This has promise for the treatment of meningitis, stroke, Alzheimer's, and brain cancers [63,65,81,87].

4.9.1 EYE ISSUES

Additionally, your eyes are shielded from outside contaminants by barriers. Drugs have a hard time reaching their targets because of these barriers. The most popular methods of administering eye medications—drops, injections, oral medications, and IVs—all encounter this issue. Nanoparticles, contact lens coatings, and implants are some of the delivery systems offered by nanomedicine to deliver medications where they are required [15]. Conjunctivitis (pinkeye), cataracts, corneal injuries, macular degeneration, and glaucoma can all be treated using nanomedicine [17].

4.9.2 INFECTIONS

Nanomedicine can administer medicines in a targeted manner and assist in the detection of bacterial infections [41]. Nanomaterials that resist germs can be used in medical equipment like catheters and heart valves to assist avoid infection [85,88,89].

4.9.3 MENOPAUSE

Some symptoms may be alleviated by hormone replacement treatment. Studies have demonstrated that administering these hormones topically is efficient and avoids some of the issues associated with medications taken orally. People have fewer adverse effects, such as rashes and blisters, when the hormones are administered via nanoparticles.

4.9.4 THE DISEASE OF THE BLOOD

Chemotherapy, bone marrow transplants, stem cell treatment, and medications have historically been used to treat diseases including leukemia, lymphoma, anemia, and hemophilia [49,90,91]. Researchers are concentrating on utilizing nanomedicine to create synthetic blood components that might replace some of the activities disrupted by blood disorders.

4.9.5 SPINAL CORD DAMAGE

When you sustain this kind of injury, the trauma starts a chain reaction that further damages your nerves. Your spinal cord has a layer of defense cells, much like your brain. To guarantee that a steroid crosses the barrier, doctors have historically utilized large dosages of the drug. However, that medication quickly degrades and can have dangerous negative effects at large dosages.

Blood arteries that are disorganized and leaky frequently develop through and off of tumors [58]. Because chemotherapy molecules are so tiny, they easily diffuse through the capillaries and leave the tumor, affecting the tissues around it. These vessels make it easy for chemotherapy medications to penetrate the tumor [71]. Larger molecules known as nanoparticles become stuck inside the tumor, where they cause all of the harm.

Nanoparticles can be made to degrade into harmless metabolites after delivering their pharmacological payload to cells. For young children who are still growing, this is especially crucial.

4.10 DRAWBACKS OF NANOMEDICINES

After intravenously injecting photosensitizers and nanocarriers into the cancer patients or animals suffering from tumors, they could build up in tumor tissue, also they have lethal effects on tumor cells and only create ROS when stimulated by light of a certain wavelength. PDT provides the following benefits and drawbacks in comparison to the current standard cancer treatments like surgery or chemotherapy because other healthy tissues that haven't been exposed to light are kept [63,75,79,92].

Chemotherapeutic medications have side effects that affect both cancer cells and healthy cells, however, photosensitizers and nanocarriers aggregate specifically in tumor sites and display cytotoxicity only in the region that has been subjected to light irradiation [26,46,59]. In patients who are ineligible for surgery, PDT can be used instead; and also in those patients who have tumor surgery for removal of tumors, light irradiation of the surgical site can lower the chance of cancer recurrence [27,63]. Combining PDT with chemotherapy provides the benefit of decreasing the dosage of anticancer medications, which reduces adverse effects [29,64,66,80].

It is difficult to afford a local treatment with a PDT in optical fiber, in contrast to systemic chemotherapy, to eradicate tumor cells that are in individuals with advanced-stage illness or alter the course of treatment outside the target region [89]. Due to endogenous molecules absorbing the light during PDT, the effectiveness of the light penetration into the deep tissue is limited. For more than 1 cm below the surface of the tumor, photosensitizers are difficult to excite effectively. PDT still has obvious limitations for treating large, deeply buried cancers, despite advancements in laparoscopic light delivery technology or microendoscopic technologies [75,82].

Most photosensitizers that have been approved for use in clinical settings are derived from the porphyrin moiety, which is a type of photosensitizer that includes dyes, chlorophylls, and porphyrins. Tetrapyrrole macrocycles porphyrins are formed when methine bridges join them. Low singlet oxygen quantum yield, water aggregation, and large dosages are needed for medicinal effectiveness. Some of the limitations of first-generation photosensitizers in clinical applications to various solid cancers include limited selectivity to the tumor location, skin photosensitivity, and extended elimination half-life [61,82].

The practical usage of the first-generation porphyrin-based photosensitizers was hampered by undesired hydrophobicity and shallow penetration. Cancer therapy has been researched using Chlorins and phthalocyanines, second-generation photo-sensitizers that are structurally similar to tetrapyrrole macro-cycles [82,84]. The addition of hydrophilic substituents to pyrrole rings increased their stability, pKa value, and water solubility. However, the enhanced water solubility's effect on renal clearance tends to reduce the photosensitizer's bioavailability.

Because the ROS produced by light irradiation are reactive and have a short half-life, one can get efficient cytotoxic effects via localizing intracellular organelles with photosensitizers including the mitochondria, lysosomes, and the nucleus [26,59]. It has been tried to modify photosensitizers by employing peptides that penetrate cells or coupling with the targeted ligands to enable the accumulation of photosensitizers in the target region in adequate quantities. Additionally, the therapeutic effectiveness of PDT is influenced by the laser's power density per unit area, photosensitizer dose, and light wavelength. The design and development of various PDT modalities have received a lot of attention during the past few decades [30].

Rapid development in the field of nanotechnology makes it easier to regulate the physicochemical characteristics of nanomaterials, like their surface, functional group, diameter, and form [41]. It has been made possible to create nanomedicines that react to stimuli like light exposure and to expand PDT tactics in combination with nanomedicine. As a result of the EPR effect, which is dependent on solid tumors' leaky vasculature, nanoparticle usage offers the advantage of prolonging circulation and accumulating at the tumor site [61]. The immune-suppressive TME is also influenced by the tumor vasculature, and cancer cells interact with immune cells and other TME constituents by overproducing vascular mediators [79,82,83]. To reduce harm to healthy cells when not intended and boost therapy efficiency, modern nanocarriers with targeting moiety grafted on them have been developed to precisely engage by having active target cargo or target cells medications [14,44,46,58].

Pharmaco-kinetics of nanomedicines are reliant on the physical and chemical properties of the nano-carriers, and encapsulating the medications within the nano-particles provides benefits in the protection of carefully regulated medication discharge from shipment. In the nanoformulation of cancer treatments to date, existing approved pharmaceuticals are preferred over recently explored therapeutic candidates [82], and FDA clearances and clinical studies for nanomedicines are still in their infancy [13,41,89]. In the therapeutic environment, nanomedicines such as PEGylated proteins, albumin-bound paclitaxel, and liposomal doxorubicin (Doxil®) are employed [55,60,64,69]. They displayed an increased maximum tolerable dosage ratio to the beginning dose than smaller molecule medications in phase I clinical investigations. It implies that using the proper preclinical model is necessary to assess the toxicity of nanomedicines [26,59].

4.11 CONCLUSION

The fact that most medications are neither specific nor water-soluble presents challenges that must be solved. The aforementioned nanocarriers were created to first solubilize medications in aqueous environments, then act as nano-vectors toward certain targets and regulate medication release [41,46,58]. The majority of currently utilized nanocarriers enable oral medication delivery [46,74]. Although these nano-vectors are intended to pass the blood-brain, lung, and digestive tract barriers, the quantity of medicine that reaches the organ is less than 1%, making advances difficult.

To maximize the benefit/risk ratio, nano-vector-drug assemblies are created, and their toxicity must be assessed by several clinical trials in addition to extended in vivo and in vitro experiments. These nanomaterials need to be defined extremely precisely and in a form that is entirely repeatable for use in biological tests. Research on the antigenicity, immunotoxicity, and potential activation of complements (a group of serum proteins that trigger inflammation [86], kill cells, and take part in opsonization), as well as their medication (drug) release rates, pharmaco-kinetics, and biodistribution, must be conducted on suitable nanocarriers (including metabolites) [26,46].

The many clinical studies of these nano-drugs are covered in several of the views listed in this introduction. Nanomedicine research is booming, but multi-phase clinical studies are exceedingly time-consuming. Only a small percentage of nano-drug candidates ultimately meet regulatory authority standards [39,41]. There is little question that future multidisciplinary partnerships involving biomedical researchers, chemists, and biophysicists will facilitate the commercialization of additional medications made with nanotechnology [25].

REFERENCES

   1. McPhee Derek J. ISM, University of Bordeaux, 351 Cours de la Libération, 33405 Talence Cedex, France, Introduction to Nanomedicine.

2. McGrady E, Conger S, Blanke S, Landry BJ. Emerging technologies in healthcare: navigating risks, evaluating rewards. J Healthc Manag. 2010 Sep–Oct;55(5):353–364; discussion 364-5. PMID: 21077584.

3. Bhaskar S, Tian F, Stoeger T, Kreyling W, de la Fuente JM, Grazú V, Borm P, Estrada G, Ntziachristos V, Razansky D. Multifunctional nanocarriers for diagnostics, drug delivery and targeted treatment across blood-brain barrier: perspectives on tracking and neuroimaging. Part Fibre Toxicol. 2010 Mar 3;7:3. doi: 10.1186/1743-8977-7-3. PMID: 20199661; PMCID: PMC2847536.

4. Sugahara KN, Teesalu T, Karmali PP, Kotamraju VR, Agemy L, Girard OM, Hanahan D, Mattrey RF, Ruoslahti E. Tissue-penetrating delivery of compounds and nanoparticles into tumors. Cancer Cell. 2009 Dec 8;16(6):510–520. doi: 10.1016/j.ccr.2009.10.013. PMID: 19962669; PMCID: PMC2791543.

5. Sabnani MK, Rajan R, Rowland B, Mavinkurve V, Wood LM, Gabizon AA, La-Beck NM. Liposome promotion of tumor growth is associated with angiogenesis and inhibition of antitumor immune responses. Nanomedicine. 2015 Feb;11(2):259–262. doi: 10.1016/j.nano.2014.08.010.

6. Shmeeda H, Amitay Y, Gorin J, Tzemach D, Mak L, Stern ST, Barenholz Y, Gabizon A. Coencapsulation of alendronate and doxorubicin in pegylated liposomes: a novel formulation for chemoimmunotherapy of cancer. J Drug Target. 2016 Nov;24(9):878–889. doi: 10.1080/1061186X.2016.1191081. Epub 2016 Jun 6. PMID: 27187807.

7. Ganesan A, Nolan L, Crabb SJ, Packham G. Epigenetic therapy: histone acetylation, DNA methylation and anti-cancer drug discovery. Curr Cancer Drug Targets. 2009 Dec;9(8):963–981. doi: 10.2174/156800909790192428. PMID: 20025605.

8. Ferrari M. Cancer nanotechnology: opportunities and challenges. Nat Rev Cancer. 2005 Mar;5(3):161–171. doi: 10.1038/nrc1566. PMID: 15738981.

9. Bhattacharya B, Roy P, Bhattacharya S, Prasad B, Mandal AK. Nanotechnology and sustainable development. In *Engineered Nanomaterials for Sustainable Agricultural Production, Soil Improvement and Stress Management* (pp. 431–445). 10.1016/B978-0-323-91933-3.00020-9

10. Vaddiraju S, Tomazos I, Burgess DJ, Jain FC, Papadimitrakopoulos F. Emerging synergy between nanotechnology and implantable biosensors: a review. Biosens Bioelectron. 2010 Mar 15;25(7):1553–1565. doi: 10.1016/j.bios.2009.12.001. Epub 2009 Dec 11. PMID: 20042326; PMCID: PMC2846767.

11. Peer D, Karp JM, Hong S, Farokhzad OC, Margalit R, Langer R. Nanocarriers as an emerging platform. Nat Nanotechnol. 2007;2:751–760. doi: 10.1038/nnano.2007.387.

12. Azhdarzadeh M, Saei AA, Sharifi S, Hajipour MJ, Alkilany AM, Sharifzadeh M, Ramazani F, Laurent S, Mashaghi A, Mahmoudi M. Nanotoxicology: advances and pitfalls in research methodology. Nanomedicine (Lond). 2015;10(18):2931–2952. doi: 10.2217/nnm.15.130. Epub 2015 Sep 15. PMID: 26370561.

13. "1. The atom's structure I: Electrons and shells". Volume 1 Introduction, Berlin, Boston: De Gruyter, 2014, 1–36. 10.1515/9783110221923.1

14. European Science Foundation. Forward Look Nanomedicine: An EMRC Consensus Opinion 2005. Available online: http://www.esf.org (accessed on 15 September 2021).

15. Decuzzi P, Pasqualini R, Arap W, Ferrari M. Intravascular delivery of particulate systems: does geometry really matter? Pharm Res. 2009 Jan;26(1):235–243. doi: 10.1007/s11095-008-9697-x. Epub 2008 Aug 20. PMID: 18712584.

16. Bailey AM, Mendicino M, Au P. An FDA perspective on preclinical development of cell-based regenerative medicine products. Nat Biotechnol. 2014 Aug;32(8):721–723. doi: 10.1038/nbt.2971. PMID: 25093890.

17. Joudeh N, Linke D. Nanoparticle classification, physicochemical properties, characterization, and applications: a comprehensive review for biologists. J Nanobiotechnol. 2022;20:262. 10.1186/s12951-022-01477-8

18. Mulvaney P. Nanoscience vs nanotechnology—defining the field. ACS Nano. 2015;9(3): 2215–2217. 10.1021/acsnano.5b01418

19. Soares S, Sousa J, Pais A, & Vitorino C. Nanomedicine: principles, properties, and regulatory issues. Front Chem. 2018. 10.3389/fchem.2018.00360

20. Adabi M, Naghibzadeh M, Adabi M, Zarrinfard MA, Esnaashari SS, Seifalian AM, Faridi-Majidi R, Tanimowo Aiyelabegan H, Ghanbari H. Biocompatibility and nanostructured materials: applications in nanomedicine. Artif Cells Nanomed Biotechnol. 2017 Jun;45(4):833–842. doi: 10.1080/21691401.2016.1178134. Epub 2016 May 31. PMID: 27247194.

21. Soares S, Sousa J, Pais A, Vitorino C. Nanomedicine: principles, properties, and regulatory issues. Front Chem. 2018 Aug 20;6:360. doi: 10.3389/fchem.2018.00360. PMID: 30177965; PMCID: PMC6109690.

22. Okano T, Yamada N, Sakai H, Sakurai Y. A novel recovery system for cultured cells using plasma-treated polystyrene dishes grafted with poly(N-isopropyl acrylamide). J Biomed Mater Res. 1993 Oct;27(10):1243–1251. doi: 10.1002/jbm.820271005. PMID: 8245039.

23. Kami D, Gojo S. Tuning cell fate: from insights to vertebrate regeneration. Organogenesis. 2014 Apr–Jun;10(2):231–240. doi: 10.4161/org.28816. Epub 2014 Apr 15. PMID: 24736602; PMCID: PMC4154958.

24. Arts JH, Hadi M, Keene AM, Kreiling R, Lyon D, Maier M, Michel K, Petry T, Sauer UG, Warheit D, Wiench K, Landsiedel R. A critical appraisal of existing concepts for the grouping of nanomaterials. Regul Toxicol Pharmacol. 2014 Nov;70(2):492–506. doi: 10.1016/j.yrtph.2014.07.025. Epub 2014 Aug 7. PMID: 25108058.

25. Albanese A, Tang PS, Chan WC. The effect of nanoparticle size, shape, and surface chemistry on biological systems. Annu Rev Biomed Eng. 2012;14:1–16. doi: 10.1146/annurev-bioeng-071811-150124. Epub 2012 Apr 18. PMID: 22524388.

26. Bawa R. Regulating nanomedicine – can the FDA handle it? Curr Drug Deliv. 2011 May;8(3):227–234. doi: 10.2174/156720111795256156. PMID: 21291376.

27. Saikiran V, Dar MH, Kuladeep R, Jyothi L, NarayanaRao D. Strategies in laser-induced synthesis of nanomaterials. In *Nanomaterials Synthesis* (pp. 149–199). 10.1016/B978-0-12-815751-0.00006-7

28. Moghimi SM, Farhangrazi ZS. Nanomedicine and the complement paradigm. Nanomedicine. 2013 May;9(4):458–460. doi: 10.1016/j.nano.2013.02.011. Epub 2013 Mar 14. PMID: 23499667.

29. Duncan R. Polymer conjugates as anticancer nanomedicines. Nat Rev Cancer. 2006;6:688–701. 10.1038/nrc1958

30. Ghajar CM, Peinado H, Mori H, Matei IR, Evason KJ, Brazier H, Almeida D, Koller A, Hajjar KA, Stainier DY, Chen EI, Lyden D, Bissell MJ. The perivascular niche regulates breast tumour dormancy. Nat Cell Biol. 2013 Jul;15(7):807–817. doi: 10.1038/ncb2767. Epub 2013 Jun 2. PMID: 23728425; PMCID: PMC3826912.

31. Poirot-Mazères I. Legal aspects of the risks raised by nanotechnologies in the field of medicine. J Int Bioethique. 2011 Mar-Jun;22(1):99–118, 212. doi: 10.3917/jib.221.0099. PMID: 21850972.

32. Bae YH, Park K. Targeted drug delivery to tumors: myths, reality and possibility. J Control Release. 2011 Aug 10;153(3):198–205. doi: 10.1016/j.jconrel.2011.06.001. Epub 2011 Jun 6. PMID: 21663778; PMCID: PMC3272876.

33. Moghimi SM. Cancer nanomedicine and the complement system activation paradigm: anaphylaxis and tumour growth. J Control Release. 2014 Sep 28;190:556–562. doi: 10.1016/j.jconrel.2014.03.051. Epub 2014 Apr 16. PMID: 24746624.

34. Petersen GH, Alzghari SK, Chee W, Sankari SS, La-Beck NM. Meta-analysis of clinical and preclinical studies comparing the anticancer efficacy of liposomal versus conventional non-liposomal doxorubicin. J Control Release. 2016 Jun 28;232:255–264. doi: 10.1016/j.jconrel.2016.04.028. Epub 2016 Apr 22. PMID: 27108612.

35. Ellis L, Atadja PW, Johnstone RW. Epigenetics in cancer: targeting chromatin modifications. Mol Cancer Ther. 2009 Jun;8(6):1409–1420. doi: 10.1158/1535-7163. MCT-08-0860. Epub 2009 Jun 9. PMID: 19509247.

36. Peer D, Karp J, Hong S, et al. Nanocarriers as an emerging platform for cancer therapy. Nature Nanotech. 2007;2:751–760. doi: 10.1038/nnano.2007.387

37. Bharali DJ, Mousa SA. Emerging nanomedicines for early cancer detection and improved treatment: current perspective and future promise. Pharmacol Ther. 2010 Nov;128(2):324–335. doi: 10.1016/j.pharmthera.2010.07.007. Epub 2010 Aug 10. PMID: 20705093.

38. Agrahari V, Hiremath P. Challenges associated and approaches for successful translation of nanomedicines into commercial products. Nanomedicine (Lond). 2017 Apr;12(8):819–823. doi: 10.2217/nnm-2017-0039. Epub 2017 Mar 24. PMID: 28338401.

39. Zanganeh S, Hutter G, Spitler R, Lenkov O, Mahmoudi M, Shaw A, Pajarinen JS, Nejadnik H, Goodman S, Moseley M, Coussens LM, Daldrup-Link HE. Iron oxide nanoparticles inhibit tumour growth by inducing pro-inflammatory macrophage polarization in tumour tissues. Nat Nanotechnol. 2016 Nov;11(11):986–994. doi: 10.1038/nnano.2016.168. Epub 2016 Sep 26. PMID: 27668795; PMCID: PMC5198777.

40. Khalil IAH, Arida IA, Ahmed M. 2020, 'Introductory Chapter: Overview on Nanomedicine Market', in IAH Khalil (ed.), *Current and Future Aspects of Nanomedicine*, London: IntechOpen. doi: 10.5772/intechopen.91890.

41. Taylor E, Webster TJ. Reducing infections through nanotechnology and nanoparticles. Int J Nanomedicine. 2011;6:1463–1473. doi: 10.2147/IJN.S22021. Epub 2011 Jul 13. PMID: 21796248; PMCID: PMC3141873.

42. Tanei T, Leonard F, Liu X, Alexander JF, Saito Y, Ferrari M, Godin B, Yokoi K. Redirecting transport of nanoparticle albumin-bound paclitaxel to macrophages enhances therapeutic efficacy against liver metastases. Cancer Res. 2016 Jan 15;76(2):429–439. doi: 10.1158/0008-5472.CAN-15-1576. Epub 2016 Jan 7. PMID: 26744528; PMCID: PMC4715951.

43. Stewart BW, Kleihues P. World Cancer Report (World Health Organization Press, Geneva, 2003).

44. Jones SW, Roberts RA, Robbins GR, Perry JL, Kai MP, Chen K, Bo T, Napier ME, Ting JP, Desimone JM, Bear JE. Nanoparticle clearance is governed by Th1/Th2 immunity and strain background. J Clin Invest. 2013 Jul;123(7):3061–3073. doi: 10.1172/JCI66895. Epub 2013 Jun 17. PMID: 23778144; PMCID: PMC3696555.

45. Gabizon AA, Patil Y, La-Beck NM. New insights and evolving role of pegylated liposomal doxorubicin in cancer therapy. Drug Resist Updat. 2016 Nov;29:90–106. doi: 10.1016/j.drup.2016.10.003. Epub 2016 Oct 29. PMID: 27912846.

46. Araújo L, Antonio G, Tedesco C. doi: 10.1016/B978-0-323-85754-3.00003-4.

47. Chanan-Khan A, Szebeni J, Savay S, Liebes L, Rafique NM, Alving CR, Muggia FM. Complement activation following first exposure to pegylated liposomal doxorubicin (Doxil): possible role in hypersensitivity reactions. Ann Oncol. 2003 Sep;14(9):1430–1437. doi: 10.1093/annonc/mdg374. PMID: 12954584.

48. Cancer Facts & Figures 2007 (American Cancer Society, Atlanta, 2007).

49. Godin B, Sakamoto JH, Serda RE, Grattoni A, Bouamrani A, Ferrari M. Emerging applications of nanomedicine for the diagnosis and treatment of cardiovascular diseases. Trends Pharmacol Sci. 2010 May;31(5):199–205. doi: 10.1016/j.tips.2010.01.003. Epub 2010 Feb 19. PMID: 20172613; PMCID: PMC2862836.

50. Weissig V, Pettinger TK, Murdock N. Nanopharmaceuticals (part 1): products on the market. Int J Nanomedicine. 2014 Sep 15;9:4357–4373. doi: 10.2147/IJN.S46900. PMID: 25258527; PMCID: PMC4172146.

51. Esteller M. Cancer epigenomics: DNA methylomes and histone-modification maps. Nat Rev Genet. 2007 Apr;8(4):286–298. doi: 10.1038/nrg2005. Epub 2007 Mar 6. PMID: 17339880.

52. Galvin P, Thompson D, Ryan KB, McCarthy A, Moore AC, Burke CS, Dyson M, Maccraith BD, Gun'ko YK, Byrne MT, Volkov Y, Keely C, Keehan E, Howe M, Duffy C, MacLoughlin R. Nanoparticle-based drug delivery: case studies for cancer and cardiovascular applications. Cell Mol Life Sci. 2012 Feb; 69(3):389–404. doi: 10.1007/s00018-011-0856-6. Epub 2011 Oct 21. PMID: 22015612.

53. Choi CH, Alabi CA, Webster P, Davis ME. Mechanism of active targeting in solid tumors with transferrin-containing gold nanoparticles. Proc Natl Acad Sci USA. 2010 Jan 19;107(3):1235–1240. doi: 10.1073/pnas.0914140107. Epub 2009 Dec 29. PMID: 20080552; PMCID: PMC2824286.

54. Astier A, Barton Pai A, Bissig M, Crommelin DJA, Flühmann B, Hecq JD, Knoeff J, Lipp HP, Morell-Baladrón A, Mühlebach S. How to select a nanosimilar. Ann NY Acad Sci. 2017 Nov;1407(1):50–62. doi: 10.1111/nyas.13382. Epub 2017 Jul 17. PMID: 28715605.

55. Markman JL, Rekechenetskiy A, Holler E, Ljubimova JY. Nanomedicine therapeutic approaches to overcome cancer drug resistance. Adv Drug Deliv Rev. 2013 Nov;65(13–14):1866–1879. doi: 10.1016/j.addr.2013.09.019. Epub 2013 Oct 10. PMID: 24120656; PMCID: PMC5812459.

56. Laffleur F, Keckeis V. Advances in drug delivery systems: work in progress still needed? Int J Pharm: X. 2020;2:100050. doi: 10.1016/j.ijpx.2020.100050.

57. Ventola CL. The nanomedicine revolution: part 1: emerging concepts. P T. 2012 Sep;37(9):512–525. PMID: 23066345; PMCID: PMC3462600.

58. Peer D, Karp JM, Hong S, Farokhzad OC, Margalit R, Langer R. Nanocarriers as an emerging platform for cancer therapy. Nat Nanotechnol. 2007;2:751–760.

59. Hazan-Halevy I, Landesman-Milo D, Rosenblum D, Mizrahy S, Ng BD, Peer D. Immunomodulation of hematological malignancies using oligonucleotides based-nanomedicines. J Control Release. 2016 Dec 28;244(Pt B):149–156. doi: 10.1016/j.jconrel.2016.07.052. Epub 2016 Aug 2. PMID: 27491881.

60. Buzea C, Pacheco II, Robbie K. Nanomaterials and nanoparticles: sources and toxicity. Biointerphases. 2, MR17 (2007). doi: 10.1116/1.2815690.

61. Rayburn ER, Ezell SJ, Zhang R. Anti-inflammatory agents for cancer therapy. Mol Cell Pharmacol. 2009;1(1):29–43. doi: 10.4255/mcpharmacol.09.05. PMID: 20333321; PMCID: PMC2843097.

62. Alharbi KK, Al-Sheikh YA. Role and implications of nanodiagnostics in the changing trends of clinical diagnosis. Saudi J Biol Sci. 2014 Apr;21(2):109–117. doi: 10.1016/j.sjbs.2013.11.001.

63. Ediriwickrema A, Saltzman WM. Nanotherapy for cancer: targeting and multi-functionality in the future of cancer therapies. ACS Biomater Sci Eng. 2015 Feb 9; 1(2):64–78. doi: 10.1021/ab500084g.

64. Moghimi SM, Farhangrazi ZS. Just so stories: the random acts of anti-cancer nanomedicine performance. Nanomedicine. 2014 Nov;10(8):1661–1666. doi: 10.101 6/j.nano.2014.04.011. PMID: 24832960.

65. Lessene G, Czabotar PE, Colman PM. BCL-2 family antagonists for cancer therapy. Nat Rev Drug Discov. 2008 Dec;7(12):989–1000. doi: 10.1038/nrd2658. PMID: 19043450.

66. Atkins J, Gershell L. Selective anticancer drugs. Nat Rev Cancer. 2002;2:645–646. doi: 10.1038/nrc900.

67. Chan VS. Nanomedicine: an unresolved regulatory issue. Regul Toxicol Pharmacol. 2006 Dec;46(3):218–224. doi: 10.1016/j.yrtph.2006.04.009. Epub 2006 Nov 1. PMID: 17081666.

68. Alharbi KK, Al-Sheikh YA. Role and implications of nanodiagnostics in the changing trends of clinical diagnosis. Saudi J Biol Sci. 2014 Apr;21(2):109–117. doi: 10.1016/j.sjbs.2013.11.001. Epub 2013 Nov 19. PMID: 24600302; PMCID: PMC3942856.

69. Huebsch N, Mooney DJ. Inspiration and application in the evolution of biomaterials. Nature. 2009 Nov 26;462(7272):426–432. doi: 10.1038/nature08601. PMID: 19940912; PMCID: PMC2848528.

70. Donovan HS, Sereika SM, Wenzel LB, Edwards RP, Knapp JE, Hughes SH, Roberge MC, Thomas TH, Klein SJ, Spring MB, Nolte S, Landrum LM, Casey AC, Mutch DG, DeBernardo RL, Muller CY, Sullivan SA, Ward SE. Effects of the WRITE symptoms interventions on symptoms and quality of life among patients with recurrent ovarian cancers: an NRG oncology/GOG study (GOG-0259). J Clin Oncol. 2022 May 1;40(13):1464–1473. doi: 10.1200/JCO.21.00656.

71. Lammers T, Kiessling F, Hennink WE, Storm G. Drug targeting to tumors: principles, pitfalls and (pre-)clinical progress. J Control Release. 2012 Jul 20;161(2):175–187. doi: 10.1016/j.jconrel.2011.09.063. Epub 2011 Sep 16. PMID: 21945285.

72. Szebeni J. Complement activation-related pseudoallergy: a new class of drug-induced acute immune toxicity. Toxicology. 2005 Dec 15;216(2-3):106–121. doi: 10.1016/j.tox.2005.07.023. Epub 2005 Sep 2. PMID: 16140450.

73. Anchordoquy TJ, Barenholz Y, Boraschi D et al. Mechanisms and barriers in cancer nanomedicine: addressing challenges, looking for solutions. CS Nano. 2017;11(1): 12–18. doi: 10.1021/acsnano.6b08244.

74. Vessillier S, Eastwood D, Fox B, Sathish J, Sethu S, Dougall T, Thorpe SJ, Thorpe R, Stebbings R. Cytokine release assays for the prediction of therapeutic mAb safety in first-in-man trials–whole blood cytokine release assays are poorly predictive for TGN1412 cytokine storm. J Immunol Methods. 2015 Sep;424:43–52. doi: 10.1016/j.jim.2015.04.020. Epub 2015 May 7. PMID: 25960173; PMCID: PMC4768082.

75. Hanahan D, Weinberg RA. Hallmarks of cancer: the next generation. Cell. 2011 Mar 4;144(5):646–674. doi: 10.1016/j.cell.2011.02.013. PMID: 21376230.

76. Arora S, Rajwade JM, Paknikar KM. Nanotoxicology and in vitro studies: the need of the hour. Toxicol Appl Pharmacol. 2012 Jan 15;258(2):151–165. doi: 10.1016/j.taap.2011.11.010. Epub 2011 Dec 2. PMID: 22178382.

77. Lund AW, Wagner M, Fankhauser M, Steinskog ES, Broggi MA, Spranger S, Gajewski TF, Alitalo K, Eikesdal HP, Wiig H, Swartz MA. Lymphatic vessels regulate immune microenvironments in human and murine melanoma. J Clin Invest. 2016 Sep 1;126(9):3389–3402. doi: 10.1172/JCI79434. Epub 2016 Aug 15. PMID: 27525437; PMCID: PMC5004967.

78. Sarkissian Carol D, What we know about nanomedicines? https://www.webmd.com/a-to-z-guides/nanomedicine-what-to-know

79. Luo J, Solimini NL, Elledge SJ. Principles of cancer therapy: oncogene and non-oncogene addiction. Cell. 2009 Mar 6;136(5):823–837. doi: 10.1016/j.cell.2009.02.024. Erratum in: Cell. 2009 Aug 21;138(4):807. PMID: 19269363; PMCID: PMC2894612.

80. Cui X, Boland T, D'Lima DD, Lotz MK. Thermal inkjet printing in tissue engineering and regenerative medicine. Recent Pat Drug Deliv Formul. 2012 Aug;6(2):149–155. doi: 10.2174/187221112800672949. PMID: 22436025; PMCID: PMC3565591.

81. Oryan A, Alidadi S, Moshiri A, Maffulli N. Bone regenerative medicine: classic options, novel strategies, and future directions. J Orthop Surg Res. 2014 Mar 17;9(1):18. doi: 10.1186/1749-799X-9-18. PMID: 24628910; PMCID: PMC3995444.

82. Hanahan D, Weinberg RA. The hallmarks of cancer. Cell. 2000 Jan 7;100(1):57–70. doi: 10.1016/s0092-8674(00)81683-9. PMID: 10647931.

83. Sajja HK, East MP, Mao H, Wang YA, Nie S, Yang L. Development of multifunctional nanoparticles for targeted drug delivery and noninvasive imaging of therapeutic effect. Curr Drug Discov Technol. 2009 Mar;6(1):43–51. doi: 10.2174/1570163 09787581066. PMID: 19275541; PMCID: PMC3108242.

84. Harding K, Sumner M, Cardinal M. A prospective, multicentre, randomised controlled study of human fibroblast-derived dermal substitute (Dermagraft) in patients with venous leg ulcers. Int Wound J. 2013 Apr;10(2):132–137. doi: 10.1111/iwj.12053. PMID: 23506344; PMCID: PMC7950758.

85. Picard FJ, Bergeron MG. Rapid molecular theranostics in infectious diseases. Drug Discov Today. 2002 Nov 1;7(21):1092–1101. doi: 10.1016/s1359-6446(02)02497-2. PMID: 12546841.

86. Bardhan R, Lal S, Joshi A, Halas NJ. Theranostic nanoshells: from probe design to imaging and treatment of cancer. Acc Chem Res. 2011;44(10):936–946. doi: 10.1021/ar200023x.

87. Seigneuric R, Markey L, Nuyten DS, Dubernet C, Evelo CT, Finot E, Garrido C. From nanotechnology to nanomedicine: applications to cancer research. Curr Mol Med. 2010 Oct;10(7):640–652. doi: 10.2174/156652410792630634. PMID: 20712588.

88. Mofazzal Jahromi MA, Sahandi Zangabad P, Moosavi Basri SM, Sahandi Zangabad K, Ghamarypour A, Aref AR, Karimi M, Hamblin MR. Nanomedicine and advanced technologies for burns: preventing infection and facilitating wound healing. Adv Drug Deliv Rev. 2018 Jan 1;123:33–64. doi: 10.1016/j.addr.2017.08.001. Epub 2017 Aug 4. PMID: 28782570; PMCID: PMC5742034.

89. Moses MA, Brem H, Langer R. Advancing the field of drug delivery: taking aim at cancer. Cancer cell, 4(5), 337–341. doi: 10.1016/S0959-437X(00)00164-7.

90. Jaklenec A, Stamp A, Deweerd E, Sherwin A, Langer R. Progress in the tissue engineering and stem cell industry "are we there yet?". Tissue Eng Part B Rev. 2012 Jun;18(3):155–166. doi: 10.1089/ten.TEB.2011.0553. Epub 2012 Feb 8. PMID: 22220809.

91. Mendelson A, Frenette PS. Hematopoietic stem cell niche maintenance during homeostasis and regeneration. Nat Med. 2014 Aug;20(8):833–846. doi: 10.1038/nm.3647. PMID: 25100529; PMCID: PMC4459580.

92. Dupont Pharmaceuticals Co., Department of Cancer Research, Glenolden, Pennsylvania 19036, USA. 10.1016/S0959-437X(00)00164-7

5 Clinical Development of Nanomedicines for Rheumatoid Arthritis

Neha Aggarwal, Sakshi Kataria, Sandrine Auger, and Jasmina Vidic

5.1 INTRODUCTION

Rheumatoid arthritis is a chronic inflammatory joint disease that can damage cartilage and bones as well as cause impairment. It mainly affects the joints, but it ought to be viewed as a disorder with extra-articular symptoms including rheumatoid nodules, pulmonary engagement, or vasculitis, as well as systemic chronicity, especially those influencing the vasculature and metabolism. The specific burden is a direct result of musculoskeletal deprivation, with accompanying declines in physiological functional ability, as well as an accumulated co-morbid threat (Smolen, J. S. et al., 2016). The provenance of RA is still unknown as numerous genetic and environmental factors for the pathogenesis of RA have been studied. Thus limiting the prevention or complete remission of the ailment. Autoantibodies to autoantigens such as citrullinated peptide (ACPA, anti-citrullinated protein antibody) (Scherer, H. U. et al., 2020) and immunoglobulin G (RF, rheumatoid factor), characterize RA. Extreme intrusion of both innate and autoantigen-specific adaptive immune cells provokes hyperplasia and upregulates proinflammatory cytokine in inflammatory joints, leading to irrevocable cartilage and bone degeneration (Malmström, V. et al., 2017). Under the stimulation of particular cytokines, macrophages, neutrophils, lymphocytes, chondrocytes, fibroblasts, and other cells may cause permanent damage and degradation of synovial membrane and cartilage in joints. As a result of the multifaceted pathogenesis, alternative treatments for RA are less effective, particularly when using a specific drug (Zhang, S. et al., 2022).

In addition to major treatments, drugs such as disease-modifying antirheumatic drugs (DMARDs), nonsteroidal anti-inflammatory drugs (NSAIDs), and glucocorti- coids (GCs) are now used to cure RA. Amidst the evident medicinal benefits, the adverse effects of these drugs, as well as their disadvantages, cannot be neglected (Smolen, J. S. et al., 2020). NSAIDs are frequently used as diagnosable drugs to alleviate swelling and inflammation in RA but do not counteract the disease's course (Wongrakpanich, S. et al., 2018). GCs can hinder the activity and multiplication of Th1 cells and thus decrease the severity of the disease by reducing the secretion of pro-inflammatory elements. However, relatively higher dosage and protracted use

DOI: 10.1201/9781003348672-5

could have negative consequences (Luís, M. et al., 2022). The most prevalently used DMARD is methotrexate (MTX), which is the most effective but it may affect the human gut microbiome and therefore the immune function (Nayak, R. R. et al., 2021). Furthermore, nucleic acid-based drugs that interrupt the expression of inflammation-related proteins, including small interfering RNA (siRNA) and small molecule RNA (microRNA, miRNA), and anti-microRNA (anti-miRNAs) are being studied to control the RA disease progression. In physiological conditions, exogenous siRNAs are easily degraded by enzymes and are unstable and can even have off-target impacts as well as immune clearing (Feng 2020; Abolmaali 2013).

Nano-delivery systems also made significant advancements in the treatment of a wide range of ailments. As a result, developing novel drugs to mitigate RA's adaptive treatment tolerance (ATT) and obtain superior therapy efficacy is extremely desirable. For this context, nanotechnology-based nanomedicines (NMs) for RA are a promising new treatment modality. Even though nanoparticles can deposit effectively in arthritic joints' inflammatory microhabitats, which are characterized by angiogenic vessels and an unusual peripheral lymphatic system (Jeong, M., & Park, J. H. 2020). Nanomedicine deposition in inflamed joints may improve anti-inflammatory intrusion and also reduce the off-target effects of several drugs by avoiding high-dose administration. Following these characteristics, non-targeted RA drugs like GCs, MTX, and nucleic acids are excellent candidates for nanomedicine-based delivery (Yu, Z. et al., 2020). Among the important tenets in developing more attainable regimens for more effective RA treatment are multifunctional NPs with targeted stimuli-responsive attributes. Since the provision of these medications at targeted sites in response to specific external or internal stimuli, these engineered NPs can effectively suspend RA advancement without any adverse effects on healthy tissue (Liu, L. et al., 2019). Among the numerous RA nanomedicines described in the literature, mainly focused on nanomedicine designed for targeted delivery to inflamed joints, stimuli-responsive drug release, and immune modulation (Jeong, M., & Park, J. H. 2020). The manipulation strategies and anti-RA effects of nanomaterials on macrophages for RA treatment are also discussed in this chapter (Li, S. et al., 2021).

5.2   EPIDEMIOLOGY

Rheumatoid arthritis (RA) is a systemic disease in which joint inflammation (arthritis) is the central hallmark. In Europe and North America, its prevalence is 0.5 to 1.0% (Garner et al., 2014). It affects at least twice as many women as men, and although it can occur at any age, the peak incidence is at the age of 50 years. There is an ongoing debate about whether the prevalence and incidence of RA are increasing or decreasing. Several groups have reported a declining incidence of RA during the second half of the 20th century (Safiriet al., 2019). By contrast, it appears that after 1995, the incidence of RA may be increasing again. One can speculate whether this change may be explained by variations in environmental risk factors, but a single culprit seems difficult to identify. RA has existed for centuries (Arima et al., 2022). One of the first extensive descriptions of the disease is from Landre-Beauvais in 1800, but paintings from an even earlier century also showed rheumatic joints. Initially, the concept of RA was much more heterogeneous than it is at present, as up until the 1950s, gout and spondylarthritis were also considered to be RA (Gönen & Bal, 2015). Since the middle of the 20th century, no large dissections in different disease entities have occurred. However, since then, the classical presentation of RA slightly changed with time, as did the classification criteria (Garner et al., 2014).

5.3 CAUSES AND GENETICS

5.3.1 Risk Factors Associated with Rheumatoid Arthritis

A number of risk factors have been suggested as important contributors to the development or progression of RA. Of these, the best studied have been genetics, infectious agents, oral contraceptive medications, smoking, and formal education (Gabriel, 2001).

5.3.2 Genetics

The familial nature of RA has long been recognized suggesting that genetic risk factors are important in the etiology of this disease. Genetic studies of RA have focused primarily on the role of the major histocompatibility locus in RA. Several investigators have demonstrated important associations between specific human leukocyte antigen (HLA) alleles (i.e., HLA-DR4 and HLA-DR1) and susceptibility to RA (Deighton et al., 1993). There is controversy, however, regarding the mode of inheritance (i.e., recessive vs dominant)and the characteristics of the association (i.e., are there specific disease susceptibility loci, or do they simply affect disease severity). Irrespective of the mode of inheritance and the role of HLA-associated susceptibility gene(s), the relation between HLA-DR alleles and RA is insufficient to explain the familial nature of the disease. The observations of high RA incidence rates, more severe clinical disease, and familial aggregation among certain North American Indian populations combined with the unusually low incidence of RA in other populations all lend support to the hypothesis of a genetic predisposition to RA (Gabriel, 2001). A study of the genetic epidemiology of RA identified variables associated with risk for RA in first-degree relatives of probands. These analyses identified gender and age at onset in the proband as important risk factors, with relatives of male probands having the greatest cumulative risk of RA. Complex segregation analyses indicated that a small proportion of all cases of RA may be attributed to a highly penetrant recessive gene. In this model, the largest proportion of genetic cases of RA would be expected to occur in men affected before the age of 40 years (Chang et al., 2008). Significant heterogeneity in the inheritance of RA and in the distribution of risk for RA among first-degree relatives was demonstrated. A recent study examined familial aggregation of RA in the Netherlands and analyzed the effect of proband characteristics on the concordance rates for RA (Heliovaara M. et al., 1993). Cross-sectional hospital-based surveys were used to identify familial RA (i.e., affected sib-pair families). The estimated prevalence for familial RA was 9.8%, and familial aggregation of RA was estimated to occur preferentially in large siblings. Probands with familial RA were more often RF-positive and had a longer follow-up period. Male gender and history of joint replacements were associated with higher concordance for RA (Ohno et al., 2020).

5.3.3 FACTORS THAT MAY INCREASE RISK OF RHEUMATOID ARTHRITIS

- **Sex.** Women are more likely than men to develop rheumatoid arthritis.
- **Age.** Rheumatoid arthritis can occur at any age, but it most commonly begins in middle age.
- **Family history.** If a member of your family has rheumatoid arthritis, you may have an increased risk of the disease.
- **Smoking.** Cigarette smoking increases your risk of developing rheumatoid arthritis, particularly if you have a genetic predisposition for developing the disease. Smoking also appears to be associated with greater disease severity.
- **Excess weight.** People who are overweight appear to be at a somewhat higher risk of developing rheumatoid arthritis.

5.4 PHYSIOPATHOLOGY OF RHEUMATOID ARTHRITIS

Pathophysiological mechanisms for RA are not fully elucidated; several hypotheses have been postulated. It has been reported that immunological processes can occur many years before symptoms of joint inflammation are noticed, the so-called pre-RA phase modification in the structure of collagen and vitamins by which the protein with arginine residue converted to citrulline by peptidyl arginine deiminases (PAD) in a post-translational modification called citrullination (Garner et al., 2014). Due to the susceptibility genes HLA-DR1 and HLA-DR4, the immune system is no longer able to recognize citrullinated protein (Scherer et al., 2020) (vimentin, collagen, histones, fibrin, fibronectin, Epstein, Barr nuclear antigen 1) as a self structure. Antigens are taken up by antigen-presenting cells (APC) which are dendritic cells that are activated to initiate an immune Response. The whole complex migrates to lymph nodes where the activation of CD4+ helper T-cells takes place. The germinal center of the lymph node contains B-cells that get activated by reciprocal and sequential signals with T-cells, an immunological process called co-stimulation. An example of co-stimulation is the interaction between CD28 and CD80/86.

Now, B-cells undergo somatic hypermutation and start to proliferate and differentiate into plasma cells, which produce autoantibodies, and memory cells. Autoantibodies are mainly proteins that are produced by an immune system that is no longer able to discriminate self from non-self structures, so self-tissues and organs are accidentally targeted. Of RF (rheumatoid factor) and ACPA (anti-citrullinated protein), RF is the most studied of the autoantibodies involved in RA. RF is an IgM antibody with a testing specificity of 85% in RA patients, which targets the Fc portion of IgG, also called the constant region. It also forms an immune complex with IgG and a complement protein, a complex able to migrate in the synovial fluid. However, ACPA is more specific for RA and targets citrullinated proteins and after their binding interactions, immune complexes are formed with an

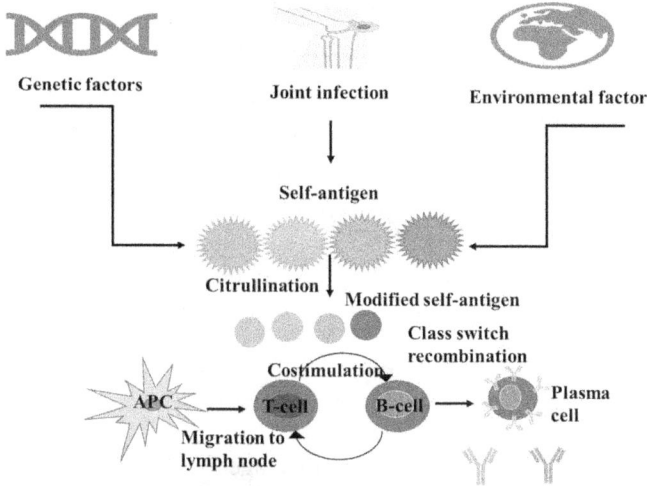

FIGURE 5.1 Immunological processes in the pre-RA phase. ACPA, anti-citrullinated protein antibodies; APC, antigen-presenting cells; RF, rheumatoid factor.

accumulation in the synovial fluid. All the features of an immune response in the pre-RA phase are summarized in Figure 5.1 (Radu, A. F., & Bungau, S. G. 2021).

ACPA, on the other hand, is more focused on RA and specifically targets citrullinated proteins. Following their binding interactions, immune complexes are formed with an accumulation in the synovial fluid. Air pollution, which is made up of a variety of suspended particulate materials (PM) of different sizes and gases (nitrates, ozone, sulfur dioxide, and carbon monoxide), has recently drawn more attention in the field of RA. Agriculture, the burning of fossil fuels, the chemical industry, the usage of solvents, volcanic eruptions, wind-borne dust, plant emissions, etc., are only a few examples of the many man-made and natural sources that emit pollutants into the air. The clinical effects of air pollution are mostly taken into account in relation to respiratory illnesses.

There have been claims that ozone can harm the alveoli, a vital component of the respiratory system that filters carbon dioxide and oxygen. By interfering with several enzymes, pollutants can potentially damage lung tissue in a secondary manner, leading to infection or pulmonary inflammation. Three significant epidemiological studies carried out in the US, Canada, and Sweden have shown that air pollution can contribute to the development of RA.

Regression modeling was used to evaluate the relationships between air pollution and RA activity. Important risk factors for the development of RA have been identified as nitrates and sulfur dioxide. A case-crossover study that evaluated a potential link between RA and air pollution in the Verona area is one of the newest research articles to be published. On a few mechanistic mechanisms, it may be possible to attribute air pollutants' role in the pathogenesis of RA. By activating nuclear factor kappa B (NF-KB), which in turn stimulates T helper type 1 (Th1), free reactive oxygen species (ROS) produced by PM inhalation can cause the production of TNF-, IL-1, and IL-6 (IL-6). These cytokines encourage the development of dormant monocytes into mature dendritic cells, which present auto-antigens to self-reactive T lymphocytes, causing them to migrate to target organs.

5.5 THERAPEUTIC STRATEGIES FOR THE TREATMENT OF RA

Pro-inflammatory cells have a strong relationship to the pathological development of RA. As a result, macrophages and synoviocytes, as well as pro-inflammatory cytokines, are the key treatment targets in arthritic joints. Activated T-cells induce infiltrating mononuclear cells to release pro-inflammatory cytokines such TNFα, IL-6, and IL-1, which ultimately activate synoviocytes in arthritic joints (Jeong, M., & Park, J. H. (2020)). The synovium lining layer contains synoviocytes, which are divided into two subsets: macrophage-like synoviocytes (MLSs) and fibroblast-like synoviocytes (FLSs) (Mathiessen, A., & Conaghan, P. G. 2017).

Interleukin (IL)-6, a key proinflammatory agent, is one of the cytokines that activated FLS secrete in order to initiate or worsen inflammation (Brennan, F. M., & McInnes, I. B. 2008). Additionally, in order to penetrate the joint cartilage, excited FLS produces mediators or extracellular enzymes including matrix metalloproteinase (MMP), aggrecanase (Bartok, B., & Firestein, G. S. 2010), and vascular adhesion molecule 1 (VCAM-1) (Müller-Ladner et al., 2007). By engaging more inflammatory responses and stimulating FLS, activated MLS primarily releases proinflammatory cytokines including IL-1 and tumor necrosis factor (TNF) to hasten the inflammatory response (Tu, J. et al., 2018). Numerous investigations have demonstrated a connection between defective synoviocytes and altered mitochondrial structure, elevated levels of mtROS (reactive oxygen species), and compromised mitochondrial function (Li, M. et al., 2021).

The signal pathway, known as NF-κB, is activated by TNFα and has an anti-apoptotic effect (Woo, C. H. et al., 2000).

TNFα and mtROS may induce the expression of anti-apoptotic protein A1, which would increase synoviocytes' vulnerability to apoptosis (Wang, C. Y. et al., 1998).

Currently, RA is still an incurable disease, and there are three classes of medications commonly used in clinics, i.e., non-steroidal anti-inflammatory drugs (NSAIDs), glucocorticoids (GCs), and disease-modifying anti-rheumatic drugs (DMARDs). Inadequate symptom control in RA patients requires the use of nonsteroidal anti-inflammatory drugs (NSAIDs) and glucocorticoids (GCs) as adjunctive therapy to reduce inflammation (Yang, Y. et al., 2021).

5.5.1 DMARDs (DISEASE-MODIFYING ANTIRHEUMATIC DRUGS)

DMARDs have a propensity for inhibiting autoimmune activity and deferring or curing joint aging. The American College of Rheumatology (ACR) has created a new class of nonbiologic DMARDs that encompasses targeted synthetic DMARDs, biologic DMARDs, and conventional synthetic DMARDs (Radu, A. F., & Bungau, S. G. 2021). By intervening with inflammatory pathways in different immune cells, synthetic and biological DMARDs delay the course of RA.

5.5.1.1   Methotrexate

Because of its dependability, efficacy, long-lasting effects, affordability, and excellent tolerability, methotrexate (MTX) is the first-line therapy for the protracted management of RA (Sepriano, A. et al., 2020). In therapeutic settings, when there is no medication response, methotrexate is used with corticosteroids, further biologic DMARDs, and NSAIDs (Rau, R., & Herborn, G. 2004). Methotrexate is an antifolate (Quéméneur, L. et al., 2003), and its effectiveness is improved when taken intramuscularly and subcutaneously because oral administration decreases its bioavailability (Li, Det al., 2016). Methotrexate is polyglutamylated, and following absorption, it becomes deposited in the tissues and endures for days to weeks (Dervieux, T. et al., 2003). Oral ulcers, cirrhosis, hepatitis, interstitial pneumonitis, and cytopenias are a few unfavorable side effects of methotrexate (Wang, W., Zhou, H., & Liu, L. 2018).

5.5.1.2   Sulfasalazine

In the 1930s, the unsubstantiated hypothesis that an infectious agent was the cause of RA led to the development and synthesis of sulfasalazine. Following absorption, the molecule is split by microorganisms in the colon into 5-aminosalicylic acid and sulfapyridine (Chatham, W. W. (2005). Through the regulation of NF-KB activation, it impairs T-cell activity, inhibits neutrophil function, and lowers immunoglobulin levels (Abbasi, M. et al., 2019). Hematologic (neutropenia, thrombocytopenia) and gastrointestinal (causing nausea, vomiting, diarrhea, and abdominal pain) are the most prevalent toxicities (Gaffo, A. et al., 2006).

5.5.1.3   Immunosuppressive Drugs

Immunomodulatory medication leflunomide is recommended, if MTX intolerance exists (Olsen, N. J., & Stein, C. M. 2004). Due to their cytotoxic nature and negative effects on the cardiovascular system, two other immunosuppressive drugs, Ciclosporin A and Azathioprine, have only a limited role in the treatment of RA (Solomon, D. H. et al., 2006).

5.5.1.4   Hydroxychloroquine

The DMARDs list was finally expanded to include the malaria medication hydroxy-chloroquine. Following the failure of MTX monotherapy, it is administered as a triple treatment along with MTX and sulfasalazine (Hazlewood, G. S. et al., 2016).

5.5.2   Non-Steroid Anti-Inflammatory Drugs (NSAIDS) and Glucocorticoids (Gc)

In accordance with ACR and EULAR recommendations, available therapies address RA from two angles: symptomatic management (NSAIDs and GCs), and disease-modifying therapy (DMARDs) (Fraenkel et al., 2021). There has been significant development in pharmacological methods for discovering a treatment for RA as a result of continuous improvement in the processes and techniques in drug design strategies. The acute phase reaction is treated with NSAIDs (naproxen, ibuprofen, and coxibs) to lessen discomfort by reducing inflammation.

Cyclooxygenase (COX), particularly COX-2, which is elevated during inflammation, is inhibited by NSAIDs, which is how they work pharmacologically. The
danger of injury should be taken into account, though, as inhibiting prostaglandins can have negative side effects that can be life-threatening, including
bleeding, gastrointestinal ulcers, renal failure, heart failure, rashes, disorientation,
confusion, seizures, etc. By utilizing COX-2-selective NSAIDs, some of the
negative effects can be avoided (celecoxib, rofecoxib valdecoxib). In placebo-
controlled trials involving individuals who had not had GC therapy, the efficacy
of NSAIDs in treating RA was established. Due to the intricate processes
underlying their anti-inflammatory and immunosuppressive actions, GCs (prednisone, hydrocortisone, prednisolone, and dexamethasone) are more potent and
effective than NSAIDs, although NSAIDs have a marginally better safety profile.
GCs can cause a variety of long-term negative effects, such as weight gain, water
retention, muscle weakness, diabetes, bone thinning, etc. They can be given
orally, intravenously, intramuscularly, or intra-particularly, and have a short-term
utility for this reason. As a bridge therapy for DMARDs before their effects start,
and as an adjuvant therapy for active RA that persists after utilizing DMARDs,
GCs play two key roles in the treatment of RA. Negative feedback in the control
of the hypothalamic-pituitary-adrenal (HPA) axis palpability makes it crucial not
to abruptly stop corticosteroid therapy.

5.5.3   Nucleic Acids: A New Strategy for the Treatment of Rheumatoid Arthritis

Broad-sense RNA interference is comprised of two mechanisms: miRNA and
siRNA. Small interfering RNA (siRNA), short hairpin RNA (shRNA), and small
molecule RNA [microRNA,(miRNA)] interfering with the translation of inflammatory mediators (proteins) are also being studied as ways to alter the RA disease
process (Courties, G. et al., 2009).

Several experimental studies have proven the potential of siRNA in RA
treatment, and siRNA-based techniques have demonstrated superior promise in
RA treatment. To achieve gene control, miRNA is a single-stranded RNA molecule
that can be coupled with its regulated mRNA via incomplete complementary
pairing, followed by various pathways: cut mRNA, diminish mRNA stability, or
hinder mRNA translation efficiency (Lu, T. X., & Rothenberg, M. E. 2018). Unlike
miRNA, siRNA is a 20–25 nucleotide double-stranded RNA fragment whose
sequence is fully complementary to the mRNA it regulates, interfering directly with
the mRNA's translation (Feng, N., & Guo, F. 2020).

TNF or signaling pathways such as NF-KB, Notch1, c-Rel, transforming growth
factor-activated kinase-1 (TAK1), C-C chemokine receptor type 5, STAT1, Polo-like
kinase-1 (PLK-1) are the most common targets for siRNA in RA (Yu, Z. et al., 2020).

Research on rheumatic illness patients' miRNA profiles demonstrated important
modifications in the expression of specific miRNAs such as miRNA-155, 146a, 326,
21, and 181 (Chen, J. Q. et al., 2016). Upregulation of miRNA-146a and miRNA-
155 has been demonstrated to increase the nuclear factor-kappa B pathway in

macrophages, as well as the release of pro-inflammatory cytokines such as TNF-, IL-1, and IL-17 (O'Connell, R. M. et al., 2012).

The importance of miRNA-155 in RA has been proven further in mice, where subcutaneous injection of collagen in miRNA-155 gene-deficient animals did not result in the development of clinical symptoms of arthritis such as increased paw edema and decreased grip strength (Blüml et al., 2011). MiRNA-155 has been discovered as a critical mediator of monocyte/macrophage apoptosis at the cellular level (Rajasekhar et al., 2017) and has been demonstrated to be overexpressed in synovial fibroblasts.

When compared to healthy controls, miRNA-16, 132, 146a, and 223 were shown to be overexpressed in patients' synovial fluid and blood plasma (Murata et al., 2010). Only miRNA-223 was increased, while miRNA-99a, -100, -125b, -199-3p, -152, and -214 were downregulated (Ogando et al., 2016). When miRNAs are down-regulated, one option is to re-equilibrate the level of miRNA by administering the necessary missing sequence. When some miRNAs are overexpressed, the best way to block their function is to create anti-miRNA oligonucleotides. Unfortunately, anti-miRNAs are extremely fragile in vivo, and physiological changes might disrupt their bioactivities, resulting in serious off-target side effects such as decreased protective immunity, fibrosis, or liver steatosis (Alivernini et al., 2018).

Among the most significant studies on the suppression of miRNA-34a, Dang et al. (2017) evaluated the impact of synthetically produced anti-miRNA-34a on RA in collagen-induced arthritis (CIA) mice model because miRNA-34a has been demonstrated to engage in cell death, immunological stimulation, and osteogenesis. The anti-miRNA-34a medication reduced arthritis symptoms and reduced joint swelling. Concurrently, the synthesis of inflammatory cytokines was suppressed. The administration of anti-miRNA-34a drastically reduced the percentage of T-cell lineages, including Th1, Th2, Th17, and regulatory T-cells. Furthermore, anti-miRNA-34a treatment of CIA mice reduced autoimmune bone loss (Dang et al., 2017).

5.6 DELIVERY STRATEGY TO INFLAMED JOINTS

The qualities of the active molecule to be delivered, the biological target, the environment before and after the target, and the environment at the target locations should all be taken into account while designing a nanoparticle system. Since inter-endothelial cell gaps are typically 1–2 nm in healthy tissue but can reach 600nmin disease, such as inflamed joints, nanomedicines can be made to prevent the therapeutic agent from degrading, stay in the bloodstream for longer, be tailored for macrophage uptake, or be targeted to specific receptors (Muller et al.). Invading into joint tissues, autoantigen-specific lymphocytes programmed by antigen-presenting cells like dendritic cells produce an inflammatory response and leukocyte activation, which creates the inflammatory status. The synovial joint's natural lining of synovial cells propagates abnormally, creating microenvironments that are deficient in oxygen and nutrients and promoting angiogenesis (Wang et al., 2020). Due to the leaky vasculature that results, macromolecules can permeate into the inflammatory joint tissues through large facades up to 600 nm. Due to the leaky vasculature, intravenously delivered nanomedicine selectively concentrates in the inflamed joints via passive targeting, considerably increasing the delivery efficacy compared to intravenous injection of free medicines (Zhao et al., 2021). The mononuclear phagocytic system (MPS), which includes the liver and spleen, continues to clear a significant quantity of nanomedicine. Size and charge, which evade the MPS and renal clearance, are the main components of nanomedicines. The indicated ideal size range for the effective delivery of nanomedicine to inflamed joints is around 200 nm, and zwitterionic surface charge—which can reduce interactions between nanomedicine and macrophages—is preferred over negative or positive surfaces (Arlt et al., 2021). Nanomedicine may include drug-loaded liposomes, nanoparticles, polymeric micelles, nanogels, and nano capsules. In addition, polymer-drug conjugate, polymer-protein conjugate are all classified as nanomedicines. The synovial tissue is infiltered by various inflammatory cells, especially macrophages, which play an important role in pathophysiological responses. The activated macrophage (M1) produced a series of inflammation cytokines such as TNFα, IL-1β, and IL-6, to sustain and aggravate joint inflammation (Grossen et al., 2017). A functional surface coating can further increase the delivery of nanomedicine to inflamed joints. It is simple for plasma proteins in the blood to opsonize nanoparticles with naked surfaces, which makes it easier for macrophages in the MPS to phagocytosis them. Stealth polymers, such as poly (ethylene glycol), were applied to the surface of nanoparticles to decrease macrophage uptake and prolong blood circulation. The blood circulation time of nanomedicine increases with increasing PEG coating density and layer thickness. Many efforts have been undertaken to create PEGylated nanoparticles for the treatment of RA because of their stealth function. PEGylated nanoparticles or conjugates increase blood circulation time and enhance drug stability, successfully delivering numerous medications such as NSAIDs, corticosteroids, DMARDs, siRNAs, therapeutic peptides, and other medications to the inflammatory tissue (Liu et al., 2008) (Table 5.1). Prednisolone phosphate and budesonide phosphate, two water-soluble corticosteroid derivatives, were included in PEGylated liposomal preparations, whilst insoluble corticosteroids were delivered via PEGylated micelles or polymer-based nanoparticles. Additionally, methotrexate was loaded into polymeric hybrid nanoparticles or PEGylated liposomes to enhance therapeutic efficacy and lessen systemic toxicity. For efficient cytosolic distribution, siRNAs were specifically encapsulated with positively charged PEGylated lipid nanoparticles. For the treatment of RA, there is no FDA-approved nanomedicine, but the PEGylated Liposomal Prednisolone Formulation is now in Clinical Phase II (NCT00241982). Certolizumab pegol, an FDA-approved PEGylated anti-TNF Fab antibody for the treatment of RA, is not a nanomedicine. Researchers discovered, however, that repeated injections of PEGylated substances stimulated the formation of antiPEG antibodies, resulting in faster blood vessel growth (Bartok & Firestein, 2010).

TABLE 5.1

Strategies for Extending the Circulation of Nanomedicines (Jeong, M., & Park, J. H. 2020)

Strategy	Formulation (size and charge)	Drug		Route
		Passive targeting		
PEGylation		NSAIDs	Indomethacin	
	Liposomes (100_400 nm and neutral/negative)		Methylprednisolone	
			budenisonide	
		Corticosteroids	dexamethasone	I.V.
			betamethasone	
		DMARDs	Methotrexate	
		Other drugs	SOD, peptide	
	Micelles (50_100 nm and neutral /negative)	Corticosterioids	Dexamethasone	I.V.
		siRNA	NF-KB siRNA	
		other drug	Campthothecin	
	Polymeric NP(50_200 nm and negative	Corticosteroids	Betamethasone	I.V.
		DMARDs	Methotrexate	
		siRNA	TNFα siRNA	
			Mcl-1 siRNA	
	Conjugate	Corticosteroids	Dexamethasone	I.V.
		DMARDs	Certolizumab	S.C
		Other drugs	Peptide2	P.O, S.C
Self-mimicking	Albumin conjugate	DMARDs	IL-1 receptorantagonist	I.V.
			Methotrexate	I.V., I.P
		Other drugs	Tacrolimus	I.V.
		Magnetic targeting		
Magnetic attraction	SPIO NP (45 nm)	siRNA	IL-2/IL-15Rβ siRNA	I.V.
	SPIO-PLGA(1_10 μm)	corticosteroids	Dexamethasone	I.A.
	Au/Fe/Au/PLGA NP (-100 nm & negative)	DMARDs	Methotrexate	I.V.

NP-Nanoparticle, NSAIDs-non steroid anti-inflammatory drugs, DMARDs-disease-modifying arthritic drugs, siRNA-small interfering RNA, SPIO-superparamagnetic iron oxides, PLGA-poly. (lactic -glycolic acid), TNF-α -tumor necrosis factor alpha, SOD-superoxide dismutase, I.V.-intravenous, I.A.-intraarticular, S.C.-subcutaneous, P.O.-oral administration, I.P.-intraperitoneal.

5.7   CLINICAL DEVELOPMENT IN NANOMEDICINES FOR THE TREATMENT OF RHEUMATOID ARTHRITIS

Currently, there are various antiarthritis groups. NSAIDs and DMARDs are examples of the therapeutics used to treat RA. DMARDs are a class of medications that also comprise biomaterials such anti-interleukin 6 (anti-IL-6) antibodies against

TNFα and receptors. Despite being regarded as powerful and effective medications, their prolonged intake could have negative side effects (Oliveira, I. M. et al., 2018). One of the primary issues with the use of these medications is their widespread availability across the body except in swollen joints and where illness is present. Because of this, numerous vital organs, including the heart and kidneys, are frequently destroyed in chronic arthritis patients. In order to maximize these medications' effectiveness in treating arthritis, it is vital to transport them to the RA sites that are inflamed effectively (Meka, R. R. et al., 2019).

Nanomedicine has evolved as a new therapeutic technique for efficient medication administration in the treatment of a variety of disorders, including cancer. Recently, there has been a fast growth in the advancement of nanomedicine in RA because nanoparticles can aggregate effectively in inflammatory niches of arthritic joints. The therapeutic targets for the therapy of RA include macrophages, T-cells, FLSs, and other pro-inflammatory cells, as well as their cytokines. In order to increase the therapeutic effectiveness of anti-rheumatic medications, nanomaterial distribution to afflicted joints and cells was suggested. (Jeong, M., & Park, J. H. 2020).

5.7.1 LIPOSOMES

Liposomes are composed of phospholipids, which are amphiphilic in nature and spontaneously self-aggregate into vesicular structures in aqueous mediums. It is a bilayer structure composed of two lipid monolayers. The hydrophilic region of liposome is in contact with the aqueous environment.

A few strategies have been implemented to enhance the in vitro and in vivo longevity of GC liposomal regimens administered intravenously, such as the integration of cholesterol, which strengthens molecular packaging inside the lipid membranes and thus increases stability. The stability of parenteral administration of liposomes can be augmented even more by integrating PEG into the liposomal bilayer, which delays endocytosis and affirmation by phagocytes of the mononuclear phagocytic system (MPS), allowing the liposomes to remain in the bloodstream for a longer duration of time. Thus, increasing the passive target genes accumulation and clinical effects (Ozbakir et al., 2014).

Following intravenous injection into rats, conventional liposomes made of 1,2-dipalmitoyl-sn-glycero-3-phosphocholine (DPPC), first used to encapsulate prednisolone palmitate (a lipidic prodrug of prednisolone), demonstrated higher anti-inflammatory activity than prednisolone hemisuccinate, using a carrageenan paw edema test (Yu, Z. et al., 2020).

Dxamethasone phosphate (DxM-P), a water-soluble corticosteroid was encapsulated in a non-PEGylated liposome formulation (Micromethason). Novosom AG (Halle, Germany) synthesized micromethason liposomes from 1,2-dipalmitoylsn-glycero-3-phosphocholine (DPPC), 1,2-dipalmitoylsn-glycero-3-(phosphor-rac-(1-glycerol))(sodium salt) (DPPG), and cholesterol (50:10:40 mol%). Liposomal DxM-P was also injected intravenously in a mouse and rat arthritis model.

The PEG-free regimens drastically decreased the dose and/or frequency needed to treat RA in both cases, with the ability to enhance or prolong tolerability whilst also limiting side effects (Anderson, R. et al., 2010).

FA-lip(DEX + GNRs/ODNs), a triple therapy-based folic acid liposome composed of Dexamethasone (DEX), gold nanorods (GNRs), and oligodeoxynucleotides (ODNs), was developed by Xue, L et al. The treatment with this FA-lip (DEX + GNRs/ODNs) demonstrated a steady decline in TNF-α, IL-6, and NO, indicating that this therapy effectively suppressed pain and swelling. FA-lip(DEX + GNRs/ODNs) + laser-treated mice had adherent cartilage, no pannus tissue intrusion, and no innate immune incursion (Xue, L. et al., 2020).

5.7.2 POLYMERIC MICELLES

Micelles are single-tailed phospholipids and glycolipids with a diameter of approximately 10 to 100 nm, typically formed by the self-aggregation of amorphous polymer in an aqueous medium. Their pivotal clustering causes the formation of a core-shell structure, with the hydrophobic part of the polymer inside (core) and the hydrophilic part on the outside (shell) (Lu, Y. et al., 2018). Entrapped hydrophobic or low water-soluble drugs, such as GCs, are typically found in the hydrophobic inner core and are released through diffusion (Amjad, M. W. et al., 2017). The hydrophilic shell and small size act as a shield by limiting opsonin adsorption and providing good stability in body fluid, allowing for a longer circulation time. PEG is commonly used as a hydrophilic block, while poly (ε-caprolactone) (Khodaverdi, E. et al., 2019) poly-L-cysteine can be used as a hydrophobic block (Kim, H. C. et al., 2017).

Until now, the potency of micelles as RA carriers has not been thoroughly investigated. Only a few amphiphilic molecules have been created and reported, capable of forming micelles including poly(ethylene glycol)-poly(ε-caprolactone) (PCL-PEG) and polysialic acid-polycaprolactone (PSA-PCL) (Wang, Q. et al., 2016, 2019; Wilson, D. R. et al., 2014). Wang et al. (2019) demonstrated that a low dose of dexamethasone could be delivered to inflamed joints using PCL-PEG. When compared to the free drug, these functional micelles with a diameter <100 nm and a high entrapment effectiveness evidenced a reasonably long perseverance of dexamethasone in plasma. In the treatment of arthritis in rats, it was found to be more effective than free dexamethasone (Wang, Q. et al., 2019).

5.7.3 LIPID NANOEMULSION (LDE)

Nanoemulsions (NE) are metastable submicron oil-in-water dispersions with droplet diameters ranging from 20 to 500 nm. Attributes such as particle stability, rheological properties, color, structure, and shelf life can all be affected by the size and polydispersity of NE (Hoscheid, J. et al., 2015). Mello et al. created an MTX-loaded lipidic nanoemulsion for the treatment of RA. In-vivo investigations demonstrated that MTX-loaded nanoemulsion was mostly absorbed by the liver, with arthritic joints absorbing twice as much as control joints. The use of MTX-loaded nanoemulsions lowers leukocyte infiltration into synovial fluid by 65% (Mello, S. B. et al., 2016).

5.7.4 Metal NPs

Metal NPs' distinct physical, biological, mechanical, thermal, and chemical properties have led to their immense use in medical and pharmaceutical domains. Metal NPs are very small <100 nm, one-dimension inorganic molecules (Kaur, M., 2020)

5.7.4.1 Gold Nanoparticles (AuNPs)

Au NPs (gold nanoparticles) have unique properties that can help with biological imaging, drug delivery, therapeutic, and diagnostic agents. For producing different sizes and shapes of Au NPs, several synthetic methods have already been reported (Sengani, M., 2017). The use of plant extract is convenient in the production of Au NPs not only because of its lower environmental impact, but also its capability of creating a large number of NPs. Plant extracts can act as both stabilizing and reducing agents in the formation of NPs (Mittal, A. K. et al., 2013; An, H. et al., 2020).

Triamcinolone–gold nanoparticle (Triam-AuNP) was developed by Park, J. Y et al. Triamcinolone (Triam) is a synthetic glucocorticoid (GC) and PEGylated AuNPs with a size of 20 nm were conjugated with clinical-grade Triam. Triam-AuNPs suppressed inflammation derived by main RA fibroblast-like synovial cells (FLSs). TriamNPs significantly promoted cartilage regeneration in a collagen-induced arthritis (CIA) mouse model by lowering the levels of significant proinflammatory cytokines in cartilage tissues (TNF-, IL-6, INF-, and IL-1) and increasing the number of M2 macrophages. While the commercial GC (Triam) only mitigates the pro-inflammatory expressions of FLS and M1 macrophages without stimulating the anti-inflammatory expressions of FLSs or repolarizing macrophages from the M1 to the M2 phenotype. Triam-AuNPs can be used to modulate dynamic immune regulation (both upregulation of anti-inflammatory responses and down-regulation of pro-inflammatory responses). Thus, the efficacy of the Triam-AuNPs surpasses that of the standard GC drug (Triam), allowing for subsequent recovery of cartilage regeneration in the inflamed synovium (Park, J. Y. et al., 2020).

5.7.4.2 Silver NPs (AgNPs)

Silver nanoparticles AgNPs are an advanced industrial nanomaterial for clinical fields because of their ease of synthesis, adaptability, and broad biological properties (Yang, Y. et al., 2021). Ag NPs are shown to be anti-inflammatory in RA patients by reducing the production of proinflammatory cytokines such as TNF-and IL-6. A factor produced by epithelial cells, vascular endothelial cells growth factor (VEGF), that intensifies pathogen responsivity, plays an important role in physiological anomalies, induces plasma proteins to overflow into the extracellular fluid, causes respiratory wall thickening, and maximizes T helper type-2 (TH2) cell-mediated inflammation (IL-9, IL-4, IL-5, and IL-13), can be reduced by Ag NPs (Agarwal, H. et al., 2019).

M1 macrophages play critical roles in the progression of RA. The invasion of these macrophages results in the release of various inflammatory cytokines. Yang et al. developed (FA-AgNPs). To strengthen the colloidal stability of NPs, the AgNPs were PEGylated and modified with folic acid (FA) to achieve active targeting towards M1 macrophages. AgNPs were highly efficient in reducing inflammation by inducing

M1 macrophage phagocytosis and M2 macrophage polarization in a coordinated way. M1 macrophage reduction followed by M2 macrophage polarization is required for successful RA therapy.

As activated macrophages are pathologically characterized by high oxidative pressure, AgNPs act as ROS scavengers to down-regulate the ROS level. Because FA-AgNPs were able to rapidly release Ag+ in response to intracellular GSH, the ROS level was significantly reduced. As a result, FA-AgNPs can elicit anti-inflammatory intrusion by modulating macrophage polarization and, as a result, regulating the expression of inflammation cytokines (Yang, Y. et al., 2021).

5.7.5 POLYMER-DRUG CONJUGATE NANOCARRIERS

Dextran (Dex) belongs to the polysaccharide family. Dex, as a suitable biopolymer, is widely used for bioengineering and drug carrier administration due to its good biological features such as favorable biocompatibility, biodegradability, and polyfunctionality (Raemdonck, K. et al., 2013). Chemical coupling is among the most efficient methods for combining pharmaceuticals and nanocarriers and producing efficient prodrugs (Ding, J. et al., 2013). Dex-g-MTX/FA, a folic acid (FA) -targeted Dex-MTX nanocomposite, and Dex-g-MTX, an untargeted MTX prodrug, were produced. In vitro analysis revealed that the release rate of MTX from Dex-g-MTX/FA was slightly slower than that of Dex-g-MTX because Dex-g-MTX/FA is hydrophobic due to the additional FA. For nonactivated cells, the aforementioned two conjugates were nearly comparable, however, Dexg-MTX/FA is more highly expressed on the FR (folic acid receptor) activated macrophages more than Dexg-MTX. Dex-g-MTX/FA had a more potent anti-arthritic effect (Yang, M. et al., 2016).

5.8 STIMULI-RESPONSIVE NANOMEDICINES

Antiinflammatory or analgesic drugs (given orally, topically, or intra-articularly), surgery, and physical therapy are currently used to treat arthritis (Wenham, C. Y., & Conaghan, P. G. 2013). Moreover, the premises of these drugs and treatments have a number of drawbacks, most of which are linked to the significantly impaired biocompatibility and low efficacy of anti-arthritic agents, including poor water solubility, low cell permeability, unpalatable pharmacokinetics, random distribution in vivo, and poorly regulated drug degeneration prior to actually achieving the intended spots (Majumder, J., & Minko, T. 2021).

Stimuli-responsive NMs can improve drug specificity and bioavailability while reducing off-target side effects by taking advantage of the inflamed articular milieu. Because of their ability to target afflicted sites and respond to internal or external stimuli, stimuli-responsive NMs can provide remarkable dynamic control of both NM accumulation and medication administration at RA locations.

There are two types of stimuli-responsive nanomaterials-

- Internal stimuli-responsive nanomaterials
- External stimuli-responsive nanomaterials

5.8.1 Internal Stimuli-Responsive Nanomaterials

By utilizing the inflammatory articular microenvironment or endogenous factors such as pH, (ROS) reactive oxygen species (hypoxia, energy depletion, redox potential) and overexpression of enzymes such as matrix metalloproteinases (MMPs) (Yang, M. et al., 2017), stimuli-responsive NMs can improve drug selectivity and bioavailability while reducing adverse effects. Here we will discuss much more about the three internal stimuli responsive nanomaterials.

5.8.1.1 pH-Responsive Nanomedicine

According to the researchers, pH-responsive nanoparticles (Table 5.2) for arthritis treatment are being developed to address three sites: articular bone, synovium, and chondrocytes. PCA (protocatechuic acid) is a phytochemical derived from plants (Kakkar, S., & Bais, S. 2014) with anti-inflammatory characteristics due to its ability to drastically downregulate inflammatory factor indicators such as inducible nitric oxide synthase (iNOS), cyclooxygenase-2 (COX2) (Yoon, C. H. et al., 2013), and a Disintegrin and metalloproteinase with thrombospondin motifs (ADAMTSs).

[MOF@HA@(PCA)] is a pH-responsive metal-organic framework (MOF) augmented by hyaluronic acid (HA) and anti-inflammatory PCA. was developed by Feng et al. that greatly slowed the course of OA by inhibiting type II collagen deterioration and the formation of IL-1-stimulated proinflammatory cytokines. It is worth mentioning that their approach expedited cartilage rejuvenation and enhanced chondrocyte growth in vivo. It also demonstrated significant drug loading (owing to the dense pore structure and large pore size), strong biocompatibility, and pH responsiveness. The release of PCA was reduced at pH 7.4 but increased when the pH was reduced to 5.6. Following that, PCA linked to CD44 on chondrocytes via HA in the carrier substance (Xiong, F. et al., 2020).

The milieu of synovial fluid is acidic, with a pH as low as 6.0, due to aberrant metabolism in inflammatory joints (Liu, Let al., 2019). TNF-α-siRNA was synthesized into nanomaterials using the polymer PLGA (poly lactic-co-glycolic acid) emulsified with stearoyl-hydrazone-polyethylene glycol 2000, a particular acid-responsive surface active agent. The PLGA NPs' PEGylation shielding was cleavable following aggregation in affected regions with acidic surroundings, resulting in the effective distribution of TNF-α-siRNA to inflamed joints (Aldayel, A. M. et al., 2016) (Figure 5.2).

5.8.1.2 Enzyme-Responsive Nanocarrier

The enzyme-responsive nano-drug (in Figure 5.3) (Table 5.2) delivery system is made up of two parts: I a nanomaterial scaffold and (ii) encapsulated therapeutic drugs coupled to the carrier (Majumder, J., & Minko, T. 2021). Some enzymes are found in high concentrations in inflammatory areas. Extracellular matrix (ECM) proteins, such as metalloproteinase (MMP), are one of the inflammation-associated enzymes that are frequently released in inflamed joints (Huber, L. C. et al., 2006; Vandooren, B. et al., 2004).

Transforming growth factor β–inducible gene h3 (βIG-H3) is an ECM protein released by various cell types in synovial tissue, including synoviocytes such as

TABLE 5.2

Strategies for Internal—Responsive Nanomaterials (Jeong, M., & Park, J. H. 2020)

Strategy	Formulation	Bioactive agent	Stimuli-responsive mechanism	Animal model
1. pH-responsive nanomaterials				
Acid-cleavable linkage	HA- MTX conjugate	MTX	Ester linkage between MTX and HA is cleaved in endosomes	CIA
Sheddable PEGylated NPs	PHC-PLGA- siRNA PHC-SLN-siRNA	TNF-α-siRNA	PHC (sheddable PEG) becomes positive and increases NP retention and uptake in inflamed joints	CIA/ CAIA
PK3 polymer NP	FA-PEGlipid/ PK3/PLGA-MTX	MTX	PK3 degrades and releases MTX in endosomes	AIA
	FA-PEGPK3/ PLGA-siRNA	Mcl-1 siRNA	PK3 degrades and releases siRNA in endosomes	AIA
Calcium phosphate coating	PEG-CAP-HANPs	MTX	Calcium phosphate degrades in endosome and releases MTX	CIA
2. Enzyme-responsive nanomaterials				
MMP cleavable peptide	dhfas-1-RGD composite peptide	dhfas-1	MMP-1 cleaves a linkage between dhfas-1 and RGD and releases dhfas1	CIA
MMP-degradable TG-18	TG-18-TA hydrogel	TA	MMP-2/3/9 degrade hydrogel and release TA	K/BxN

NP, nanoparticle; DDS, drug delivery system; PK3, polyketal polymer; MMP, matrix metalloproteinase; HA, hyaluronic acid; FA, folic acid; SLN, solid lipid nanoparticle; CAP, calcium phosphate; PHC, polyethylene glycol hydrazone conjugate; TG-18, triglycerol monostearate; CIA, collagen-induced arthritis; CAIA, collagen antibody-induced arthritis; AIA, adjuvantinduced arthritis; K/BxN, K/BxN serum-transfer arthritis

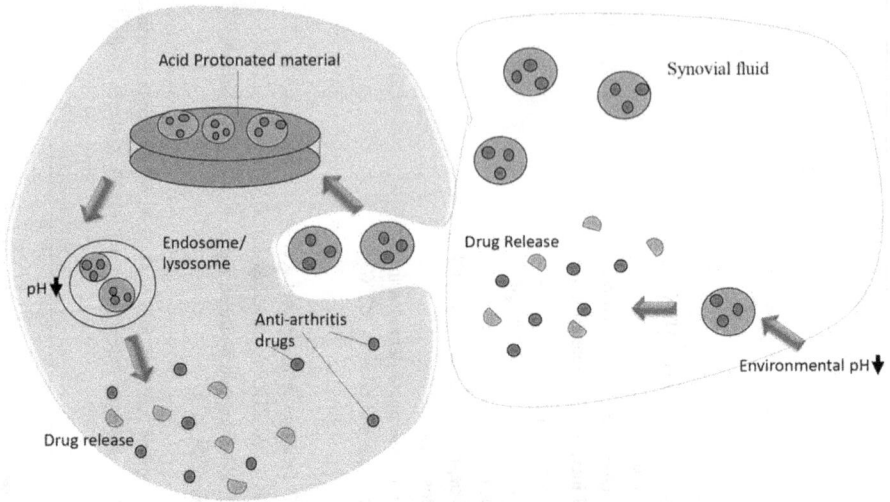

FIGURE 5.2 Extracellular drug release in acidic synovial fluid or acidic subchondral bone, microenvironment from pH-responsive materials; Intracellular drug release in endosomes and lysosomes from pH-responsive materials.

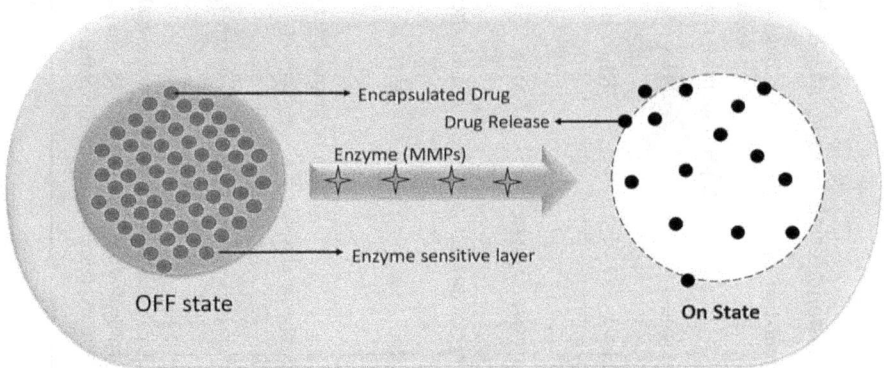

FIGURE 5.3 Enzyme-responsive drug delivery system. OFF-state: before enzyme action, and ON-state: after enzyme action.

FLS, and is significantly prevalent in rheumatoid synovium (Nam, E. J. et al., 2006). The βIG-H3 protein, which is made up of four homologous fas-1 domains and an Arg-Gly-Asp (RGD) motif at the carboxyl terminus, governs cellular adhesion, emigration, proliferation, differentiation, and viability, and hence modulates inflammatory pathways and tumor progression (Kim, H. J. et al., 2009). Each fas-1 domain has two highly conserved 10-amino acid sequences with H1 and H2 motifs at both ends and one YH18 motif with at least 18 amino acids between tyrosine and histidine (Kim, J. E. et al., 2002).

Nam et al. created the MFK-24 peptide, which is a composite peptide made up of dhfas-1 and RGD peptides joined by MMP-1 substrate. MMP-1 potentially cleaves MFK24 after it binds to integrins on the invasive front of FLS. Dhfas-1 strongly decreased synovial fibroblast adhesion, and the recombinant RGD peptide hindered cell attachment, migration, proliferation, and differentiation. Furthermore, the RGD peptide can directly induce apoptosis by activating procaspase 3 and suppressing inflammation, proliferation, and cell adhesion. As a result, the MFK-24 peptide functions as an anti-inflammatory nanocarrier (Nam, E. J. et al., 2013).

5.8.1.3 ROS-Responsive Drug Delivery

Under standard circumstances, a normal cell produces low level of reactive oxygen species (ROS), primarily through NADPH oxidase (Saita, M. et al., 2016). ROS engages in intracellular signaling mechanisms and regulates cartilage metabolism by modulating osteocyte apoptosis, gene expression, ECM formulation and malfunction, and cytokine secretion. ROS has two aspects: oxidative stress and redox signaling, both of which contribute to normal and dysfunctional cellular processes (Sies, H., 2015). Oxidative stress is defined as elevated intracellular ROS levels, whereas redox signaling is defined as reduced cytoplasmic ROS levels ("oxidative eustress") that trigger signaling pathways to initiate biological processes. Overexpression of ROS diminished antioxidative enzyme processing, and the appearance of lipid peroxide products in synovial fluid in Osteoarthritis (OA) chondrocytes indicate a role for oxidative stress in OA pathogenesis (Lepetsos, P. et al., 2019).

Many ROS-responsive materials have been investigated in drug delivery applications, including those containing thioether propylene sulfide (PPS), boronic ester, selenium/tellurium, peroxalate ester, thioketal, aminoacrylate, polysaccharide, polyproline (Liang, J., & Liu, B. 2016). The redox-responsive material (Figure 5.4) responds to stimuli while also effectively protecting cells from oxidative stress by removing the associated oxidants. The constituents of redox-responsive materials are released in two ways: phase transition and bond breaking (Zhang, M. et al., 2022). When ROS-responsive materials oxidize, the hydrophobic form transforms into the hydrophilic form (He, Q. et al., 2020).

PPS, for example, is often used to create thioether-based polymers, that are exploited as a type of drug transporter and following ROS exposure, its molecular characteristic alters. When PPS is oxidized, the hydrophobic sulfide group is structurally converted to a hydrophilic group. For example, in an H_2O_2rich environment, the sulfide group of PPS forms hydrophilic polysulfoxide, and at low levels of H_2O_2 concentration with low temperature or in response to strong oxidative acids such as organic peroxyacids, sulfone is formed. Thus releasing the analgesics. (Lee, J. B. et al., 2018).

CLT/BRNP are PEGylated nanoparticles in which bilirubin has been PEGylated and self-assembled into nanoparticles (BRNP) and celastrol has been loaded into BRNP. Hence CLT/BRNP has been formed. After being efficiently internalized by activated macrophages, CLT/BRNP demonstrated the ability to scavenge intracellular ROS and lower the level of nitric oxide. BRNP is primarily deposited in inflamed joints, relieving joint swelling and bone degeneration and drastically

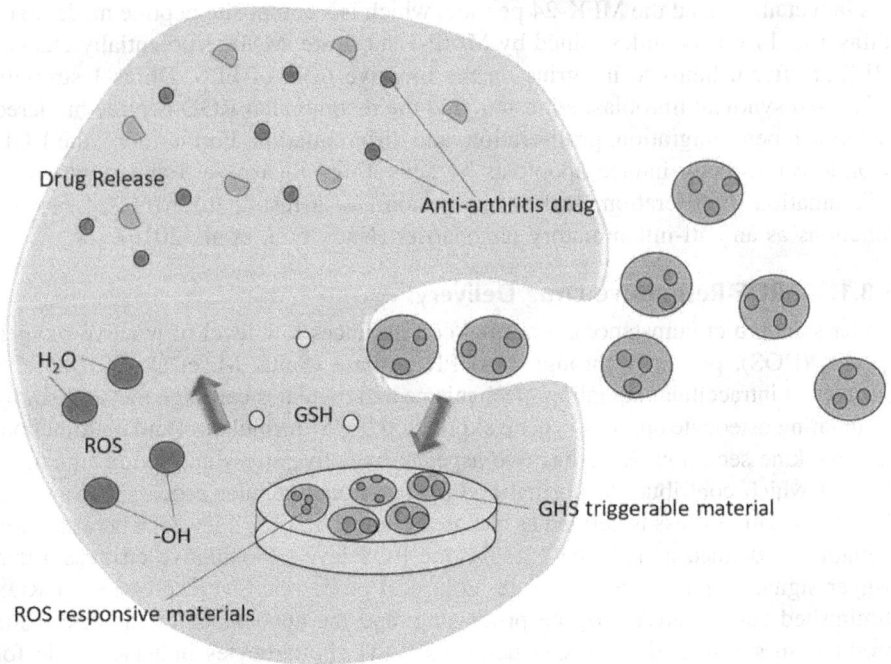

FIGURE 5.4 Redox-responsive material drug release, caused by abnormal signals resulting from an imbalance in the intracellular redox system.

reducing pro-inflammatory cytokine release to limit RA development. When compared to free celastrol, CLT/BRNP significantly increased its anti-arthritic impact and decreased its toxic effect (Zhao, X. et al., 2022).

5.8.2 EXTERNAL STIMULI RESPONSIVE NANOMATERIALS

Nanomaterials that are responsive to exogenous stimuli (such as temperature, light (in Table 5.3), ultrasound, and magnet) have just been developed to accomplish more precise and on-demand medication delivery adjustment (Liu, D. et al., 2016), as well as to enhance the efficiency of drug carrier platform because Endogenous stimuli research is challenging, and internal stimuli are fairly complex and unpredictable (Raza, A. et al., 2019). These external stimuli-responsive nanomaterials will be thoroughly discussed.

5.8.2.1 Temperature-Responsive Nanocarriers

When compared to other stimuli, temperature is one of the most favorable and efficient elements for controlling medication administration. Generally, temperature in pathological situations such as inflammation and malignancies is greater than those in healthy cells (Shi, Y. et al., 2015). When the loaded pharmaceuticals are released, the chemical and physical characteristics of thermo-responsive nano-carriers at the specific site change substantially (in Figure 5.5). At 37 degrees

TABLE 5.3
External Stimuli-Responsive Nano-Drug Delivery Systems (Zhang, M. et al., 2022)

External stimuli	Formulation	Bioactive Agent	Target cell	Effects	Animal model
Temperature	F127/COS/ KGNDCF nanospheres	KGN, DCF	Macrophagechondrocyte, MSC	Promote chondrogenic differentiation of MSCs, induce cartilage regeneration, and reduce inflammation	U937 macrophage-like cells, primary human chondrocytes, hBMSC, rat models of ACLT and DMM
	ELP-based fusion proteins	IL-1Ra	Chondrocyte, fibroblast	Inhibit the progression of OA and relieve the pain and swelling of joint	Canine models of ACLTinduced OA
Light	MTX PEGPLGA-Au	MTX	Macrophage	Significantly reduce inflammatory cytokines IL1β, IL-6 and TNF-α	THP1 differentiated macrophages
	MNPs	MTX	Macrophage	Suppress serum levels of pro-inflammatory cytokines and anti-CII IgG, reduce inflammation and prevent bone erosion in the joints	FLS, rat model of CIA

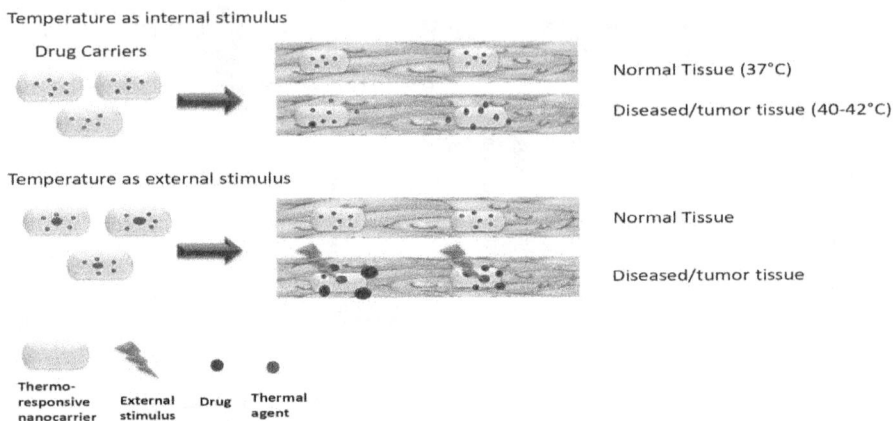

Temperature as internal stimulus

Drug Carriers

Normal Tissue (37°C)

Diseased/tumor tissue (40-42°C)

Temperature as external stimulus

Normal Tissue

Diseased/tumor tissue

Thermo-
responsive   External   Drug   Thermal
nanocarrier   stimulus   agent

FIGURE 5.5 Schematic presentation of drug release activated by temperature-responsive nanocarriers through temperature as an internal and external stimulus.

Celsius, the load of these substances ought to be stable, but reactive to and susceptible to small temperature variations (such as changing from hydrophilic to hydrophobic) (Zhou, M. et al., 2017).

poly N-isopropyl acrylamide (PNIPAM) (Mi, P. et al., 2010), poly amidoamine (PAMAM) (Kono, K. et al., 2011), poly 2-oxazoline (POxs) (Osawa, S. et al., 2017), and poly[2-(2-methoxyethoxy) ethyl methacrylate]-b-poly(2-hydroxyethyl methacrylate) (PMEO$_2$MA-b-PHEMA) (Yang, J. et al., 2010) are some of the thermo-responsive nanocarriers (Zhang, M. et al., 2022). The most prominent polymer is poly (N-isopropyl acrylamide) (PNIPAM), which transforms from arbitrary coils to globules at 33°C, i.e. the lowest critical solution temperature (LCST). The LCST can be tweaked by adding the hydrophilic moiety to increase it and the hydrophobic moiety to lower it (Dimitrov, I. et al., 2007).

Kang et al., particularly, created a class of thermoresponsive nanospheres (F127/ COS/KGNDCF) from poly (ethyleneoxide)-block-poly (oxypropylene)-block-poly (ethylene oxide) (PEOxPPOy-PEOz) loaded with diclofenac (DCF) and kartogenin to stimulate articular rejuvenation in OA (KGN). The size of the nanospheres ranged from 305 nm at 37°C to 650 nm at 4°C, indicating that the framework of the nanospheres was open and the medication was released more quickly at 4°C. This suggested that local freezing therapy could increase drug delivery from nanospheres, improving the therapeutic impact (Kang, M. L. et al., 2016).

5.8.2.2   Photo/Light-Responsive Nanomedicines

External light illumination has the potential to stimulate drug release at the appropriate location using light-responsive devices. Photon piercing characteristic is a feasible form of energy in constructing stimuli-responsive biomaterials that may be regulated with great temporal and spatial accuracy by modulating the intensity, frequency, polarization, and photo-direction (Lee, H. P., & Gaharwar, A. K. 2020). Different wavelength ranges of light [ultraviolet, visible, and near-infrared (NIR)] have been proposed to be employed for medication distribution regulation.

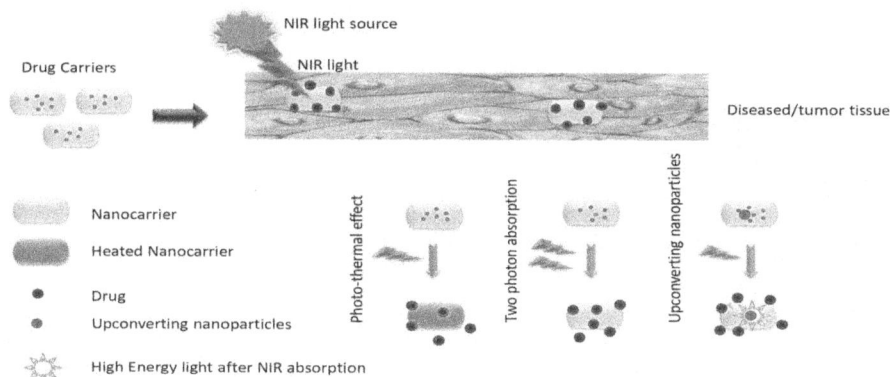

FIGURE 5.6 Mechanisms of drug release through NIR responsive DDSs.

Nevertheless, UV and visible light are not generally reliable for in vivo therapeutic uses because of poor dermal absorption, whereas the NIR range is a possible illumination source for modulating therapeutic effects due to safety and greater tissue penetration (Xiang, J. et al., 2018).

Photoisomerization, photolysis, photo-crosslinking, photo-redox [which can be used in photodynamic therapy (PDT)] (Karimi, M. et al., 2017), and photothermal trigger [which is associated with photothermal therapy (PTT)] all can plausibly stimulate photo-sensitive groups of photo-responsive nanomaterials to trigger drug delivery (Zhang, M. et al., 2022). Yin, X. et al. generated pDA/MTX@ZIF-8 NPs that demonstrated good photothermal effects under NIR irradiation (Yin, X. et al., 2022).

Methotrexate (MTX)-loaded poly(ethylene glycol)-poly(lactic-co-glycolic acid) (PLGA) nanoparticles were created by Ha, Y. J et al, resulting in MTX-loaded MNPs (Multifunctional naoparticles) (Kim, H. J. et al., 2015). MTX is liberated from PLGA nanoparticles when exposed to NIR light (Figure 5.6). In vitro studies revealed that MTX-loaded MNPs with NIR irradiation had better clinical efficiency than chemotherapy alone. In vivo NIR illustrations of MTX-loaded MNPs revealed that the MNPs were delivered effectively to the inflamed joints. Furthermore, in collagen-induced arthritic (CIA) mice, MTX-loaded MNPs carrying MTX solution (repeated-dose injection) demonstrated therapeutic benefits comparable to standard MTX solution treatment (Ha, Y. J. et al., 2020).

5.8.2.3 Magnetic-Responsive Nanomaterials

Magnetic flux may permeate body cells and is extensively used in MRI for body scanning. Besides scanning, applied magnetic field stimulation has been used to regulate drug delivery from magnetic field-sensitive transporters (Thirunavukkarasu, G. K. et al., 2018). Freeman et al. first proposed the utilizing of magnetic fields as an external trigger to release medications in 1960 (Karimi, M. et al., 2016). Controlling drug delivery in the blood circulation and nanoparticle diffusion are critical challenges for the nano platform employed in. intravenous infusion. Magnetic flux offers enormous potential for controlling medication delivery in the bloodstream (Lee, J. H. et al., 2007). Following intravenous administration, a specific magnetic

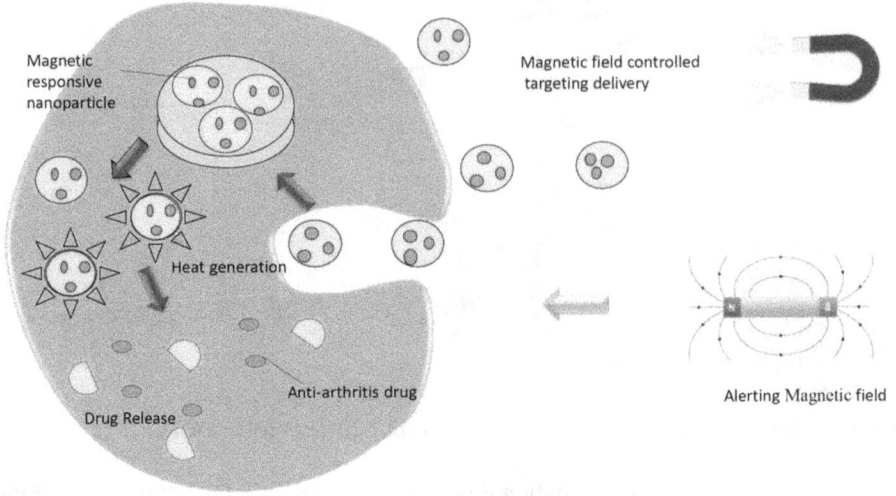

FIGURE 5.7 Drug release from magnetic-responsive materials induced by magnetic guidance or magnetocaloric effect.

field is applied at a particular target to increase the deposition of NPs (Figure 5.7) at the intended site via magnetic guiding, hence increasing the drug's therapeutic effectiveness to a certain level (Hu, X. et al., 2018). As of now, magnetic nanocomposites have included cobalt oxide, iron oxide (Fe3O4, Fe2O3), nickel oxide NPs, and others, with superparamagnetic iron oxide nanoparticles (SPION) being widely used in biological applications (Lee, J. H. et al., 2013).

The external magnetic field is classified into two types: continuous magnetic field and alternating magnetic fields (AMF) (Mura, S. et al., 2013). For example, when the iron gel constituted of superparamagnetic iron oxide NPs and Pluronic-F127 micelles is exposed to a permanent magnetic field, the micelles get squeezed and Pluronic-F127 releases along with the iron oxide NPs (Mdlovu, N. V. et al., 2019). Because of its heating properties, AMF is tightly linked to magnetic hyperthermia therapy. Applying an alternating magnetic field (AMF) at 4.4 kW was found to raise the temperature of a medium containing nanoparticles by 5.2 degrees Celsius (from 37°C to 42.2°C) (Wang, Y. et al., 2018). Energy emitted by AMF induces an alteration in the structure of the nanoparticles, such as an increase in shell or double-layer pores, dissolution of the Fe3O4 core, or distortion of the single crystal nanoshell lattice, and thus releases the drug (Hu, S. H. et al., 2008).

However, no magnetic responsive nanocarriers for the treatment of rheumatoid arthritis are now available; those that have been designed are for tumor treatment. Its application in the treatment of arthritis is fairly limited.

5.9 ANTIGEN-SPECIFIC IMMUNOTHERAPEUTIC NANOMEDICINES

In the pathophysiology of RA, autoantigen-specific immunity is already established systemically before it localizes in a particular area. The presence of a regulatory immune system directed against autoantigens is not sufficient to control the generation of autoantibodies during the autoantigen-specific immune response. The regulatory immune system has been the subject of numerous studies aiming at boosting it against autoantigens, but most of them have been limited by the antigen non-specificity of the immune system. By modifying the autoantigen-specific regulatory immune system, Clemente-Casares et al. developed iron oxide nanoparticles attached with MHC II tetramers containing autoantigen peptides (pMHCII) to cure autoimmune disorders, including RA. Due to their small size—less than 50 nm—systemically given nanoparticles were successfully located in the peripheral lymph nodes. In the lymph nodes, pMHCII-nanoparticles directly bind to the TCR of T-cells and increase regulatory TR1-like CD4+ T-cells, suppressing dendritic cells laden with autoantigens and differentiating cognate B-cells into regulatory B-cells that are specific to autoantigens. Thus, the autoantigen-specific decrease of RA autoimmune symptoms was achieved by the pMHCII-nanoparticles. According to this study, secondary lymphoid organs including the spleen and lymph nodes can be targeted by nanomedicine to modify the regulatory immune system particular to RA.

5.10 DISCUSSION

RA is a complex autoimmune disease in which many immune cells, synovial cells, and intracellular signaling pathways are activated. The NF-KB signaling pathway is considered to be the most significant in the inflammatory process because it governs the initiation of numerous other inflammatory signaling pathways and factors, including the JAK-STAT pathway, the MAPKs pathway, the c-JUN N-terminal kinase (JNK), the p38 and AP1 transcription factors, and others (Yang et al., 2018). RA symptoms worsen by Proinflammatory proteins that are stimulated by the NF-KB signaling pathway. TNF-α, for instance, has been shown to elicit autophagy in several RA-related cells that result in synovial cell apoptosis and synovium hyperplasia (Vomero et al., 2018).

MTX is considered one of the most efficient medications for the treatment of RA but it has certain drawbacks. Even in patients with normal renal and hepatic functionality, the pharmacokinetics of oral low-dose MTX seem to be varied and generally unexpected. MTX also causes gastrointestinal toxicities (stomatitis, nausea, and abdominal pain), baldness, bone marrow suppression, and hepatotoxicity (Ha, Y. J. et al., 2020).

To enhance the pharmacological score of MTX, so many drug carrier framework have been developed. Liposomes, dendrimers, human serum albumin, solid lipid nanoparticles, polymeric nanoparticles and micelles, carbon nanotubes, and magnetic and gold nanoparticles are among these systems. Since most research findings were pre-clinical screening studies, assessing the benefits of one framework over others is difficult at this stage (Abolmaali, S. S. et al., 2013). When MTX-loaded MNPs were illuminated with NIR, they increased delivery to inflamed joints and promoted sustained release(Ha, Y. J. et al., 2020). The potential advantages of LDE-MTX are its lack of immunogenicity and toxicity related to nanotechnological products (Mello, S. B. et al., 2016).

Free GCs, specifically DxM-P, have been shown to reduce the number of circulating lymphocytes through two mechanisms; 1) redistribution to the spleen, lymph nodes (LN,) bone marrow, and perivascular compartments; and 2) induction of cell apoptosis. However, after treatment with liposomal DxM-P, there were substantially fewer lymphocytes in lymphoid organs, implying that redistribution to spleen and LN either didn't happen or was stable by enhanced local lymphocyte apoptosis (Anderson, R. et al., 2010).

Monotherapies have been shown in clinical practise to be ineffective for many patients. Combined therapies can act through multiple mechanisms and have shown benefits in the treatment of failed monotherapy cases (Sarzi-Puttini, P. et al., 2019). Even so, various clinical agents typically have different physicochemical properties and pharmacokinetics in vivo, making synchronous influx and intervention of consolidated chemotherapeutics to the targeted tissues impossible. Due to the hydrophobic and hydrophilic regions and ease of functionalization, liposomes are ideal carriers for multiple therapeutic agents to improve the efficacy of combined therapy for RA (Du, B. et al., 2015).

DEX is a hydrophobic drug that can be encapsulated in the liposomal lipid. GNRs/ODNs are well suspended in solution and encapsulated in the liposomes' hydrophilic core. ODNs are double-stranded oligodeoxynucleotides that are readily deteriorated by DNase in in vitro and in vivo. GNRs absorb ODN, protect it and increase its encapsulation efficacy to liposomes. As a result of combining DEX, ODNs, and GNRs via liposomes, simultaneous delivery and action can be achieved, resulting in significantly enhanced anti-inflammatory efficacy in vitro and in vivo. (Xue, L. et al., 2020).

5.11 CONCLUSION

The application of nanotechnology empowers significantly improved delivery of MTX, GCs, and nucleic acids. Endeavors to articulate these drugs in the same carrier are alluring, but more research is needed. siRNA delivery was primarily investigated in mouse models with the goal of lowering TNF-α levels, which play a significant role in RA. Only a few studies have looked into the possibilities of using miRNA or anti-miRNA (Yu, Z. et al., 2020).

A co-administration of MTX-loaded MNPs and NIR irradiation demonstrated long-term and significant therapeutic effectiveness for rheumatoid remission in a finite amount of MTX (Ha, Y. J. et al., 2020).

This literature also discusses targeted therapies for nano-based co-delivery systems in combination with photothermal agents, or phototherapeutic agents, that provide standard co-delivery with light-responsive drug release and have promising applications. The co-delivery system can be useful for more than inflammation treatment like in the treatment of neurodegenerative diseases, tumor, and cancer (Yu, Z. et al., 2020).

NMs-based RA therapy approaches are new but promising, and they may make a substantial contribution to the market for articular diseases. Until there is clinical application, the novel NMs will remain theoretical. Nonetheless, we have evidence to believe that synthetic NMs will have a significant impact on RA treatment(Liu, L. et al., 2019).

REFERENCES

Abbasi, M., Mousavi, M. J., Jamalzehi, S., Alimohammadi, R., Bezvan, M. H., Mohammadi, H., & Aslani, S. (2019). Strategies toward rheumatoid arthritis therapy: the old and the new. *Journal of cellular physiology*, *234*(7), 10018–10031.

Abolmaali, S. S., Tamaddon, A. M., & Dinarvand, R. (2013). A review of therapeutic challenges and achievements of methotrexate delivery systems for treatment of cancer and rheumatoid arthritis. *Cancer chemotherapy and pharmacology*, *71*(5), 1115–1130.

Agarwal, H., Nakara, A., & Shanmugam, V. K. (2019). Anti-inflammatory mechanism of various metal and metal oxide nanoparticles synthesized using plant extracts: a review. *Biomedicine & pharmacotherapy*, *109*, 2561–2572.

Aldayel, A. M., Naguib, Y. W., O'mary, H. L., Li, X., Niu, M., Ruwona, T. B., & Cui, Z. (2016). Acid-sensitive sheddable PEGylated PLGA nanoparticles increase the delivery of TNF-α siRNA in chronic inflammation sites. *Molecular therapy-nucleic acids*, *5*, e340.

Alivernini, S., Gremese, E., McSharry, C., Tolusso, B., Ferraccioli, G., McInnes, I. B., & Kurowska-Stolarska, M. (2018). MicroRNA-155—at the critical interface of innate and adaptive immunity in arthritis. *Frontiers in immunology*, *8*, 1932.

Amjad, M. W., Kesharwani, P., Amin, M. C. I. M., & Iyer, A. K. (2017). Recent advances in the design, development, and targeting mechanisms of polymeric micelles for delivery of siRNA in cancer therapy. *Progress in polymer science*, *64*, 154–181.

An, H., Song, Z., Li, P., Wang, G., Ma, B., & Wang, X. (2020). Development of biofabricated gold nanoparticles for the treatment of alleviated arthritis pain. *Applied nanoscience*, *10*(2), 617–622.

Anderson, R., Franch, A., Castell, M., Perez-Cano, F. J., Bräuer, R., Pohlers, D., & Kinne, R. W. (2010). Liposomal encapsulation enhances and prolongs the anti-inflammatory effects of water-soluble dexamethasone phosphate in experimental adjuvant arthritis. *Arthritis research & therapy*, *12*(4), 1–15.

Arima, H., Koirala, S., Nema, K., Nakano, M., Ito, H., Poudel, K. M., Pandey, K., Pandey, B. D., & Yamamoto, T. (2022). High prevalence of rheumatoid arthritis and its risk factors among Tibetan highlanders living in Tsarang. Mustang district of Nepal. *Journal of physiological anthropology*, *41*(1), 12.

Arlt, C. R., Brekel, D., Neumann, S., Rafaja, D., & Franzreb, M. (2021). Continuous size fractionation of magnetic nanoparticles by using simulated moving bed chromatography. *Frontiers of chemical science and engineering*, *15*(5), 1346–1355.

Bartok, B., & Firestein, G. S. (2010). Fibroblast-like synoviocytes: key effector cells in rheumatoid arthritis. *Immunological reviews*, *233*(1), 233–255.

Blüml, S., Bonelli, M., Niederreiter, B., Puchner, A., Mayr, G., Hayer, S., ... & Redlich, K. (2011). Essential role of microRNA-155 in the pathogenesis of autoimmune arthritis in mice. *Arthritis & rheumatism*, *63*(5), 1281–1288.

Brennan, F. M., & McInnes, I. B. (2008). Evidence that cytokines play a role in rheumatoid arthritis. *The journal of clinical investigation*, *118*(11), 3537–3545.

Chang, M., Rowland, C. M., Garcia, V. E., Schrodi, S. J., Catanese, J. J., Van Der Helm-van Mil, A. H. M., Ardlie, K. G., Amos, C. I., Criswell, L. A., Kastner, D. L., Gregersen, P. K., Kurreeman, F. A. S., Toes, R. E. M., Huizinga, T. W. J., Seldin, M. F., & Begovich, A. B. (2008). A large-scale rheumatoid arthritis genetic study identifies association at chromosome 9q33.2. *PLoS genetics*, *4*(6), e1000107.

Chatham, W. W. (2005). Traditional disease modifying antirheumatic drugs. *Koopman WJ, Moreland LW. Arthritis and allied conditions*. 15th ed. Philadelphia: Lippincott, Williams and Wilkins, 915–944.

Chen, J. Q., Papp, G., Szodoray, P., & Zeher, M. (2016). The role of microRNAs in the pathogenesis of autoimmune diseases. *Autoimmunity reviews*, *15*(12), 1171–1180.

Courties, G., Presumey, J., Duroux-Richard, I., Jorgensen, C., & Apparailly, F. (2009). RNA interference-based gene therapy for successful treatment of rheumatoid arthritis. *Expert opinion on biological therapy*, *9*(5), 535–538.

Dang, Q., Yang, F., Lei, H., Liu, X., Yan, M., Huang, H., & Li, Y. (2017). Inhibition of microRNA-34a ameliorates murine collagen-induced arthritis. *Experimental and therapeutic medicine*, *14*(2), 1633–1639.

Deighton, C. M., Cavanagh, G., Rigby, A. S., et al. (1993). Both inherited HLA-haplotypes are important in the predisposition to rheumatoid arthritis. *British journal of rheumatology*, *32*, 893–898.

Dervieux, T., Orentas Lein, D., Marcelletti, J., Pischel, K., Smith, K., Walsh, M., & Richerson, R. (2003). HPLC determination of erythrocyte methotrexate polyglutamates after low-dose methotrexate therapy in patients with rheumatoid arthritis. *Clinical chemistry*, *49*(10), 1632–1641.

Dimitrov, I., Trzebicka, B., Müller, A. H., Dworak, A., & Tsvetanov, C. B. (2007). Thermosensitive water-soluble copolymers with doubly responsive reversibly interacting entities. *Progress in polymer science*, *32*(11), 1275–1343.

Ding, J., Li, D., Zhuang, X., & Chen, X. (2013). Self-assemblies of pH-activatable PEGylated multiarm poly(lactic acid-co-glycolic acid)-doxorubicin prodrugs with improved long-term antitumor efficacies. *Macromolecular bioscience*, *13*(10), 1300–1307.

Du, B., Han, S., Li, H., Zhao, F., Su, X., Cao, X., & Zhang, Z. (2015). Multi-functional liposomes showing radiofrequency-triggered release and magnetic resonance imaging for tumor multi-mechanism therapy. *Nanoscale*, *7*(12), 5411–5426.

Feng, N., & Guo, F. (2020). Nanoparticle-siRNA: a potential strategy for rheumatoid arthritis therapy? *Journal of controlled release*, *325*, 380–393.

Fraenkel, L., Bathon, J. M., England, B. R., et al. (2021). American college of rheumatology guideline for the treatment of rheumatoid arthritis. *Arthritis care research*, *73*, 924–939.

Gabriel, S. E. (2001). The epidemiology of rheumatoid arthritis. *Rheumatic disease clinics of North America*, *27*(2), 269–281.

Gaffo, A., Saag, K. G., & Curtis, J. R. (2006). Treatment of rheumatoid arthritis. *American journal of health-system pharmacy*, *63*(24), 2451–2465.

Garner, R., Ding, T., & Deighton, C. (2014). Management of rheumatoid arthritis. *Medicine (United Kingdom)*, *42*(5), 237–242.

Gönen, E., & Bal, A. (2015). Rheumatoid arthritis. *Musculoskeletal research and basic science*, *2016*, 517–544.

Grossen, P., Witzigmann, D., Sieber, S., & Huwyler, J. (2017). PEG-PCL-based nanomedicines: a biodegradable drug delivery system and its application. *Journal of controlled release*, *260*, 46–60.

Hazlewood, G. S., Barnabe, C., Tomlinson, G., Marshall, D., Devoe, D. J., & Bombardier, C. (2016). Methotrexate monotherapy and methotrexate combination therapy with traditional and biologic disease modifying anti-rheumatic drugs for rheumatoid arthritis: a network meta-analysis. *Cochrane database of systematic reviews*, *2016*(8), CD010227.

Ha, Y. J., Lee, S. M., Mun, C. H., Kim, H. J., Bae, Y., Lim, J. H., & Park, Y. B. (2020). Methotrexate-loaded multifunctional nanoparticles with near-infrared irradiation for the treatment of rheumatoid arthritis. *Arthritis research & therapy*, *22*(1), 1–13.

He, Q., Chen, J., Yan, J., Cai, S., Xiong, H., Liu, Y., & Liu, Z. (2020). Tumor microenvironment responsive drug delivery systems. *Asian journal of pharmaceutical sciences*, *15*(4), 416–448.

Heliovaara, M., Aho, K., Aromaa, A., et al. (1993). Smoking and risk of rheumatoid arthritis. *Journal of rheumatol*, *20*, 1830–1835.

Hoscheid, J., Outuki, P. M., Kleinubing, S. A., Silva, M. F., Bruschi, M. L., & Cardoso, M. L. C. (2015). Development and characterization of Pterodon pubescens oil nanoemulsions as a possible delivery system for the treatment of rheumatoid arthritis. *Colloids and surfaces A: Physicochemical and engineering aspects, 484,* 19–27.

Huber, L. C., Distler, O., Tarner, I., Gay, R. E., Gay, S., & Pap, T. (2006). Synovial fibroblasts: key players in rheumatoid arthritis. *Rheumatology, 45*(6), 669–675.

Hu, S. H., Chen, S. Y., Liu, D. M., & Hsiao, C. S. (2008). Core/single-crystal-shell nanospheres for controlled drug release via a magnetically triggered rupturing mechanism. *Advanced materials, 20*(14), 2690–2695.

Hu, X., Li, F., Wang, S., Xia, F., & Ling, D. (2018). Biological stimulus-driven assembly/disassembly of functional nanoparticles for targeted delivery, controlled activation, and bioelimination. *Advanced healthcare materials, 7*(20), 1800359.

Jeong, M., & Park, J. H. (2020). Nanomedicine for the treatment of rheumatoid arthritis. *Molecular pharmaceutics, 18*(2), 539–549.

Kakkar, S., & Bais, S. (2014). A review on protocatechuic acid and its pharmacological potential. *International scholarly research notices, 2014,* 952943.

Kang, M. L., Kim, J. E., & Im, G.I. (2016). Thermoresponsive nanospheres with independent dual drug release profiles for the treatment of osteoarthritis. *Acta biomaterialia, 39,* 65–78.

Karimi, M., Ghasemi, A., Zangabad, P. S., Rahighi, R., Basri, S. M. M., Mirshekari, H., & Hamblin, M. R. (2016). Smart micro/nanoparticles in stimulus-responsive drug/gene delivery systems. *Chemical society reviews, 45*(5), 1457–1501.

Karimi, M., Sahandi Zangabad, P., Baghaee-Ravari, S., Ghazadeh, M., Mirshekari, H., & Hamblin, M. R. (2017). Smart nanostructures for cargo delivery: uncaging and activating by light. *Journal of the American chemical society, 139*(13), 4584–4610.

Kaur, M. (2020). Impact of response surface methodology–optimized synthesis parameters on in vitro anti-inflammatory activity of iron nanoparticles synthesized using Ocimum tenuiflorum Linn. *BioNanoScience, 10*(1), 1–10.

Khodaverdi, E., Tayarani-Najaran, Z., Minbashi, E., Alibolandi, M., Hosseini, J., Sepahi, S., … & Hadizadeh, F. (2019). Docetaxel-loaded mixed micelles and polymersomes composed of poly (caprolactone)-poly (ethylene glycol)(PEG-PCL) and poly (lactic acid)-poly (ethylene glycol)(PEG-PLA): preparation and in-vitro characterization. *Iranian Journal of pharmaceutical research: IJPR, 18*(1), 142.

Kim, H. C., Kim, E., Ha, T. L., Lee, S. G., Lee, S. J., & Jeong, S. W. (2017). Highly stable and reduction responsive micelles from a novel polymeric surfactant with a repeating disulfide-based gemini structure for efficient drug delivery. *Polymer, 133,* 102–109.

Kim, H. J., Kim, P. K., Bae, S. M., Son, H. N., Thoudam, D. S., Kim, J. E., … & Kim, I. S. (2009). Transforming growth factor-β–induced protein (TGFBIp/β ig-h3) activates platelets and promotes thrombogenesis. *Blood, The journal of the American society of hematology, 114*(25), 5206–5215.

Kim, H. J., Lee, S. M., Park, K. H., Mun, C. H., Park, Y. B., & Yoo, K. H. (2015). Drug-loaded gold/iron/gold plasmonic nanoparticles for magnetic targeted chemo-photothermal treatment of rheumatoid arthritis. *Biomaterials, 61,* 95–102.

Kim, J. E., Jeong, H. W., Nam, J. O., Lee, B. H., Choi, J. Y., Park, R. W., & Kim, I. S. (2002). Identification of motifs in the fasciclin domains of the transforming growth factor-β–induced matrix protein βig-h3 that interact with the αvβ5 integrin. *Journal of biological chemistry, 277*(48), 46159–46165.

Kono, K., Murakami, E., Hiranaka, Y., Yuba, E., Kojima, C., Harada, A., & Sakurai, K. (2011). Thermosensitive molecular assemblies from poly (amidoamine) dendron-based lipids. *Angewandte Chemie, 123*(28), 6456–6460.

Lee, H. P., & Gaharwar, A. K. (2020). Light-responsive inorganic biomaterials for biomedical applications. *Advanced science, 7*(17), 2000863.

Lee, J. B., Shin, Y. M., Kim, W. S., Kim, S. Y., & Sung, H. J. (2018). ROS-responsive biomaterial design for medical applications. *Biomimetic medical materials*, *1064*, 237–251.

Lee, J. H., Huh, Y. M., Jun, Y. W., Seo, J. W., Jang, J. T., Song, H. T., & Cheon, J. (2007). Artificially engineered magnetic nanoparticles for ultra-sensitive molecular imaging. *Nature medicine*, *13*(1), 95–99.

Lee, J. H., Kim, J. W., & Cheon, J. (2013). Magnetic nanoparticles for multi-imaging and drug delivery. *Molecules and cells*, *35*(4), 274–284.

Lepetsos, P., Papavassiliou, K. A., & Papavassiliou, A. G. (2019). Redox and NF-κB signaling in osteoarthritis. *Free radical biology and medicine*, *132*, 90–100.

Li, D., Yang, Z., Kang, P., & Xie, X. (2016, June). Subcutaneous administration of methotrexate at high doses makes a better performance in the treatment of rheumatoid arthritis compared with oral administration of methotrexate: A systematic review and meta-analysis. In Hochberg MC (ed.), *Seminars in arthritis and rheumatism* (Vol. 45, No. 6, pp. 656–662). WB Saunders.

Li, M., Luo, X., Long, X., Jiang, P., Jiang, Q., Guo, H., & Chen, Z. (2021). Potential role of mitochondria in synoviocytes. *Clinical rheumatology*, *40*(2), 447–457.

Li, S., Su, J., Cai, W., & Liu, J. X. (2021). Nanomaterials manipulate macrophages for rheumatoid arthritis treatment. *Frontiers in pharmacology*, *12*, 699245.

Liang, J., & Liu, B. (2016). ROS-responsive drug delivery systems. *Bioengineering & translational medicine*, *1*(3), 239–251.

Liu, D., Yang, F., Xiong, F., & Gu, N. (2016). The smart drug delivery system and its clinical potential. *Theranostics*, *6*(9), 1306.

Liu, L., Guo, W., & Liang, X. J. (2019). Move to nano-arthrology: targeted stimuli-responsive nanomedicines combat adaptive treatment tolerance (ATT) of rheumatoid arthritis. *Biotechnology journal*, *14*(1), 1800024.

Liu, X. M., Quan, L. D., Tian, J., Alnouti, Y., Fu, K., Thiele, G. M., & Wang, D. (2008). Synthesis and evaluation of a well-defined HPMA copolymer-dexamethasone conjugate for effective treatment of rheumatoid arthritis. *Pharmaceutical research*, *25*(12), 2910–2919.

Lu, T. X., & Rothenberg, M. E. (2018). MicroRNA. *Journal of allergy and clinical immunology*, *141*(4), 1202–1207.

Lu, Y., Zhang, E., Yang, J., & Cao, Z. (2018). Strategies to improve micelle stability for drug delivery. *Nano research*, *11*(10), 4985–4998.

Luís, M., Boers, M., Saag, K., Buttgereit, F., & da Silva, J. A. (2022). The safety of glucocorticoids in the treatment of inflammatory rheumatic disease: new evidence. *Current opinion in rheumatology*, *34*(3), 179–186.

Malmström, V., Catrina, A. I., & Klareskog, L. (2017). The immunopathogenesis of seropositive rheumatoid arthritis: from triggering to targeting. *Nature reviews immunology*, *17*(1), 60–75.

Mathiessen, A., & Conaghan, P. G. (2017). Synovitis in osteoarthritis: current understanding with therapeutic implications. *Arthritis research & therapy*, *19*(1), 1–9.

Majumder, J., & Minko, T. (2021). Multifunctional and stimuli-responsive nanocarriers for targeted therapeutic delivery. *Expert opinion on drug delivery*, *18*(2), 205–227.

Mdlovu, N. V., Mavuso, F. A., Lin, K. S., Chang, T. W., Chen, Y., Wang, S. S. S., ... & Lin, Y. S. (2019). Iron oxide-pluronic F127 polymer nanocomposites as carriers for a doxorubicin drug delivery system. *Colloids and surfaces A: Physicochemical and engineering aspects*, *562*, 361–369.

Meka, R. R., Venkatesha, S. H., Acharya, B., & Moudgil, K. D. (2019). Peptide-targeted liposomal delivery of dexamethasone for arthritis therapy. *Nanomedicine*, *14*(11), 1455–1469.

Mello, S. B., Tavares, E. R., Guido, M. C., Bonfá, E., & Maranhão, R. C. (2016). Anti-inflammatory effects of intravenous methotrexate associated with lipid nanoemulsions on antigen-induced arthritis. *Clinics*, *71*, 54–58.

Mi, P., Ju, X. J., Xie, R., Wu, H. G., Ma, J., & Chu, L. Y. (2010). A novel stimuli-responsive hydrogel for K+-induced controlled-release. *Polymer*, *51*(7), 1648–1653.

Mittal, A. K., Chisti, Y., & Banerjee, U. C. (2013). Synthesis of metallic nanoparticles using plant extracts. *Biotechnology advances*, *31*(2), 346–356.

Müller-Ladner, U., Ospelt, C., Gay, S., Distler, O., & Pap, T. (2007). Cells of the synovium in rheumatoid arthritis. Synovial fibroblasts. *Arthritis research & therapy*, *9*(6), 1–10.

Mura, S., Nicolas, J., & Couvreur, P. (2013). Stimuli-responsive nanocarriers for drug delivery. *Nature materials*, *12*(11), 991–1003.

Murata, K., Yoshitomi, H., Tanida, S., Ishikawa, M., Nishitani, K., Ito, H., & Nakamura, T. (2010). Plasma and synovial fluid microRNAs as potential biomarkers of rheumatoid arthritis and osteoarthritis. *Arthritis research & therapy*, *12*(3), 1–14.

Nam, E. J., Sa, K. H., You, D. W., Cho, J. H., Seo, J. S., Han, S. W., ... & Kang, Y. M. (2006). Up-regulated transforming growth factor β–inducible gene h3 in rheumatoid arthritis mediates adhesion and migration of synoviocytes through αvβ3 integrin: regulation by cytokines. *Arthritis & rheumatism*, *54*(9), 2734–2744.

Nam, E. J., Kang, J. H., Sung, S., Sa, K. H., Kim, K. H., Seo, J. S., ... & Kang, Y. M. (2013). A matrix metalloproteinase 1–cleavable composite peptide derived from transforming growth factor β–inducible gene h3 potently inhibits collagen-induced arthritis. *Arthritis & rheumatism*, *65*(7), 1753–1763.

Nayak, R. R., Alexander, M., Deshpande, I., Stapleton-Gray, K., Rimal, B., Patterson, A. D., ... & Turnbaugh, P. J. (2021). Methotrexate impacts conserved pathways in diverse human gut bacteria leading to decreased host immune activation. *Cell host & microbe*, *29*(3), 362–377.

O'Connell, R. M., Rao, D. S., & Baltimore, D. (2012). microRNA regulation of inflammatory responses. *Annual review of immunology*, *30*, 295–312.

Ogando, J., Tardáguila, M., Díaz-Alderete, A., Usategui, A., Miranda-Ramos, V., Martínez-Herrera, D. J., & Mañes, S. (2016). Notch-regulated miR-223 targets the aryl hydrocarbon receptor pathway and increases cytokine production in macrophages from rheumatoid arthritis patients. *Scientific reports*, *6*(1), 1–12.

Ohno, T., Aune, D., & Heath, A. K. (2020). Adiposity and the risk of rheumatoid arthritis: a systematic review and meta-analysis of cohort studies. *Scientific reports*, *10*(1), 1–12.

Oliveira, I. M., Gonçalves, C., Reis, R. L., & Oliveira, J. M. (2018). Engineering nanoparticles for targeting rheumatoid arthritis: past, present, and future trends. *Nano research*, *11*(9), 4489–4506.

Olsen, N. J., & Stein, C. M. (2004). New drugs for rheumatoid arthritis. *New England journal of medicine*, *350*(21), 2167–2179.

Osawa, S., Ishii, T., Takemoto, H., Osada, K., & Kataoka, K. (2017). A facile amino-functionalization of poly (2-oxazoline)s' distal end through sequential azido end-capping and Staudinger reactions. *European polymer journal*, *88*, 553–561.

Ozbakir, B., Crielaard, B. J., Metselaar, J. M., Storm, G., & Lammers, T. (2014). Liposomal corticosteroids for the treatment of inflammatory disorders and cancer. *Journal of controlled release*, *190*, 624–636.

Park, J. Y., Kwon, S., Kim, S. H., Kang, Y. J., & Khang, D. (2020). Triamcinolone–gold nanoparticles repolarize synoviocytes and macrophages in an inflamed synovium. *ACS applied materials & interfaces*, *12*(35), 38936–38949.

Quéméneur, L., Gerland, L. M., Flacher, M., Ffrench, M., Revillard, J. P., & Genestier, L. (2003). Differential control of cell cycle, proliferation, and survival of primary T lymphocytes by purine and pyrimidine nucleotides. *The journal of immunology*, *170*(10), 4986–4995.

Radu, A. F., & Bungau, S. G. (2021). Management of rheumatoid arthritis: an overview. *Cells, 10*(11), 2857.

Raemdonck, K., Martens, T. F., Braeckmans, K., Demeester, J., & De Smedt, S. C. (2013). Polysaccharide-based nucleic acid nanoformulations. *Advanced drug delivery reviews, 65*(9), 1123–1147.

Rajasekhar, M., Olsson, A. M., Steel, K. J., Georgouli, M., Ranasinghe, U., Read, C. B., ... & Taams, L. S. (2017). MicroRNA-155 contributes to enhanced resistance to apoptosis in monocytes from patients with rheumatoid arthritis. *Journal of autoimmunity, 79*, 53–62.

Rau, R., & Herborn, G. (2004). Benefit and risk of methotrexate treatment in rheumatoid arthritis. *Clinical and experimental rheumatology, 22*, S83–S94.

Raza, A., Rasheed, T., Nabeel, F., Hayat, U., Bilal, M., & Iqbal, H. M. (2019). Endogenous and exogenous stimuli-responsive drug delivery systems for programmed site-specific release. *Molecules, 24*(6), 1117.

Safiri, S., Kolahi, A. A., Hoy, D., et al. (2019). Global, regional and national burden of rheumatoid arthritis 1990–2017: a systematic analysis of the global burden of disease study 2017. *Annals of the rheumatic diseases, 78*, 1463–1471.

Saita, M., Kaneko, J., Sato, T., Takahashi, S. S., Wada-Takahashi, S., Kawamata, R., & Nagasaki, Y. (2016). Novel antioxidative nanotherapeutics in a rat periodontitis model: reactive oxygen species scavenging by redox injectable gel suppresses alveolar bone resorption. *Biomaterials, 76*, 292–301.

Sarzi-Puttini, P., Ceribelli, A., Marotto, D., Batticciotto, A., & Atzeni, F. (2019). Systemic rheumatic diseases: from biological agents to small molecules. *Autoimmunity reviews, 18*(6), 583–592.

Scherer, H. U., Häupl, T., & Burmester, G. R. (2020). The etiology of rheumatoid arthritis. *Journal of autoimmunity, 110*, 102400.

Sengani, M. (2017). Identification of potential antioxidant indices by biogenic gold nanoparticles in hyperglycemic Wistar rats. *Environmental toxicology and pharmacology, 50*, 11–19.

Sepriano, A., Kerschbaumer, A., Smolen, J. S., Van Der Heijde, D., Dougados, M., Van Vollenhoven, R., ... & Landewé, R. (2020). Safety of synthetic and biological DMARDs: a systematic literature review informing the 2019 update of the EULAR recommendations for the management of rheumatoid arthritis. *Annals of the rheumatic diseases, 79*(6), 760–770.

Shi, Y., Cardoso, R. M., Van Nostrum, C. F., & Hennink, W. E. (2015). Anthracene functionalized thermosensitive and UV-crosslinkable polymeric micelles. *Polymer chemistry, 6*(11), 2048–2053.

Sies, H. (2015). Oxidative stress: a concept in redox biology and medicine. *Redox biology, 4*, 180–183.

Smolen, J. S., Aletaha, D., & McInnes, I. B. (2016). Rheumatoid arthritis. *Lancet (London, England), 388*(10055), 2023–2038.

Smolen, J. S., Landewé, R. B., Bijlsma, J. W., Burmester, G. R., Dougados, M., Kerschbaumer, A., ... & Van Der Heijde, D. (2020). EULAR recommendations for the management of rheumatoid arthritis with synthetic and biological disease-modifying antirheumatic drugs: 2019 update. *Annals of the rheumatic diseases, 79*(6), 685–699.

Solomon, D. H., Avorn, J., Katz, J. N., Weinblatt, M. E., Setoguchi, S., Levin, R., & Schneeweiss, S. (2006). Immunosuppressive medications and hospitalization for cardiovascular events in patients with rheumatoid arthritis. *Arthritis & rheumatism: Official journal of the American college of rheumatology, 54*(12), 3790–3798.

Thirunavukkarasu, G. K., Cherukula, K., Lee, H., Jeong, Y. Y., Park, I. K., & Lee, J. Y. (2018). Magnetic field-inducible drug-eluting nanoparticles for image-guided thermo-chemotherapy. *Biomaterials, 180*, 240–252.

Tu, J., Hong, W., Zhang, P., Wang, X., Körner, H., & Wei, W. (2018). Ontology and function of fibroblast-like and macrophage-like synoviocytes: how do they talk to each other and can they be targeted for rheumatoid arthritis therapy? *Frontiers in immunology*, *9*, 1467.

Vandooren, B., Kruithof, E., Yu, D. T., Rihl, M., Gu, J., De Rycke, L., & Baeten, D. (2004). Involvement of matrix metalloproteinases and their inhibitors in peripheral synovitis and down-regulation by tumor necrosis factor α blockade in spondylarthropathy. *Arthritis & rheumatism: Official journal of the American college of rheumatology*, *50*(9), 2942–2953.

Vomero, M., Barbati, C., Colasanti, T., Perricone, C., Novelli, L., Ceccarelli, F., & Alessandri, C. (2018). Autophagy and rheumatoid arthritis: current knowledges and future perspectives. *Frontiers in immunology*, *9*, 1577.

Wang, C. Y., Mayo, M. W., Korneluk, R. G., Goeddel, D. V., & Baldwin Jr, A. S. (1998). NF-κB antiapoptosis: induction of TRAF1 and TRAF2 and c-IAP1 and c-IAP2 to suppress caspase-8 activation. *Science*, *281*(5383), 1680–1683.

Wang, P., Li, A., Yu, L., Chen, Y., & Xu, D. (2020). Energy conversion-based nanotherapy for rheumatoid arthritis treatment. *Frontiers in bioengineering and biotechnology*, *8*, 652.

Wang, Q., Jiang, J., Chen, W., Jiang, H., Zhang, Z., & Sun, X. (2016). Targeted delivery of low-dose dexamethasone using PCL–PEG micelles for effective treatment of rheumatoid arthritis. *Journal of controlled release*, *230*, 64–72.

Wang, Q., Li, Y., Chen, X., Jiang, H., Zhang, Z., & Sun, X. (2019). Optimized in vivo performance of acid-liable micelles for the treatment of rheumatoid arthritis by one single injection. *Nano research*, *12*(2), 421–428.

Wang, W., Zhou, H., & Liu, L. (2018). Side effects of methotrexate therapy for rheumatoid arthritis: a systematic review. *European journal of medicinal chemistry*, *158*, 502–516.

Wang, Y., Li, B., Xu, F., Han, Z., Wei, D., Jia, D., & Zhou, Y. (2018). Tough magnetic chitosan hydrogel nanocomposites for remotely stimulated drug release. *Biomacromolecules*, *19*(8), 3351–3360.

Wenham, C. Y., & Conaghan, P. G. (2013). New horizons in osteoarthritis. *Age and ageing*, *42*(3), 272–278.

Wilson, D. R., Zhang, N., Silvers, A. L., Forstner, M. B., & Bader, R. A. (2014). Synthesis and evaluation of cyclosporine A-loaded polysialic acid–polycaprolactone micelles for rheumatoid arthritis. *European journal of pharmaceutical sciences*, *51*, 146–156.

Wongrakpanich, S., Wongrakpanich, A., Melhado, K., & Rangaswami, J. (2018). A comprehensive review of non-steroidal anti-inflammatory drug use in the elderly. *Aging and disease*, *9*(1), 143.

Woo, C. H., Eom, Y. W., Yoo, M. H., You, H. J., Han, H. J., Song, W. K., & Kim, J. H. (2000). Tumor necrosis factor-α generates reactive oxygen species via a cytosolic phospholipase A2-linked cascade. *Journal of biological chemistry*, *275*(41), 32357–32362.

Xiang, J., Tong, X., Shi, F., Yan, Q., Yu, B., & Zhao, Y. (2018). Near-infrared light-triggered drug release from UV-responsive diblock copolymer-coated upconversion nanoparticles with high monodispersity. *Journal of materials chemistry B*, *6*(21), 3531–3540.

Xiong, F., Qin, Z., Chen, H., Lan, Q., Wang, Z., Lan, N., & Kai, D. (2020). pH-responsive and hyaluronic acid-functionalized metal–organic frameworks for therapy of osteoarthritis. *Journal of nanobiotechnology*, *18*(1), 1–14.

Xue, L., Wang, D., Zhang, X., Xu, S., & Zhang, N. (2020). Targeted and triple therapy-based liposomes for enhanced treatment of rheumatoid arthritis. *International journal of pharmaceutics*, *586*, 119642.

Yang, J., Zhang, P., Tang, L., Sun, P., Liu, W., Sun, P., & Liang, D. (2010). Temperature-tuned DNA condensation and gene transfection by PEI-g-(PMEO2MA-b-PHEMA) copolymer-based nonviral vectors. *Biomaterials*, *31*(1), 144–155.

Yang, M., Ding, J., Zhang, Y., Chang, F., Wang, J., Gao, Z., & Chen, X. (2016). Activated macrophage-targeted dextran–methotrexate/folate conjugate prevents deterioration of collagen-induced arthritis in mice. *Journal of materials chemistry B*, *4*(12), 2102–2113.

Yang, M., Feng, X., Ding, J., Chang, F., & Chen, X. (2017). Nanotherapeutics relieve rheumatoid arthritis. *Journal of controlled release*, *252*, 108–124.

Yang, S., Wang, J., Brand, D. D., & Zheng, S. G. (2018). Role of TNF–TNF receptor 2 signal in regulatory T cells and its therapeutic implications. *Frontiers in immunology*, *9*, 784.

Yang, Y., Guo, L., Wang, Z., Liu, P., Liu, X., Ding, J., & Zhou, W. (2021). Targeted silver nanoparticles for rheumatoid arthritis therapy via macrophage apoptosis and Re-polarization. *Biomaterials*, *264*, 120390.

Yin, X., Ran, S., Cheng, H., Zhang, M., Sun, W., Wan, Y., & Zhu, Z. (2022). Polydopamine-modified ZIF-8 nanoparticles as a drug carrier for combined chemo-photothermal osteosarcoma therapy. *Colloids and surfaces B: Biointerfaces*, *216*, 112507.

Yoon, C. H., Chung, S. J., Lee, S. W., Park, Y. B., Lee, S. K., & Park, M. C. (2013). Gallic acid, a natural polyphenolic acid, induces apoptosis and inhibits proinflammatory gene expressions in rheumatoid arthritis fibroblast-like synoviocytes. *Joint bone spine*, *80*(3), 274–279.

Yu, Z., Reynaud, F., Lorscheider, M., Tsapis, N., & Fattal, E. (2020). Nanomedicines for the delivery of glucocorticoids and nucleic acids as potential alternatives in the treatment of rheumatoid arthritis. *Wiley interdisciplinary reviews: Nanomedicine and nanobiotechnology*, *12*(5), e1630.

Zhang, M., Hu, W., Cai, C., Wu, Y., Li, J., & Dong, S. (2022). Advanced application of stimuli-responsive drug delivery system for inflammatory arthritis treatment. *Materials today biology*, *14*, 100223.

Zhang, S., Zhang, M., Li, X., Li, G., Yang, B., Lu, X., & Sun, F. (2022). Nano-based co-delivery system for treatment of rheumatoid arthritis. *Molecules*, *27*(18), 5973.

Zhao, J., Chen, X., Ho, K. H., Cai, C., Li, C. W., Yang, M., & Yi, C. (2021). Nanotechnology for diagnosis and therapy of rheumatoid arthritis: evolution towards theranostic approaches. *Chinese chemical letters*, *32*(1), 66–86.

Zhao, X., Huang, C., Su, M., Ran, Y., Wang, Y., & Yin, Z. (2022). Reactive oxygen species–responsive celastrol-loaded. *The AAPS journal*, *24*(1), 1–13.

Zhou, M., Wen, K., Bi, Y., Lu, H., Chen, J., Hu, Y., & Chai, Z. (2017). The application of stimuli-responsive nanocarriers for targeted drug delivery. *Current topics in medicinal chemistry*, *17*(20), 2319–2334.

6 Development of Personalized Medicine

Challenges and Therapeutic Applications

*Tanushri Chatterji, Namrata Khanna,
Mansi Kumari, Arun Kumar Singh,
Neelam Thakur, and Umesh Kumar*

6.1 INTRODUCTION

Accuracy in targeted therapy has been an elusive factor in modern clinical practice, though in recent years genomics has paved the way for development of new strategies that are recasting conventional treatment and healthcare procedures by facilitating management and diagnosis of diseases in an individual through precise targeting. Many expressions have been used to describe the above concept, such as personalized medicine, stratified medicine, individualized medicine, and precision medicine (Figure 6.1).

The term individualized medicine was first coined in 2003, when it described individual drug metabolism in relation to pharmacogenomics.[1] Recently conducted studies define individualized medicine with reference to treatment strategies that use an individual's own cellular material to evolve a therapeutic plan that is specific to the patient from whom the material has been extracted. This includes stem cell therapy,[2] vaccines against malignancies,[3] and complicated cancer types with variation in molecular profiles.[4] These strategies can revolutionize the treatment of diseases where an effective treatment is elusive. However, these therapies are not yet ready for acceptance and for regular treatment in clinics.

Precision medicine was a term first used by Boguski *et al* in 2009 and was described with three essential characteristics: a comprehension of the cause of a disease; the ability to detect these disease-causing agents; and the ability to effectively treat the exact cause.[5]

The term "stratified medicine" was first coined by Trusheim *et al* in the year 2007.[6] They defined it as a treatment "where therapies are matched with specific patient population characteristics using clinical biomarkers." The term "stratified medicine" was coined on the basis that every patient can be related to a cohort (or similar groups of patients), which shows a certain response, by using a biomarker specifically related to that particular response.

DOI: 10.1201/9781003348672-6

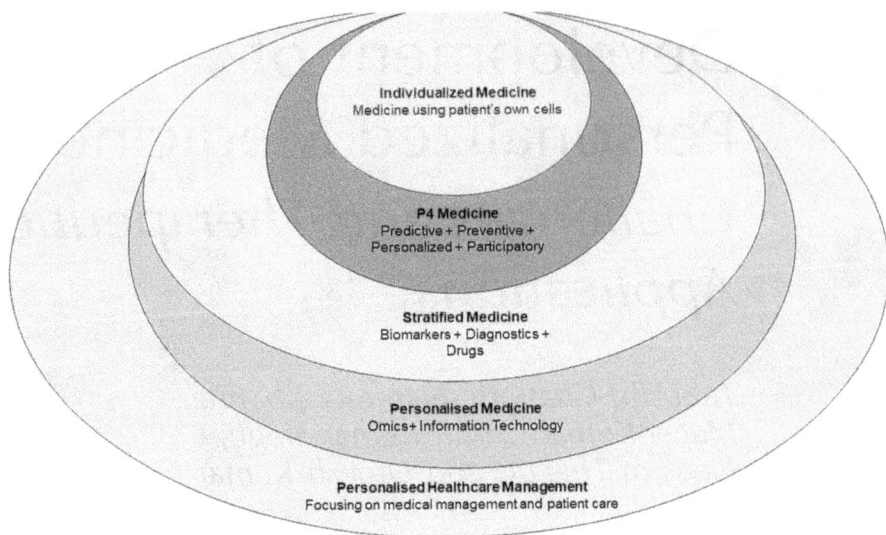

FIGURE 6.1   Correlation between personalized healthcare, personalized medicine, stratified medicine, precision medicine, individualized medicine, and P4 medicine.

The term "P4 medicine" was coined in 2008 by Leroy Hood and was based on the evolution of systems biology.[7] P4 stands for predictive, personalized, preventive, and participatory, and denotes a radical shift in clinical treatment from reactive to preventive. Hood stated that in systems biology the study of correlations in a whole system, with respect to genetic or environmental variations is dealt with, which would facilitate a more integrated approach. In the first place, molecular understanding of disease mechanisms would stratify complex diseases and facilitate novel drug discovery. Secondly, availability of more information through the internet would increase the energetic involvement of patients and individuals toward their health.

The term "personalized medicine" was used as early as 1971 by Gibson.[8] The term "personalized medicine" reappeared 30 years later as an application of pharmacogenomics in medicinal practice.[9] Since then, personalized medicine has encompassed various concepts, though most researchers use it as "human genome deciphering and the resulting sudden increase in the understanding of disease causes and therapeutic options."[10] Meyer described personalized medicine as "a comprehensive, prospective approach to preventing, diagnosing and treating diseases in order to achieve the optimal result for an individual."[11]

More recently, personalized medicine or precision therapy describes the procedure for treatment, with the objective of enhancing the effectiveness of therapy, reducing the difference between actual result and the expected response. Personalized treatment involves precisely targeted and regulated therapies that avert, halt, or decelerate progression of the disease, which is dependent on the individual's molecular configuration.[12] The approach one size fits all is rarely accepted clinically, specifically for treatment of diseases with enhanced heterogeneity in etiology and physiological

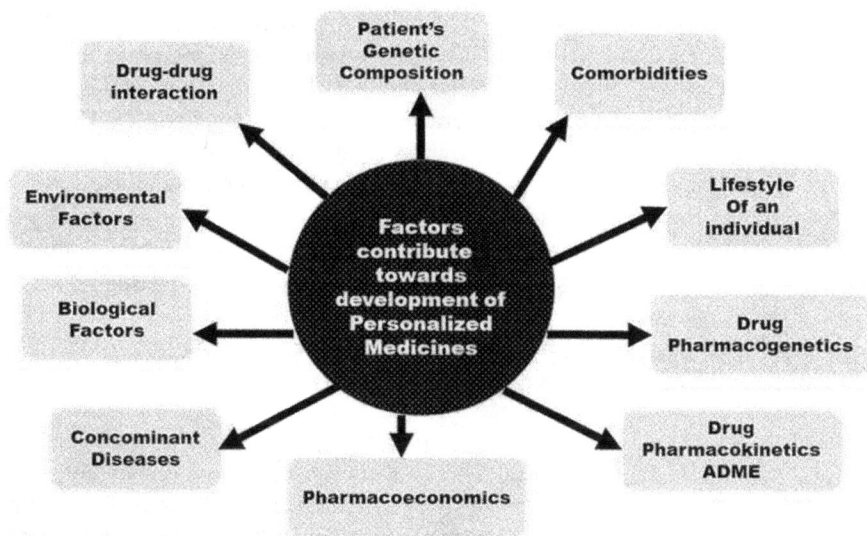

FIGURE 6.2   Factors contributing toward development of personalized medicines.

symptoms. Heterogeneity in the mechanism of disease progression and the individual's response to therapy leads to development of precision medicine. Variation in individuals' responses to a similar therapy plan is dependent on both genetic and environmental factors. Figure 6.2 represents various factors that have led to development of personalized therapeutic approaches for treatment of several diseases.

Nanomedicine, the extended branch of nanoscience, was introduced in the 1990s. The potential of nanoparticles (1–1000 nm in size) is used for diagnosis, treatment, and prevention of various diseases. Therapeutic action of nanoparticles is made possible through optimum concentration at the target over a certain time period.[13] The branch of nanomedicine is a combination of nanomaterial and nanosystems, which constitutes nanodrugs, nanocarriers, nanoconstructs, nanoparticles, nanomaterials, or nanotherapeutics. On the basis of target sites, the bioavailability of therapeutics, novel approaches of therapeutic action, and nanostructured surfaces, innovative strategies have been devised for the development of personalized medicines.

The idea of nanomedicine was conceptualized a century ago by Paul Ehrlich as "Magic Bullet," with the ability to detect the target site and deliver therapeutic action. The concept of "Magic bullet" is currently being implemented in the form of nanomedicine. During the course of development, it was observed that nanomedicines can also be related with "precision medicine," which provides accurate diagnosis and targeted treatment for various diseases.

Versatility, unique physicochemical properties, and biocompatibility of nanoparticles (NPs) make them potent therapeutic agents in the clinical world.[14] They have a high degree of multifunctionality in treatment as well as in drug development. It is concluded from various clinical studies that NPs give promising results in the treatment of cancer and other diseases, with negligible or minimal side effects.[15] Furthermore, nanobiotechnologies develop novel treatment strategies through personalized medicine. In this treatment approach, the therapeutic is customized to accommodate the specific characteristics of individual patients.[16]

Personalized medicines are customized on the basis of an individual's body type and according to the specific disease characteristic to that individual.[17,18] Therefore, considering the inter-individual variability in therapeutic response, a patient-specific treatment produces better therapeutic outcomes, along with reduction of patient discomfort and undesirable side effects.[19]

Personalized medicine-based treatment strategy is quite promising in treating life-threatening diseases like cancer but has a few adverse effects also.[17]

6.2 CHARACTERISTIC FEATURES OF NANOPARTICLES IN PERSONALIZED MEDICINES

Personalized medicine is the development of a unique therapy for an individual or a group of individuals, on the basis of genetic, phenotypic, and environmental features that could affect the effectiveness and safety of the treatment. Nanomedicines have been used for the development of personalized medicines by treating each patient or group of patients with similar characteristics (cohort) through studies on specific requirements described in their genome.[20] In this chapter, we discuss the use of nanoparticles as therapeutic agents, especially for developing personalized treatment. Although many different types of nanomedicines are in use, i.e., nanopolymers, magnetic NPs, and liposomes (Figure 6.3), all exhibit increased efficacy over conventional therapies through modification of the pharmacokinetics and pharmaco-dynamics (pK/pD) of the drug.[21]

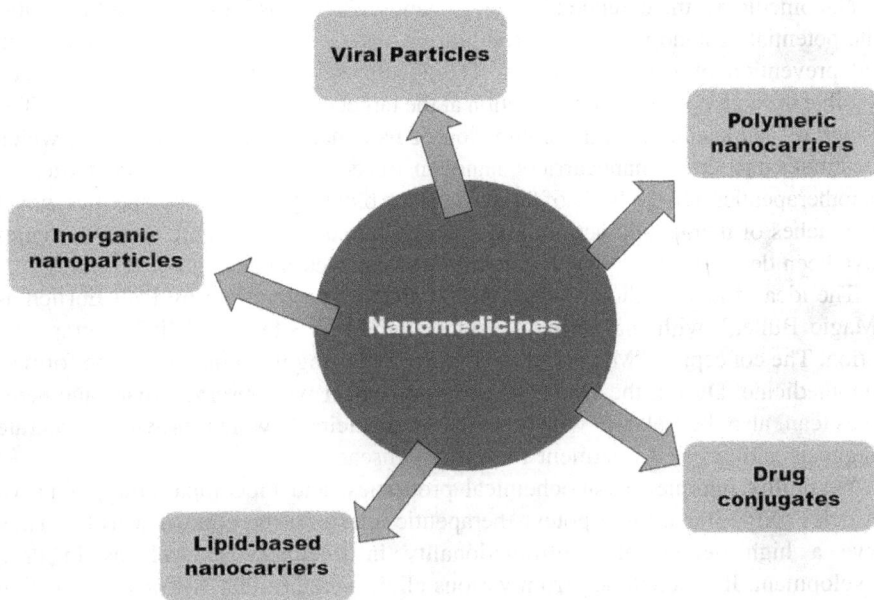

FIGURE 6.3 Types of nanomedicines for use in personalized therapy.

TABLE 6.1

Major Advantages of Nanomedicines in Personalized (Precision) Medicine[24]

S No.	Advantages of Nanomaterials in Personalized Therapy
1	Nano-sized dimensions
2	Flexibility/versatility
3	Employing labile molecules (e.g. siRNA)
4	Enclosed and protected active principles
5	Modification of pharmacokinetics
6	Capable of being targeted towards specific organs
7	Capable of adapting to a similar cohort of individuals
8	Capable of adapting to specific treatment plans in a cohort (e.g. dosage and its duration)

6.3 ADVANTAGES OF NANOMEDICINES OVER CONVENTIONAL THERAPIES

Specifically, the advantages of nanomedicines over conventional medicines depend on the following (Table 6.1):

i. The size of nanomaterials (1–1000 nm), which is very small and results in a high surface-to-volume ratio, has the advantage of improved sensing and biological recognition

ii. The opposite activities of lipophilic and hydrophilic nature can be enclosed within the same nanostructure, facilitating the administration of doses higher than in conventional therapies

iii. Protection of encapsulated drugs from exposure to surrounding nucleases and light

iv. Modification of pharmacokinetics by facilitating regulated release of the drug, which helps decrease the dosage frequency and enhances the activity and effectiveness of therapy

v. The active movement of the drug toward the target tissue, hence generating a favorable localized outcome, enhancing drug efficacy, and decreasing adverse reactions

vi. The presence of many different types of nanosystems provides the flexibility and choice of planning an appropriate treatment plan for designing a personalized therapeutic strategy.[22,23]

6.4 MECHANISM OF ACTION OF PERSONALIZED MEDICINES

The basic action of any drug is to generate a response against a particular disease and treat the state. The process is described in Figure 6.4. The complete mechanism is known as "pharmacokinetics" and is regulated by a set of genes, collectively known as drug-metabolizing enzymes. As the drug enters the body, it starts interacting with the target site to elicit a response known as pharmacodynamic effects. These effects

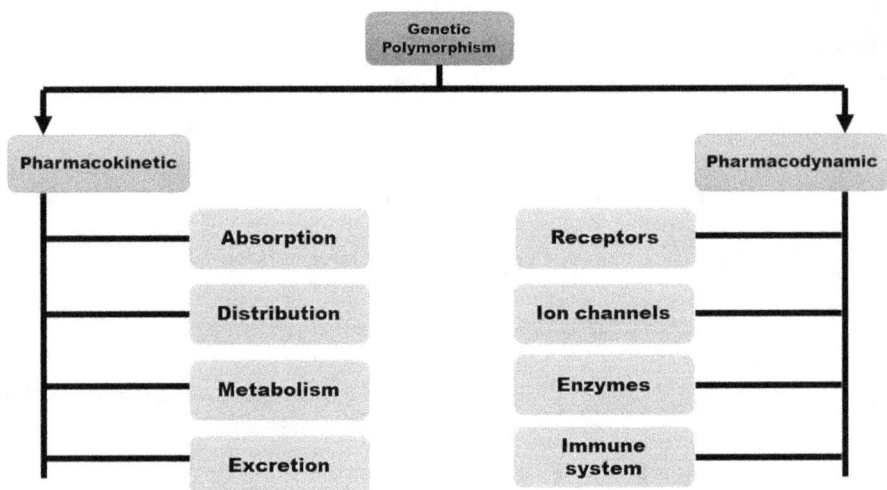

FIGURE 6.4   Representation of drug action in personalized therapy.

describe the affinity of a drug for the target, ability for modulation, or its efficacy, potency, dosage for inducing effects on the target tissue.[25]

Pharmacokinetics includes four processes: absorption, distribution, metabolism, and excretion, which are frequently represented as **ADME**. **Absorption** describes the process of drug entry into the bloodstream after intake of a drug; intravenous administration gets past absorption as the drug directly enters circulation. **Distribution** outlines the target that the drug reaches after absorption and the concentration of the drug at the target site. A few drugs cannot cross the blood-brain barrier (BBB). **Metabolism** encompasses the process of breakdown of drugs in the body, which occurs instantly through enzyme action in the GIT and may necessitate the formation of end products, which have their inherent pharmacologic activity. Eventually, **excretion** details the mechanism of elimination of drugs from the body, either by urine, bile, or, sometimes through exhalation.

- A-Absorption of the drug by body
- D-Dispersion of the drug throughout the body
- M-Biotransformation and metabolization into useful components for elicitation
- E- Excretion of remaining amounts

6.5 CURRENT PERSONALIZED THERAPEUTICS IN CLINICAL PRACTICE

The Food and Drug Administration (FDA) defined 486 drugs that demanded specific tests based on pharmacogenesis. Individual drugs have their own biomarkers for prediction of the response according to the genetic makeup of the patient and in many cases the drug use or its dosage is in accordance with the biomarker responses.

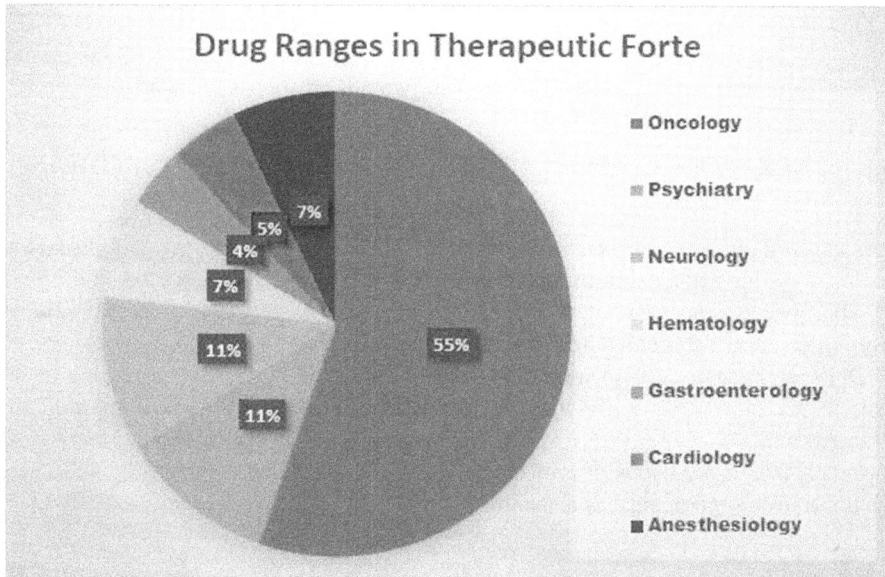

Drug Ranges in Therapeutic Forte

- Oncology
- Psychiatry
- Neurology
- Hematology
- Gastroenterology
- Cardiology
- Anesthesiology

7% · 5% · 4% · 7% · 11% · 11% · 55%

FIGURE 6.5 Percentage of personalized drugs in different therapeutic areas.

Personalized medicine includes several spheres of clinical areas, like oncology, neurology, psychiatry, anesthesiology, hematology, cardiology, and gastroenterology as depicted in Figure 6.5.[26]

Most drug biomarkers are associated with polymorphisms in cytochrome P450 (CYP) enzyme systems, resulting in various metabolic activities. The majority of CYP modifications are observed in CYP2D6 and CYP2C9, which are associated with anesthesiology; CYP2D6, CYP2C19, CYP2C9, and CYP3A5 are correlated with cardiology; CYP2C9 with hematology and CYP2D6 with oncology.

The second phase drug metabolizing enzymes are also employed as biomarkers, for example, transferases that include uridine diphosphate glucuronosyltransferase (UGTs). UGTs are endoplasmic reticulum-bound enzymes and are significant for phase II drug metabolism, essential for glucuronidation that involves 22 distinct functional enzymes. Furthermore, glutathione S-transferases (GSTs) and sulfotransferases (SULTs) are significant enzymes mediating conjugation in phase II reactions. In addition, cytosolic biomarkers like N-acetyltransferases 1 and 2 (NAT1 and NAT2) enzymes mediate acetylation reactions. Further, thiopurine S-methyltransferase (TPMT) is a cytosolic enzyme catalyzing the S-methylation reactions in drugs. ATP-binding cassette (ABC) and solute-linked carrier (SLC) proteins act as efflux transporters and may act as biomarkers associated with a few therapeutics used in cardiology, neurology, and oncology.[27]

The majority of personalized drugs related to biomarkers are anticancer therapeutics (206 drugs) (Figure 6.5) and constitute 55% of total precision therapeutics. For example, 20 anticancer drugs act against the ERBB2(HER2) gene.

Warfarin is a drug extensively used as a blood thinner, with a high risk of adverse drug reaction (ADR). The drug targets the VKORC1 gene and is metabolized by

CYP2C9 enzyme.[25] Natural genetic modification in both the VKORC1 and CYP2C9 genes leads to variation in the pharmacodynamic and pharmacokinetic characteristics of Warfarin, eventually causing variation in patients' responses to warfarin.

6.6 THERAPEUTIC APPLICATIONS OF PERSONALIZED MEDICINE IN CANCER

Personalized medicine plays a significant role in the field of oncology, with promising results in the long run, exhibiting minimal or no side effects. It is designed on the basis of appropriate selection of patients, recognition of prognostic and predictive biomarkers, and culminates into a precise target treatment (Table 6.2).

DNA of normal cells is modified into malignant cells due to variations in the genetic makeup of an individual. A few of these perturbations are sporadically attained, while others are transmitted in the carcinogenic genes. Hence, there is an approach where predisposition of cancer genes is identified followed by screening for appropriate therapeutic intervention.

6.6.1 BREAST CANCER

Mutations in BRCA 1 or BRCA 2 genes are responsible for causing breast cancer. These genes are also responsible for ovarian, colon, and prostate cancer. Conventional

TABLE 6.2

Few Cancer Types Summarized with Molecular Targets for Personalized Therapeutics

S No.	Type of Cancer	Target Cell	Targeted Agent	Class of Agent
1	Breast	HER2	Trastuzumab	Monoclonal antibody against HER2/Neu (EGFR2)
2	Colorectal	KRAS	Cetuximab	Monoclonal antibody against EGFR
3	Chronic myeloid leukemia	BCR-ABL fusion protein	Imatinib	Receptor tyrosine kinase inhibitor
4	Gastrointestinal stromal tumors	c-KIT	Imatinib	Receptor tyrosine kinase inhibitor
5	Non-small-cell lung cancer	EGFR	Erlotinib and gefitinib	Receptor tyrosine kinase inhibitor
6	Non-small-cell lung cancer	EML4-ALK fusion protein	EML4-ALK fusion protein	Receptor tyrosine kinase inhibitor
7	Metastatic malignant melanoma	BRAF V600E	Vemurafenib	B-raf/MEK/ERK pathway inhibitor
8	Ovarian, breast, and prostate cancer (under investigation)	BRCA1, BRCA2	Olaparib	Poly (ADP-ribose) polymerase (PARP) inhibitor

treatment strategy involves the removal of breast tissue through surgery, oophorectomy, or chemical estrogen deprivation. Breast cancer cases become complex with increased penetration in tissues, in such cases there is enhanced surgical risk.[28,29] In order to overcome this situation trastuzumab is used as a personalized medicine. In this humanized IgG1 monoclonal antibody is used against the breast cancer oncogene (HER2). This gene proliferates and is over-expressed in 20–25% of breast cancer patients. Therefore, the target gene HER2 predicts trastuzumab response. Trastuzumab-based personalized medicine exhibited reduction in the number of recurrent cases of breast cancer, though cardiotoxicity is observed as an ADR.[30,31]

6.6.2 COLON CANCER

Colorectal cancer (CRC) is caused by a series of germline mutations. Some bowel malignancies arise as a genetic disorder caused by familial adenomatous polyposis coli (FAP) owing to mutation in the adenomatous polyposis coli (APC) gene. Due to alterations in the APC gene, there is a loss of the Wnt negative regulator, which leads to enhanced activation of the Wnt signaling pathway, causing uncontrolled cellular proliferation in CRC.[32]

Overexpression of epidermal growth factor receptor (EGFR) leads to dysregulation of cellular proliferation in CRC. Personalized medicines are used to target and inhibit the EGFR gene. Cetuximab, a monoclonal antibody used against EGFR, over-expresses wild-type KRAS gene, which in turn downregulates EGFR synthesis. Randomized clinical trials with cetuximab therapy, exhibited better quality of life in CRC patients and an overall increase in progression-free survival was observed.[33,34]

6.6.3 CHRONIC MYELOID LEUKEMIA

In chronic myeloid leukemia (CML), translocation occurs between the long arms of chromosomes 9 and 22. This phenomenon of translocation forms the Philadelphia chromosome. The consequences of this chromosomal abnormality are expressions of BCR-ABL fusion oncoprotein with constitutive tyrosine kinase (TK) activity. TK activity enhances cellular proliferation and necessitates a tumor-selective, molecular-targeted therapy. The TK inhibitor (TKI) imatinib generates a hematological response in these patients, which leads to suppression of CML and extends the survival rate.[35,36]

6.6.4 METASTATIC MALIGNANT MELANOMA

The maximum number of cases of malignant melanomas occur due to mutation in BRAF V600 oncogene leading to substitution of a single amino acid. The genetic alteration results in the severity of the disease and there is a reduced response to conventional cytotoxic chemotherapy.[37] Vemurafenib is used as a precision therapeutic, which specifically binds to the ATP-binding site of the enzyme BRAF kinase to inhibit its activity. This may inhibit an over-activated MAPK signaling pathway downstream in tumor cells and reduce cellular proliferation. This reduces the mortality rate by 63% and the risk of disease progression by 74% in patients.[38,39]

6.7 PERSONALIZED MEDICINE IN NEUROLOGICAL DISORDERS

Neurodegenerative disorders involve an array of age-related neurological diseases, depicted by continual wasting or loss of neuronal function in particular areas of the nervous system. Alzheimer's disease (AD) and Parkinson's disease (PD) are the most studied neurodegenerative disorders. After cancer, neurological diseases provide the most favorable circumstances to accomplish precision therapy, owing to rapid advancement in gene discovery. Classification of individuals on the basis of their susceptibility to neurodegenerative disorders through application of data and genomics has led to the development of precision medicine in such disorders. Various neurodegenerative diseases, like Alzheimer's disease (AD), Parkinson's disease (PD), amyotrophic lateral sclerosis (ALS), are clinically heterogeneous diseases with a strong genetic background.[40–42] Furthermore, gene polymorphism has a unique activity in stroke and epilepsy.[43] These diseases result from complex interactions between multiple genes and the environment.[44] Although the study of clinically relevant genetic polymorphisms continues to be a challenge, established examples are being used to sub-classify groups of patients to design optimum treatment strategies through personalized therapy.[45]

6.7.1 PERSONALIZED MEDICINE IN PARKINSON'S DISEASE (PD)

Investigations to target PD genetic biomarkers and their protein products are in progress[46] LRRK2 gene codes for a large multidomain and multifunctional protein expressed mainly by microglia and macrophages. It is also observed in the kidney, lungs, and to a lesser degree in the brain. LRRK2 contributes significantly to processes like inflammation,[47] trafficking of dopamine receptor,[48] endocytosis of the synaptic vesicle,[49] and degradation of protein.[50] Many variants of the LRRK2 gene may be responsible for triggering the risk of PD.[51] The G2019S variant is most common and is responsible for 1% sporadic and 4% familial PD.[52–54] In addition, other LRRK2 variants associated with PD are R1441G/C/H, Y1699C/G,[55,56] R1628P,[57] G2385R,[58] and I2020T.[59] A few of the above genetic variants exhibit diverse penetrance on the basis of ethnicity and residence of the individual, emphasizing that genetic and environmental factors responsible for disease development are yet to be identified. Increased LRRK2 levels in the CSF are observed in PD patients with the G2019S variant.[60] The recent clinical trials on PD patients primarily aim for inhibition of LRRK2 levels[61] and are also based on a study describing enhanced activity of wild-type LRRK2 kinase, as observed in idiopathic PD.[62] There are various mechanisms defining PD progression, for example, a few studies suggest that reducing elevated LRRK2 levels in neurons can restrict PD continuance, though expression of LRRK2 has been observed more in immune cells of the brain and also in peripheral organs.[47] Furthermore, extended studies are required to understand the multiple functions of LRRK2 and the role of each protein domain related to it.

A recently concluded double-blinded, phase Ib drug trial by Denali Therapeutics, targeting elevated LRRK2 activity in PD, was done on an LRRK2 inhibitor DNL201. Inhibition of phosphorylated (p) LRRK2 (pS935) by 50% was observed in blood, indicating a direct estimate of activity, and also of pRAB10, an LRRK2 downstream target in mononuclear cells of peripheral blood in individuals suffering from idiopathic PD. A reduction of 20–60% in lysosomal biomarker bis-monoacylglycerol phosphate (BMP) was observed in urine. This was followed by another trial of the small molecule LRRK2 inhibitor DNL151, which exhibits a relatively safe profile and a significant inhibitory outcome on pS935 LRRK2 and pRAB10, along with reduced levels of BMP in urine. Ionis Pharmaceuticals is currently testing the LRRK2 antisense oligonucleotide drug BIIB094, which is being tested through intrathecal administration, in a placebo-controlled phase I trial, for evaluation of the ADR safety profile. The ongoing clinical trials on PD patients are studying the effects of LRRK2 inhibitors, in presence or absence of LRRK2 risk variants. Further studies on non-risk variants with base levels of LRRK2 need to be conducted to elevate the degree of precision in PD therapy.[63]

The enzyme glucocerebrosidase (GCase) is coded by the GBA gene that expedites the breakdown of sphingolipids in the lysosomes, for example, glucosylceramide is degraded into glucose and ceramide. This is observed in many cells, particularly in the macrophages and other immune cells.[64] The typical swollen macrophages called the Gaucher cells, accumulate glucosylceramide and invade organs, leading to organomegaly in Gaucher disease.[65] Further investigations reveal substantial participation of the adaptive immune system, which involves B- and T-cell recruitment and maturation.[66] In Gaucher's disease, approximately 300 GBA variants have been observed[67] with diversified proportions of nervous system intervention.[68] PD risk has been associated with approximately 130 GBA variants,[69] with varied effects depending on the severity of mutation.[70] A few GBA variants can also affect the development of Lewy body dementia.[71] Approximately 5–20% of idiopathic PD cases are attributed to GBA variants.[72] The GBA variants associated with PD risk have been related to reduced GCase activity. GCase activity may be inhibited by different GBA variants through distinct pathways, which may include direct loss of enzyme activity, failure to act in accordance with endoplasmic reticulum (ER) quality control leading to proteasomal degradation, which disturbs trafficking towards lysosome, owing to ER or Golgi retention or the ineffectiveness of appropriate connection with the lysosomal transporter LIMP2 or the lysosomal activator protein Saposin C.[73] Inhibited GCase activity has been observed in several areas of the brain and in the CSF of some idiopathic PD patients.[74]

Current therapeutic applications to rectify these aberrations involve pharmaceutical chaperones, gene therapy, enzyme activation, and substrate reduction. Treatment of Gaucher's disease through enzyme replacement or GCase activators has exhibited promising results, however, for PD treatment, these therapies have a major limitation in their incapacity to cross the hurdle of blood-brain barrier (BBB). Hence, a very high dosage of these drugs will be required in PD as compared to the treatment of Gaucher's disease, to make certain that adequate drugs are able to cross the BBB, which may result in acute ADR.

6.7.2 Clinical Trials on Drugs Targeting GBA Aberrations in PD

The pharmaceutical company PRO.MED.CSA has recently completed a non-randomized and non-controlled phase II clinical trial of the mucolytic and GCase chaperone Ambroxol, which has been approved by the FDA.[75] They detected Ambroxol in the blood and CSF of PD patients after 186 days of oral administration, in the absence of any noticeable adverse reaction. This was accompanied by a slight decrease in GCase activity within the CSF, which resulted from the inhibitory effects exerted by Ambroxol at neutral pH. They also detected increased α-syn in CSF and reduced tau in serum, with simultaneous amelioration in the total MDS-UPDRS score and a decline in the NMSS score. Though, these tests were inconclusive because of the absence of a placebo group. Another drug trial involving Ambroxol was designed as a double-blinded and placebo-controlled study and was commenced by the Weston Brain Institute, London Health Sciences Center, University of Western Ontario.[76] Further, there are many ongoing clinical trials that are targeting GBA, for example, Sanofi's glucosylceramide synthase inhibitor GZ/SAR402671, is currently in a phase II double-blinded and placebo-controlled trial and resTORbio's TORC1 inhibitor RTB101, which is a phase Ib/IIa trial. RTB101 is also under trial in association with rapamycin; intervening results indicate that the drugs can permeate through the BBB and are well endured. Prevail therapeutics has initiated a phase I/II double-blinded and sham-procedure controlled test, which involves intracisternal administration of GBA-coding AAV9 viral vector PR001A. Lysosomal therapeutics is conducting a trial involving a small molecule GCase activator LTI-291 in a phase Ib test. The finished clinical trials with Ambroxol, tested PD patients in the presence or absence of GBA risk variants. These trials are similar to the current tests, which are investigating effects of GZ/SAR402671 and RTB101, while the trials involving PR001A and LTI-291 are recruiting PD patients with GBA risk variants only. Including PD patients with GBA risk variants in a trial is as challenging as inclusion of PD patients with LRRK2 risk variants, such as decreased frequency of risk variant carriers and trouble in identifying individuals with identical risk variants.[63] Further, including GCase levels in carriers without GBA risk variant would be more pertinent to improve the development of precision therapy.

6.7.3 PERSONALIZED MEDICINE IN ALZHEIMER'S DISEASE

Alzheimer's disease (AD) is a global cause of concern and the major difficulties in fighting the disease are because of the complex symptoms and etiology, poor knowledge of its mechanisms, and the existence of a latent, asymptomatic, preclinical stage. Although many drugs are continuously screened in clinical studies for the treatment of Alzheimer's disease, the unexpected lack of patient response and sometimes the important adverse effects make it a potential field of application for personalized medicine. AD, with its complexity and lack of effective treatments, represents a very interesting field for precision medicine application.

Research in bionanosensors is already providing examples with high sensitivity for core and new biomarkers for AD. In therapy the functionalization of nanoparticle surfaces can add specificity for biological recognition or for improving bioavailability. This would allow the administration of lower doses with fewer adverse effects due to the local targeting.[77]

The restricted development of drugs for AD treatment is by and large due to incomplete understanding of the fundamental pathologic mechanisms responsible for disease progression. AD progression involves a complex set of mechanisms, from an initial latency phase (where pathophysiologic activities are in action but symptoms are absent), through a prodromal phase (when mild cognitive disabilities begin to appear) to the entire clinical manifestation. Clinical manifestations include a progressive decline in cognitive abilities, behavior, and function, finally resulting in complete debility and death. Significant clinical manifestations in the brain involve intracellular accumulation of tau proteins, which are hyperphosphorylated in neurofibrillary tangles, and of extracellular β-amyloid (Aβ) protein in diffuse and amyloid/neuritic plaques, produced by sequential breakdown of the amyloid precursor protein (APP) in presence of β- (BACE1) and Υ-secretase. Furthermore, neuronal and synaptic loss along with activated microglia are widely distributed and frequently observed.[78] In addition to the above complications, continual super-imposed clinical and pathological ramifications are also observed, particularly Lewy Body disease (LBD) and cerebrovascular diseases.[79,80]

These clinical and pathological complications are projected by the considerable genetic variation related with AD progression. Over the past few years, extensive genome-wide association studies (GWAS), whole exome sequencing (WES), and whole genome sequencing (WGS) have resulted in considerable progress for identification of the AD genetic variants, through mapping of 27 loci (Table 6.3).[44,81–92]

TABLE 6.3

Molecular Pathways and Genes Involved in Progression of Alzheimer's Disease Identified via Genomic Studies[93]

S No.	Pathway	Gene
1.	Amyloid pathway	APOE, CLU, CR1, SORL1, PICALM, ABCA7, BIN1, CASS4, PLD3
2.	Inflammatory/Immune response	CLU, CR1, EPHA1, ABCA7, MS4A4A/MS4A6E, CD33, CD2AP, HLA-DRB5/DRB1, INPP5D, MEF2C, TREM2/TREML2
3.	Metabolic pathways and transport of lipids	APOE, CLU, ABCA7, SORL1
4.	Endocytosis and functioning of synaptic cell	CLU, PICALM, BIN1, EPHA1, MS4A4A/MS4A6E, CD33, CD2AP, PTK2B, SORL1, SLC24A4/RIN3, MEF2C
5.	Tau pathology	BIN1, CASS4, FERMT2
6.	Migration of cells	PTK2B
7.	Synaptic function of the hippocampus	MEF2C, PTK2B
8.	Cytoskeletal function and transport across axons	CELF1, NME8, CASS4
9.	Function of the microglial and myeloid cells	INPPD5
10.	Ubiquitination dependent on phosphorylation	FBXL7

These loci precisely define specific metabolic pathways, especially APP metabolism, endocytosis, inflammatory and immune responses, and lipid metabolic processes. AD being a genetically complicated disease, each of the genetic variants, when considered individually, exert little effect on disease risk (Odds Ratio= 1.1–1.3). Despite the considerable progress in genetic studies, a significant part of AD remains associated with a rare set of unknown genetic factors.[93] To identify and isolate these rare gene variants, current researchers are largely focused on targeted resequencing of known risk loci, along with WGS and WES. This would lead to improved understanding of the fundamental pathogenic mechanisms, proteins, and metabolic pathways for development of precision therapy.

The hypothesized mechanisms explaining AD progression have led to the development of drugs that have been through elaborate trials, though the results have not been promising and the ongoing treatment procedures have very little effect. This has motivated researchers to initiate therapeutic intervention earlier during the course of progression but a significant reason for the failure to find an efficient treatment plan is the reflection of AD as a disease that is homogenous. The molecular and risk profiles of individuals afflicted with AD exhibit a wide variation, and the profiles and parameters of such patients cannot be treated as a single unit as a few groups of patients may respond to a particular treatment strategy. Thus, precision medicine is applicable to AD and any other disease that has heterogeneous molecular and clinical profiles.

6.8   MAJOR LIMITATIONS IN DEVELOPMENT OF PERSONALIZED MEDICINES

Nanomedicines are being rapidly developed as therapeutics in personalized therapy, but their clinical application is poor, suggesting various limitations that need to be addressed before introducing nano therapy for clinical application. The main challenges in the clinical application of nanomedicines are associated with their biological safety and the cost incurred in production and therapy. Likewise, precision medicine identifies and targets an individual's genome for a specific disease and has social, ethical, and legal implications.[94] Toxicity induced by nanomedicines, cannot be determined by a standard parameter. Nanomedicines can be a safety threat to biological systems, as the morphology and physicochemical features have an impact on the distribution of NPs and their interaction with the membranes in circulation. Acute toxicity is observed as inflammation, oxidative stress, hemolysis, and other effects specific to the organ affected, while chronic toxicity happens after a long time and is generally not treated.[95] Successful implementation of the therapeutic and an assessment of their toxicity can be related to the physicochemical features of both NP and the drug, along with the chemicals and processes used for their synthesis. Nanomedicine has a complex three-dimensional composition with multiple constituents, each of which serves different functions. Their complex constitution necessitates the requirement of advanced analytical tests for comprehensive detection, characterization, and measurement of each component, along with evaluation of the interrelationship between the nanocarrier and drug and also between the drug-loaded nanocarrier and the biological environment. Additionally, the stability and storage of these NPs-based therapeutics needs to be assessed; hence, the lipids and polymers required for their synthesis need investigation.[96] Translation of nanomedicine into a personalized drug requires extensive synthesis, along with a high level of reproducibility. Generally, nanocarriers loaded with drugs are produced in laboratories for clinical studies. Moreover, extensive production is hampered by the complicated configuration of different NPs, even the minutest aberration in production can lead to critical modifications in the specific characteristics of these NPs. An appropriate ratio of the NP, loaded drug, crosslinking agent, organic solvent, emulsifier, temperature, and pH must be maintained. Furthermore, large-scale production of personalized nanomedicines requires an expensive multistep process, costly even for clinical research. Approval for new nanomedicines by regulatory authorities is another challenge, especially if therapeutics with similar efficacy are commercially available and researchers are more focused on ameliorating the biodistribution, availability, and effectiveness of conventional drugs.[97] Moreover, deficient practices in manufacturing NPs, poor quality control, safety, and efficacy evaluation make their implementation as a therapeutic more challenging. The expenses required for developing a precision medicine are also very high and the process requires long-term funding with very few chances of success. The techniques required for DNA sequencing and designing a nanomedicine add to the expenses. The molecular and genetic causes of the disease need to be interpreted for designing a personalized treatment plan, which reduces the chances of failure and also improves the comprehension of an individual's state.[25,98] Clinical trials for the development of a precision and personalized treatment plan should be individualized to match the dynamic pattern of diseases. These personalized therapies, though new, have exhibited promising results in the treatment of epilepsy, cystic fibrosis, a few types of cancer, and diseases with genetic etiology. More clinical trials need to be conducted to test the efficacy of precision medicine, with simultaneous gene sequencing for identifying various subtypes of the disease. Smaller clinical trials are more efficient for testing the effects of a precision medicine. Researchers investigated a small group of individuals suffering from a specific disease and proposed that the efficacy of a precision therapy varied and chances of failure were high in a regular clinical trial. For example, a drug used in cystic fibrosis, ivacaftor (Kalydeco), was approved in 2012 for specific genetic mutations but was effective in only about 4% of the patients. Hence, clinical trials on smaller specific groups may give effective results and quick approval of the drug. Studies on defining and designing improved randomized studies are necessary to increase the commercial translation of precision medicine. Innovative strategies have been developed to collect genomic data effectively and actively, which is essential for matching specific genomic modifications with distinct therapies. These strategies include studies with adaptive designs, umbrella trials, basket trials, and platform trials. Adaptive clinical trials are designed to adjust to the data analyzed, with the objective of changing one or more specific parameters of the research design. Likewise, an umbrella design or a master trial is a design in which patients are included on the basis of a specific tumor, which is sub-classified by virtue of specific molecular changes coordinated with various anticancer therapies. On the contrary, in a basket trial, different tumor types with a common molecular alteration are identified and treated with the same matched therapy. The platform trials gauge different therapeutics or target groups specific for one or more diseases by continuing changes in sub-studies.[99,100]

6.9 CONCLUSION

The emerging field of personalized/precision medicine employs an accurate and personalized diagnosis based on the genetic/molecular profile of an individual and the therapeutic strategy is targeted for that specific pathologic condition. It reviews the genetic and environmental features of an individual or a cohort of such individuals for the development of an effective treatment plan with minimal adverse reactions.

Personalized medicine exploits use of nanomaterials for enhancing drug binding affinity; for improved compatibility and bioavailability; and for achieving maximum efficacy along with a regulated drug release to facilitate accuracy in drug targeting.

With the development of genetic/molecular therapeutics, our knowledge about drug action and pathophysiology has increased significantly. Drugs act at the molecular level, which is the key for development of an effective and personalized precision therapy. In the last few decades, molecular advancements have enabled researchers to develop an optimal treatment plan with effective results, especially in oncology. The enhanced awareness of the human genome and use of next-generation sequencing (NGS) have significantly boosted the development of precision therapeutics. Though in routine clinical practice, genetic sequencing plays a minuscule role and requires extensive trials before translating into commercial application. NGS will undoubtedly have an increased usage in personalized therapy, not only with respect to specific genetic panels but also with reference to whole exome and whole genome sequencing. Another emerging technique is the use of "liquid biopsies," in which cell-free DNA (cfDNA) procured from plasma is analyzed. cfDNA analysis can change both drug development and clinical care, especially in oncology. With enhanced knowledge of molecular processes and disease heterogeneity, a novel assay may be developed, which can amalgamate different types of "omics" data, like proteomics, genomics, micro-biomics, and metabolomics into a "composite biomarker." This strategy can merge several pathophysiological elements and the mechanisms of drug action. Though such trials will face many challenges with respect to development, validation, and interpretation of results, as well as with regard to its clinical implementation.

Personalized/precision medicine evolves from the idea of refining and customizing pharmacotherapy. In pharmacotherapeutics, we have observed that one size does not fit all, and Langreth and Waldholz named the endeavors of individualizing treatment as personalized medicine. The attempts to reach the objective of "targeting drugs for each unique genetic profile" will proceed with enhanced perseverance in years to come.

REFERENCES

1. Srivastava P. Drug metabolism and individualized medicine. *Curr Drug Metab.* 2005;4(1):33–44. doi:10.2174/1389200033336829

2. Baker M. Reprogramming Rx. *Nat Med.* 2011;17(3):243. doi:10.1038/NM0311-241
3. Gravitz L. A fight for life that united a field. *Nature.* 2011;478(7368):163–164. doi: 10.1038/478163A
4. Graham-Rowe D. Overview: multiple lines of attack. *Nature.* 2011;480(7377): S34–S35. doi:10.1038/480s34a
5. Boguski MS, Arnaout R, Hill C. Customized care 2020: how medical sequencing and network biology will enable personalized medicine. *F1000 Biol Rep.* 2009;1. doi:10.3410/B1-73
6. Trusheim MR, Berndt ER, Douglas FL. Stratified medicine: strategic and economic implications of combining drugs and clinical biomarkers. *Nat Rev Drug Discov.* 2007;6(4):287–293. doi:10.1038/nrd2251
7. Hood L. A personal journey of discovery: developing technology and changing biology. *Annu Rev Anal Chem.* 2008;1:1–43. doi:10.1146/ANNUREV.ANCHEM.1 .031207.113113
8. Gibson WM. Can personalized medicine survive? *Can Fam Physician.* 1971; 17(8):29. Accessed December 14, 2022. https://www.ncbi.nlm.nih.gov/pmc/articles/ PMC2370041/
9. Gupta R, Kim J, Spiegel J, Ferguson SM. Developing products for personalized medicine: NIH Research Tools Policy applications. *Per Med.* 2004;1(1):115–124. doi:10.1517/17410541.1.1.115
10. Burke W, Psaty BM. Personalized medicine in the era of genomics. *JAMA.* 2007;298(14):1682–1684. doi:10.1001/JAMA.298.14.1682
11. Meyer UA. Personalized medicine: a personal view. *Clin Pharmacol Ther.* 2012;91(3):373–375. doi:10.1038/CLPT.2011.238
12. Sieber BA, Landis S, Koroshetz W, et al. Prioritized research recommendations from the National Institute of Neurological Disorders and Stroke Parkinson's Disease 2014 conference. *Ann Neurol.* 2014;76(4):469–472. doi:10.1002/ANA.24261
13. Bobo D, Robinson KJ, Islam J, Thurecht KJ, Corrie SR. Nanoparticle-based medicines: a review of FDA-approved materials and clinical trials to date. *Pharm Res.* 2016;33(10):2373–2387. doi:10.1007/S11095-016-1958-5
14. Nikzamir M, Akbarzadeh A, Panahi Y. An overview on nanoparticles used in biomedicine and their cytotoxicity. *J Drug Deliv Sci Technol.* 2021;61. doi:10.1016/ J.JDDST.2020.102316
15. Davis ME, Chen Z, Shin DM. Nanoparticle therapeutics: an emerging treatment modality for cancer. *Nat Rev Drug Discov.* 2008;7(9):771–782. doi:10.1038/ nrd2614
16. Kalia M. Personalized oncology: recent advances and future challenges. *Metabolism.* 2013;62(Suppl 1). doi:10.1016/J.METABOL.2012.08.016
17. Roller BT, McNeeley KM, Bellamkonda R. Multifunctional nanoparticles for personalized medicine. In *Multifunctional Nanoparticles for Drug Delivery Applications.* 2012:277–293. doi:10.1007/978-1-4614-2305-8_13
18. Ryu JH, Lee S, Son S, et al. Theranostic nanoparticles for future personalized medicine. *J Control Release.* 2014;190:477–484. doi:10.1016/J.JCONREL.2014.04.027
19. Jokerst JV, Gambhir SS. Molecular imaging with theranostic nanoparticles. *Acc Chem Res.* 2011;44(10):1050–1060. doi:10.1021/AR200106E
20. Zhang XQ, Xu X, Bertrand N, Pridgen E, Swami A, Farokhzad OC. Interactions of nanomaterials and biological systems: implications to personalized nanomedicine. *Adv Drug Deliv Rev.* 2012;64(13):1363–1384. doi:10.1016/J.ADDR.2012.08.005
21. Arachchige MCM, Reshetnyak YK, Andreev OA. Advanced targeted nanomedicine. *J Biotechnol.* 2015;202:88–97. doi:10.1016/J.JBIOTEC.2015.01.009
22. Mitragotri S, Anderson DG, Chen X, et al. Accelerating the translation of nanomaterials in biomedicine. *ACS Nano.* 2015;9(7):6644. doi:10.1021/ACSNANO.5B03569

23. Jiang W, von Roemeling CA, Chen Y, et al. Designing nanomedicine for immuno-oncology. *Nat Biomed Eng.* 2017;1(2):1–11. doi:10.1038/s41551-017-0029

24. Fornaguera C, García-Celma MJ. Personalized nanomedicine: a revolution at the nanoscale. *J Pers Med.* 2017;7(4). doi:10.3390/JPM7040012

25. Goetz LH, Schork NJ. Personalized medicine: motivation, challenges, and progress. *Fertil Steril.* 2018;109(6):952–963. doi:10.1016/J.FERTNSTERT.2018.05.006

26. Alghamdi MA, Fallica AN, Virzì N, Kesharwani P, Pittalà V, Greish K. The promise of nanotechnology in personalized medicine. *J Pers Med.* 2022;12(5). doi:10.3390/JPM12050673

27. Li Y, Meng Q, Yang M, et al. Current trends in drug metabolism and pharmaco-kinetics. *Acta Pharm Sin B.* 2019;9(6):1113–1144. doi:10.1016/j.apsb.2019.10.001

28. Rahman N, Stratton MR. The genetics of breast cancer susceptibility. *Annu Rev Genet.* 1998;32:95–121. doi:10.1146/ANNUREV.GENET.32.1.95

29. Chen S, Parmigiani G. Meta-analysis of BRCA1 and BRCA2 penetrance. *J Clin Oncol.* 2007;25(11):1329–1333. doi:10.1200/JCO.2006.09.1066

30. Goldenberg MM. Trastuzumab, a recombinant DNA-derived humanized mono-clonal antibody, a novel agent for the treatment of metastatic breast cancer. *Clin Ther.* 1999;21(2):309–318. doi:10.1016/S0149-2918(00)88288-0

31. Moja L, Tagliabue L, Balduzzi S, et al. Trastuzumab containing regimens for early breast cancer. *Cochrane Database Syst Rev.* 2012;2012(4). doi:10.1002/14651858.CD006243.PUB2

32. Pineda M, González S, Lázaro C, Blanco I, Capellá G. Detection of genetic alterations in hereditary colorectal cancer screening. *Mutat Res – Fundam Mol Mech Mutagen.* 2010;693(1–2):19–31. doi:10.1016/J.MRFMMM.2009.11.002

33. Karapetis CS, Khambata-Ford S, Jonker DJ, et al. K-ras mutations and benefit from cetuximab in advanced colorectal cancer. *N Engl J Med.* 2008;359(17):1757–1765. doi:10.1056/NEJMOA0804385

34. Wheeler DL, Dunn EF, Harari PM. Understanding resistance to EGFR inhibitors-impact on future treatment strategies. *Nat Rev Clin Oncol.* 2010;7(9):493–507. doi: 10.1038/NRCLINONC.2010.97

35. Smith BD. Imatinib for chronic myeloid leukemia: the impact of its effectiveness and long-term side effects. *J Natl Cancer Inst.* 2011;103(7):527–529. doi:10.1093/JNCI/DJR073

36. Is Imatinib Still an AccepTable 6. First-Line Treatment for CML in Chronic Phase? Accessed December 14, 2022. https://www.cancernetwork.com/view/imatinib-still-accepTable6.-first-line-treatment-cml-chronic-phase

37. Tsai J, Lee JT, Wang W, et al. Discovery of a selective inhibitor of oncogenic B-Raf kinase with potent anti melanoma activity. *Proc Natl Acad Sci U S A.* 2008;105(8):3041–3046. doi:10.1073/PNAS.0711741105

38. Chapman PB, Hauschild A, Robert C, et al. Improved survival with vemurafenib in melanoma with BRAF V600E mutation. *N Engl J Med.* 2011;364(26):2507–2516. doi:10.1056/NEJMOA1103782

39. Jackson SE, Chester JD. Personalised cancer medicine. *Int J Cancer.* 2015;137(2):262–266. doi:10.1002/IJC.28940

40. Gatz M, Reynolds CA, Fratiglioni L, et al. Role of genes and environments for explaining Alzheimer's disease. *Arch Gen Psychiatry.* 2006;63(2):168–174. doi:10.1001/ARCHPSYC.63.2.168

41. Montine TJ, Montine KS. Precision medicine: clarity for the clinical and biological complexity of Alzheimer's and Parkinson's diseases. *J Exp Med.* 2015;212(5):601–605. doi:10.1084/JEM.20150656

42. Zou ZY, Liu CY, Che CH, Huang HP. Toward precision medicine in amyotrophic lateral sclerosis. *Ann Transl Med.* 2016;4(2):27. doi:10.3978/j.issn.2305-5839. 2016.01.16

43. Berkovic SF, Scheffer IE, Petrou S, et al. A roadmap for precision medicine in the epilepsies. *Lancet Neurol.* 2015;14(12):1219–1228. doi:10.1016/S1474-4422(15) 00199-4

44. Seshadri S, Fitzpatrick AL, Ikram MA, et al. Genome-wide analysis of genetic loci associated with Alzheimer's disease. *JAMA.* 2010;303(18):1832–1840. doi:10.1001/ JAMA.2010.574

45. Collins FS, Varmus H. A new initiative on precision medicine. *N Engl J Med.* 2015;372(9):793–795. doi:10.1056/NEJMP1500523

46. Titova N, Chaudhuri KR. Personalized medicine in Parkinson's disease: Time to be precise. *Mov Disord.* 2017;32(8):1147–1154. doi:10.1002/MDS.27027

47. Shutinoski B, Hakimi M, Harmsen IE, et al. Lrrk2 alleles modulate inflammation during microbial infection of mice in a sex-dependent manner. *Sci Transl Med.* 2019;11(511):eaas9292–eaas9292. doi:10.1126/SCITRANSLMED.AAS9292

48. Rassu M, del Giudice MG, Sanna S, et al. Role of LRRK2 in the regulation of dopamine receptor trafficking. *PLoS One.* 2017;12(6):e0179082–e0179082. doi:1 0.1371/JOURNAL.PONE.0179082

49. Shin N, Jeong H, Kwon J, et al. LRRK2 regulates synaptic vesicle endocytosis. *Exp Cell Res.* 2008;314(10):2055–2065. doi:10.1016/J.YEXCR.2008.02.015

50. Tong Y, Yamaguchi H, Giaime E, et al. Loss of leucine-rich repeat kinase 2 causes impairment of protein degradation pathways, accumulation of alpha-synuclein, and apoptotic cell death in aged mice. *Proc Natl Acad Sci U S A.* 2010;107(21): 9879–9884. doi:10.1073/PNAS.1004676107

51. Trabzuni D, Ryten M, Emmett W, et al. Fine-mapping, gene expression and splicing analysis of the disease associated LRRK2 locus. *PLoS One.* 2013;8(8):e70724. doi: 10.1371/JOURNAL.PONE.0070724

52. Nichols WC, Pankratz N, Hernandez D, et al. Genetic screening for a single common LRRK2 mutation in familial Parkinson's disease. *Lancet.* 2005;365(9457): 410–412. doi:10.1016/S0140-6736(05)17828-3

53. di Fonzo A, Rohé CF, Ferreira J, et al. A frequent LRRK2 gene mutation associated with autosomal dominant Parkinson's disease. *Lancet.* 2005;365(9457):412–415. doi:10.1016/S0140-6736(05)17829-5

54. Gilks WP, Abou-Sleiman PM, Gandhi S, et al. A common LRRK2 mutation in idiopathic Parkinson's disease. *Lancet.* 2005;365(9457):415–416. doi:10.1016/ S0140-6736(05)17830-1

55. Funayama M, Hasegawa K, Kowa H, Saito M, Tsuji S, Obata F. A new locus for Parkinson's disease (PARK8) maps to chromosome 12p11.2-q13.1. *Ann Neurol.* 2002;51(3):296–301. doi:10.1002/ANA.10113

56. Zimprich A, Biskup S, Leitner P, et al. Mutations in LRRK2 cause autosomal-dominant parkinsonism with pleomorphic pathology. *Neuron.* 2004;44(4):601–607. doi:10.1016/j.neuron.2004.11.005

57. Ross OA, Wu YR, Lee MC, et al. Analysis of Lrrk2 R1628P as a risk factor for Parkinson's disease. *Ann Neurol.* 2008;64(1):88–92. doi:10.1002/ANA. 21405

58. Tan EK, Peng R, Wu YR, et al. LRRK2 G2385R modulates age at onset in Parkinson's disease: a multi-center pooled analysis. *Am J Med Genet B Neuropsychiatr Genet.* 2009;150B(7):1022–1023. doi:10.1002/AJMG.B.30923

59. Gloeckner CJ, Kinkl N, Schumacher A, et al. The Parkinson's disease causing LRRK2 mutation I2020T is associated with increased kinase activity. *Hum Mol Genet.* 2006;15(2):223–232. doi:10.1093/HMG/DDI439

60. Mabrouk OS, Chen S, Edwards AL, Yang M, Hirst WD, Graham DL. Quantitative measurements of LRRK2 in human cerebrospinal fluid demonstrates increased levels in G2019S patients. *Front Neurosci.* 2020;14:526. doi:10.3389/FNINS.2020.00526/BIBTEX

61. Tolosa E, Vila M, Klein C, Rascol O. LRRK2 in Parkinson disease: challenges of clinical trials. *Nat Rev Neurol.* 2020;16(2):97–107. doi:10.1038/S41582-019-0301-2

62. di Maio R, Hoffman EK, Rocha EM, et al. LRRK2 activation in idiopathic Parkinson's disease. *Sci Transl Med.* 2018;10(451). doi:10.1126/SCITRANSLMED.AAR5429

63. von Linstow CU, Gan-Or Z, Brundin P. Precision medicine in Parkinson's disease patients with LRRK2 and GBA risk variants – Let's get even more personal. *Transl Neurodegener.* 2020;9(1). doi:10.1186/S40035-020-00218-X

64. Parkin JL, Brunning RD. Pathology of the Gaucher cell. *Prog Clin Biol Res.* 1982;95:151–175. Accessed December 14, 2022. https://europepmc.org/article/med/7122633

65. Stirnemann JÔ, Belmatoug N, Camou F, et al. A review of gaucher disease pathophysiology, clinical presentation and treatments. *Int J Mol Sci.* 2017;18(2). doi:10.3390/IJMS18020441

66. Liu J, Halene S, Yang M, et al. Gaucher disease gene GBA functions in immune regulation. *Proc Natl Acad Sci U S A.* 2012;109(25):10018–10023. doi:10.1073/PNAS.1200941109

67. O'Regan G, Desouza RM, Balestrino R, Schapira AH. Glucocerebrosidase mutations in Parkinson's disease. *J Parkinsons Dis.* 2017;7(3):411–422. doi:10.3233/JPD-171092

68. Hruska KS, LaMarca ME, Scott CR, Sidransky E. Gaucher disease: mutation and polymorphism spectrum in the glucocerebrosidase gene (GBA). *Hum Mutat.* 2008;29(5):567–583. doi:10.1002/HUMU.20676

69. Goker-Alpan O, Schiffmann R, LaMarca ME, Nussbaum RL, McInerney-Leo A, Sidransky E. Parkinsonism among Gaucher disease carriers. *J Med Genet.* 2004;41(12):937–940. doi:10.1136/JMG.2004.024455

70. Liu G, Boot B, Locascio JJ, et al. Specifically neuropathic Gaucher's mutations accelerate cognitive decline in Parkinson's. *Ann Neurol.* 2016;80(5):674. doi:10.1002/ANA.24781

71. Guerreiro R, Ross OA, Kun-Rodrigues C, et al. Investigating the genetic architecture of dementia with Lewy bodies: a two-stage genome-wide association study. *Lancet Neurol.* 2018;17(1):64–74. doi:10.1016/S1474-4422(17)30400-3

72. Sidransky E, Nalls MA, Aasly JO, et al. Multicenter analysis of glucocerebrosidase mutations in Parkinson's disease. *N Engl J Med.* 2009;361(17):1651–1661. doi:10.1056/NEJMOA0901281

73. Do J, McKinney C, Sharma P, Sidransky E. Glucocerebrosidase and its relevance to Parkinson disease. *Mol Neurodegener.* 2019;14(1). doi:10.1186/s13024-019-0336-2

74. Alcalay RN, Levy OA, Waters CC, et al. Glucocerebrosidase activity in Parkinson's disease with and without GBA mutations. *Brain.* 2015;138(Pt 9):2648–2658. doi:10.1093/BRAIN/AWV179

75. Mullin S, Smith L, Lee K, et al. Ambroxol for the treatment of patients with Parkinson disease with and without glucocerebrosidase gene mutations: a nonrandomized, noncontrolled trial. *JAMA Neurol.* 2020;77(4):427–434. doi:10.1001/JAMANEUROL.2019.4611

76. Silveira CRA, MacKinley J, Coleman K, et al. Ambroxol as a novel disease-modifying treatment for Parkinson's disease dementia: protocol for a single-centre, randomized, double-blind, placebo-controlled trial. *BMC Neurol.* 2019;19(1). doi: 10.1186/S12883-019-1252-3

77. de Matteis L, Martín-Rapún R, de la Fuente JM. Nanotechnology in personalized medicine: a promising tool for Alzheimer's disease treatment. *Curr Med Chem.* 2018;25(35):4602–4615. doi:10.2174/0929867324666171012112026

78. Duyckaerts C, Delatour B, Potier MC. Classification and basic pathology of Alzheimer's disease. *Acta Neuropathol.* 2009;118(1):5–36. doi:10.1007/S00401-009-0532-1

79. Dugger BN, Serrano GE, Sue LI, et al. Presence of striatal amyloid plaques in Parkinson's disease dementia predicts concomitant Alzheimer's disease: usefulness for amyloid imaging. *J Parkinsons Dis.* 2012;2(1):57–65. doi:10.3233/JPD-2012-11073

80. Attems J, Jellinger KA. The overlap between vascular disease and Alzheimer's disease – lessons from pathology. *BMC Med.* 2014;12(1). doi:10.1186/S12916-014-0206-2

81. Ertekin-Taner N. Genetics of Alzheimer's disease: a centennial review. *Neurol Clin.* 2007;25(3):611–667. doi:10.1016/J.NCL.2007.03.009

82. Kim M, Suh J, Romano D, et al. Potential late-onset Alzheimer's disease-associated mutations in the ADAM10 gene attenuate α-secretase activity. *Hum Mol Genet.* 2009;18(20):3987–3996. doi:10.1093/HMG/DDP323

83. Lambert JC, Heath S, Even G, et al. Genome-wide association study identifies variants at CLU and CR1 associated with Alzheimer's disease. *Nat Genet.* 2009;41(10):1094–1099. doi:10.1038/NG.439

84. Harold D, Abraham R, Hollingworth P, et al. Genome-wide association study identifies variants at CLU and PICALM associated with Alzheimer's disease. *Nat Genet.* 2009;41(10):1088–1093. doi:10.1038/NG.440

85. Naj AC, Jun G, Beecham GW, et al. Common variants at MS4A4/MS4A6E, CD2AP, CD33 and EPHA1 are associated with late-onset Alzheimer's disease. *Nat Genet.* 2011;43(5):436–443. doi:10.1038/NG.801

86. Cruchaga C, Chakraverty S, Mayo K, et al. Rare variants in app, PSEN1 and PSEN2 increase risk for AD in late-onset Alzheimer's disease families. *PLoS One.* 2012;7(2):e31039. doi:10.1371/JOURNAL.PONE.0031039

87. Lambert JC, Ibrahim-Verbaas CA, Harold D, et al. Meta-analysis of 74,046 individuals identifies 11 new susceptibility loci for Alzheimer's disease. *Nat Genet.* 2013;45(12):1452–1458. doi:10.1038/NG.2802

88. Guerreiro R, Wojtas A, Bras J, et al. TREM2 variants in Alzheimer's disease. *N Engl J Med.* 2013;368(2):117–127. doi:10.1056/NEJMOA1211851

89. Jonsson T, Stefansson H, Steinberg S, et al. Variant of TREM2 associated with the risk of Alzheimer's disease. *N Engl J Med.* 2013;368(2):107–116. doi:10.1056/NEJMOA1211103

90. Cruchaga C, Karch CM, Jin SC, et al. Rare coding variants in the phospholipase D3 gene confer risk for Alzheimer's disease. *Nature.* 2014;505(7484):550–554. doi:10.1038/NATURE12825

91. Logue MW, Schu M, Vardarajan BN, et al. Two rare AKAP9 variants are associated with Alzheimer's disease in African Americans. *Alzheimers Dement.* 2014;10(6):609–618.e11. doi:10.1016/J.JALZ.2014.06.010

92. Tosto G, Fu H, Vardarajan BN, et al. F-box/LRR-repeat protein 7 is genetically associated with Alzheimer's disease. *Ann Clin Transl Neurol.* 2015;2(8):810–820. doi:10.1002/ACN3.223

93. Reitz C. Genetic loci associated with Alzheimer's disease. *Future Neurol.* 2014; 9(2):119–122. doi:10.2217/FNL.14.1

94. Liu X, Luo X, Jiang C, Zhao H. Difficulties and challenges in the development of precision medicine. *Clin Genet.* 2019;95(5):569–574. doi:10.1111/CGE.13511/

95. Metselaar JM, Lammers T. Challenges in nanomedicine clinical translation. *Drug Deliv Transl Res.* 2020;10(3):721–725. doi:10.1007/s13346-020-00740-5

96. Hua S, de Matos MBC, Metselaar JM, Storm G. Current trends and challenges in the clinical translation of nanoparticulate nanomedicines: Pathways for translational development and commercialization. *Front Pharmacol.* 2018;9(JUL). doi:10.3389/FPHAR.2018.00790/FULL

97. Wu LP, Wang D, Li Z. Grand challenges in nanomedicine. *Mater Sci Eng C Mater Biol Appl.* 2020;106. doi:10.1016/J.MSEC.2019.110302

98. McGrath SP, Peabody AE, Walton D, Walton N. Legal challenges in precision medicine: what duties arising from genetic and genomic testing does a physician owe to patients? *Front Med (Lausanne).* 2021;8. doi:10.3389/FMED.2021.663014/FULL

99. Garralda E, Dienstmann R, Piris-Giménez A, Braña I, Rodon J, Tabernero J. New clinical trial designs in the era of precision medicine. *Mol Oncol.* 2019;13(3):549–557. doi:10.1002/1878-0261.12465

100. Li A, Bergan RC. Clinical trial design: past, present, and future in the context of big data and precision medicine. *Cancer.* 2020;126(22):4838–4846. doi:10.1002/CNCR.33205

7 Nanotherapeutics and Rheumatoid Arthritis

Different Types of Nanomedicines Used in Arthritis

Monika Rani, Kumar Rakesh Ranjan, and Vivek Mishra

7.1 INTRODUCTION: OVERVIEW OF RHEUMATOID ARTHRITIS

The term arthritis is derived from the Greek word for "joint inflammation." The most prevalent type of arthritis, osteoarthritis, is caused by the breakdown of the cartilage that covers the bones in the joints. Rheumatoid arthritis (RA) is a condition in which the immune system attacks the joints, starting with the joint lining as the body interprets this soft lining as a threat, similar to virus or bacteria (Figure 7.1). Osteoarthritis typically develops later in life, after years of mechanical wear and strain on the cartilage that lines and cushions the joints. RA is an autoimmune illness, which means that the immune system unintentionally attacks healthy cells in the body, that can strike at any age. Clinically, RA may be distinguished from osteoarthritis (OA) because RA affects the proximal interphalangeal (PIP) and metacarpophalangeal (MP) joints, whereas OA commonly affects the distal interphalangeal (DIP) joint[1,2]. Another distinguishing feature is that RA patients have chronic morning stiffness for at least one hour. Morning stiffness is common in OA patients, although it usually fades or reduces within 20–30 minutes.

Dr. Augustin Jacob Landré-Beauvais (1772–1840) of Paris published the first accepted description of RA in 1800[3]. It is named after the Greek word for fluid and inflamed joints. RA is a symmetrical, long-lasting, autoimmune condition, leading to inflammation (painful swelling) in the area of the body affected. The body fails to distinguish between self and foreign substances. Studies[4] over the years have identified multiple cells types (including T and B cells) as key regulators of immunologic events in RA. The involvement of B cells has lately[5] received a lot of interest because it was discovered that B-cell-depleting medication (anti-CD20 monoclonal antibodies or rutiximab) is effective in RA. T cells, too, have been identified as important mediators in the pathophysiology of RA. T cells are abundant in the synovium of RA patients, and they contribute to the inflammatory

DOI: 10.1201/9781003348672-7

143

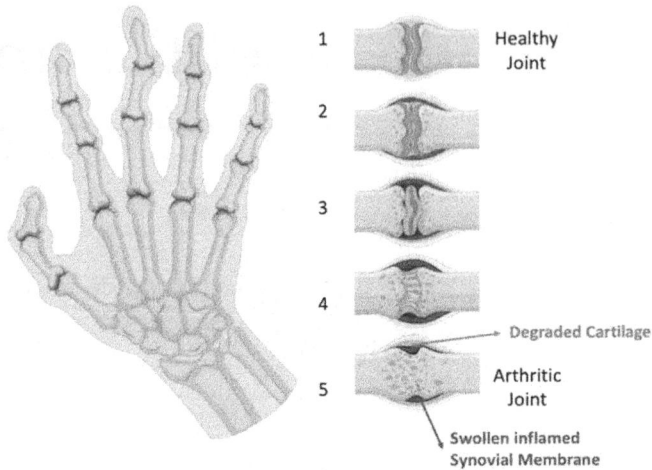

FIGURE 7.1   Rheumatoid arthritis schematic illustration.

response by producing cytokines and interacting with other cells that promote inflammation and joint destruction. RA is initially inflammatory beginning with minor joints, expanding to larger joints, and subsequently the kidneys, lungs, heart, skin, and eyes in severe cases. This results in long-term incapacity, an inability to engage fully in social interactions and day-to-day activities, and a rise in mortality rates, all of which have a significant negative influence on the patient's quality of life. It affects 1% of the general population worldwide, with women two to four times as likely as men to develop the disease[6]. While RA affects a number of organs and lymphoid tissues on a systemic level, the synovium in inflamed joints is the site of inflammation (Figure 7.1) (Synovium tissue: a connective tissue layer that lines the bursae (fluid-filled sacs between tendons and bones), tendon sheaths, and joint cavities. The lubricating synovial fluid is produced by the synovial membrane. RA increases the risk of developing osteoporosis: a condition that weakens bones and makes them prone to fracture), rheumatoid nodules (firm bumps of tissue), Sjogren's syndrome (a disorder that decreases moisture in eyes and mouth), etc (Figure 7.2).

The onset of disease differs between patients depending on the type, number, and sequence of joint involvement. The severity of the inflammatory process and the presence or absence of several variables, such as genetic background, frequency of swollen joints, autoantibodies in the serum, may also influence the course of the disease. Environmental factors including smoking, dust inhalation, and microbiota infection may potentially hasten the onset of RA in addition to increased immunological reactivity[7]. To relieve the inflammatory response and pathological progression of RA symptoms, therapeutic medication, surgical treatment, and routine adjustments such as moderate exercise and nutritional supplements are generally used, depending on the severity of the symptoms. The purposes of therapy for RA are to minimize joint inflammation and discomfort, enhance joint function, and avoid joint deterioration and deformities.

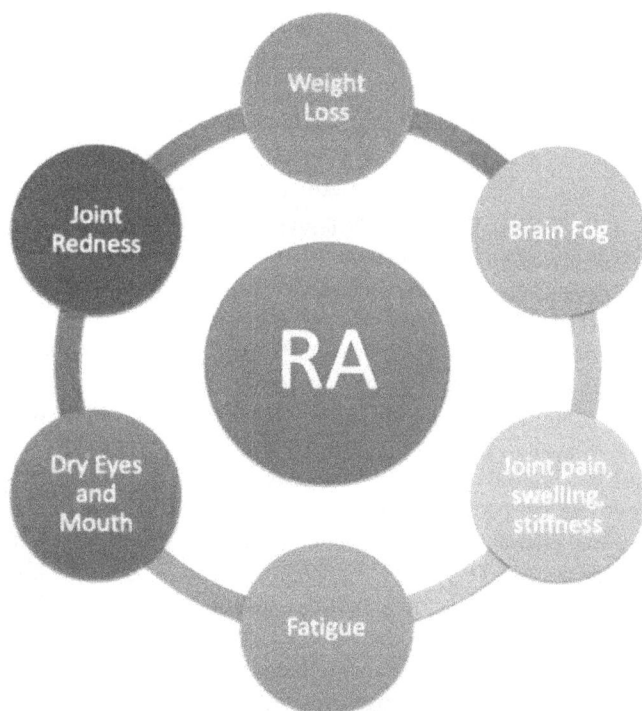

FIGURE 7.2   Symptoms and effects of RA.

Early diagnosis is considered to be the primary advancement indicator for attaining the most positive consequences (i.e., reduced joint destruction, less radiologic progression, no functional disability, and disease-modifying anti-rheumatic drug (DMARD)-free remission) as well as cost-effectiveness, as the first 12 weeks following the onset of early symptoms are regarded as the optimal therapeutic window[8,9]. However, early diagnosis remains difficult because it is predominantly dependent on clinical information gleaned from the subject's history and physical examination, which is supplemented by blood tests and imaging studies. While there is presently no cure for RA, the treatment plan attempts to accelerate diagnosis and attain a low disease activity level as quickly as possible (LDAS). This chapter highlights the use of nanomedicines in the treatment of RA.

7.2   CURRENT DIAGNOSIS AND TREATMENTS FOR RA

Early diagnosis and treatment of RA can alter the course of the disease, stop joint erosions from developing, or slow the course of erosive disease. However, in patients with early disease, it can be challenging to distinguish the joint manifestations from other types of inflammatory polyarthritis. The more recogniz-able symptoms of RA, such as joint erosions and rheumatoid nodules, are typically absent at the time of initial presentation and are more common in people with long-term, poorly controlled disease. The lack of an independent gold standard in RA diagnosis research is a concern[10]. There are no disease-specific clinical, radiological, or immunological characteristics of RA. Currently, it is advised that practitioners follow the RA classification standard for diagnosis that was released by the ACR/EULAR[11] in 2010 and the American College of Rheumatology (ACR) in 1987. However, such a diagnosis is primarily based on physical examination and observation of recognizable symptoms, like pain, morning stiffness, and swelling of several joints in bilaterally symmetrical patterns[12]. This makes early RA diagnosis nearly hard because a true clinical diagnosis can only be made once a disease has developed for six months to a year. The 2018 Chinese guideline for the diagnosis and management of RA was created in consideration of this by the Chinese Rheumatology Association. The most common techniques involve imaging methods and serological examinations. The early diagnosis and prognosis of RA can both benefit greatly from RA-specific antibodies. The autoantibodies against antigens containing one or more citrulline residues (cyclic citrulline peptides, CCP)—the anti-CCP antibodies—are the most promising candidates among the antibodies identified in recent years. Recent studies[13] have demonstrated that they are crucial to the diagnosis, prognosis, and treatment of RA patients. The anti-CCP will likely become a crucial serologic marker in the future due to its high specificity, capacity to detect RA early in its development, and ability to distinguish it from other types of non-erosive arthritis. On the contrary, imaging techniques might help us comprehend the mechanisms that happen in the joint(s) during inflammatory arthritis. Conventional radiography, ultrasonography, computed tomography, and magnetic resonance imaging are among the imaging diagnostic techniques for RA (MRI). More information about the examination for RA can be found elsewhere[14,15].

The primary goals of treatment for RA patients are to reduce pain and inflammation, and the ultimate objective is for all patients to achieve remission or at the least, minimal disease activity. According to data from several observational cohorts and clinical studies, starting therapy during the first 12 weeks after the commencement of the disease is particularly successful at reducing disease activity and improving mid- and long-term outcomes[16]. Early 20th-century treatments for RA were mostly based on gold therapy[17], which involved administering gold salts orally or by injection. In the mid-20th century, Penicillamine, a penicillin derivative, was first shown to reduce RA disease activity when compared to a placebo, making it another potential force. Although these treatment options for RA were effective, they were also frequently associated with harmful side effects[18]. The treatment is complicated, encompassing not only many medication classes with various modes of administration, but also nonpharmacologic therapies A comprehensive approach that combines medical, social, and emotional care for the patient is necessary for the best treatment of RA.. Treatments are typically tailored to the needs of the patient and are based on their overall health. Patient education is the most critical, followed by exercise and physical and occupational treatment. Because smoking, hyperlipidaemia, hypertension, and obesity are risk factors for coronary atherosclerosis, efforts should be taken to minimize them. The European League Against Rheumatism (EULAR) has created 10 global recommendations on how to manage patients in this situation[19].

Non-steroidal anti-inflammatory drugs (NSAIDs), corticosteroids, and disease-modifying anti-rheumatic therapies (DMARDs) are the three main groups of

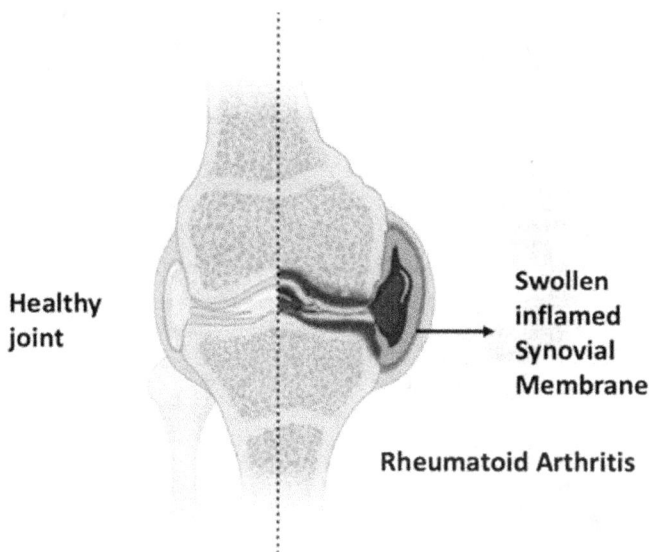

Healthy joint

Swollen inflamed Synovial Membrane

Rheumatoid Arthritis

FIGURE 7.3   Healthy joint vs RA affected joint.

medications frequently used to treat rheumatoid arthritis, alongside small molecule drugs and biologics (Figure 7.3).

While DMARDs can take weeks or months to have a clinical effect, NSAIDs and corticosteroids have a quick beginning of action. Due to NSAIDs' potent anti-inflammatory and analgesic properties, they are frequently used in rheumatology. They mainly work by preventing cyclooxygenase (COX) enzyme activity; however, there are drawbacks, such as organ toxicity and the lack of a disease-progression effect. The chemical class of NSAIDs varies greatly, but they all have the property of inhibiting prostaglandin synthesis (PGs). These include aspirin, ibuprofen (commercially sold as Advil, Motrin), naproxen (Aleve), etc. Conventional synthetic DMARDs, such as methotrexate, targeted synthetic DMARDs, such as Janus kinase inhibitors, and biological DMARDs are the three categories of DMARDs (biological medicines or bDMARD). However, long-term use of DMARDs frequently causes kidney, skin, and mucous membrane toxicity as well as infection brought on by immunosuppression. The most widely used DMARDs is methotrexate (MTX), which is frequently recommended as a first-line treatment for RA. Other review papers[20,21] offer more specific information on each drug category. RA patients take corticosteroids like prednisolone, dexamethasone, and betamethasone as anti-inflammatory medications. Leukocyte migration is inhibited, and the production of inflammatory cytokines is downregulated, according to the known mechanism of action. Biological treatments come in a vast variety, but their relative efficacy is still up for debate. Three TNF inhibitors, etanercept, infliximab, and adalimumab, are the best-selling medications in any class, with $26.5 billion in estimated sales in 2012[22]. Unfortunately, major complications from the usage of these biologics may occur, leaving patients susceptible to severe infections like tuberculosis.

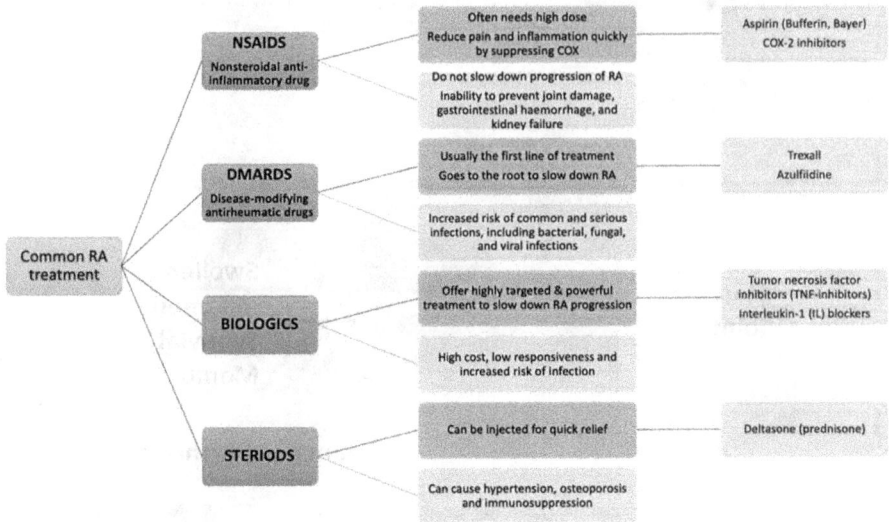

FIGURE 7.4   Common RA treatments with their pros and cons.

Despite expanding treatment choices (Figure 7.4), RA remains a difficult illness to treat since currently prescribed regimens seldom result in a cure (remission) and are frequently linked with the development of drug resistance and side effects and only a minority of patients attain and maintain disease remission without the requirement for ongoing immunosuppressive therapy.

Traditional Chinese medicine (TCM), which includes preparations including sinomenine, total glycosides of paeony, and preparations derived from the plant Tripterygium, has been used to treat RA in China. There are demonstrable therapeutic benefits and a low frequency of negative effects associated with the use of TCM substances in clinical practise. TCM substances have the ability to lessen toxicity and improve therapy efficacy through drug compatibility. However, the substantial variations in the ingredients and dose of various formulations make their use more challenging. Therefore, it's critical to find ways to circumvent these drugs' drawbacks for treating RA. Recent studies[23] have demonstrated that different nanomaterials can transport anti-RA medications by modulating macrophages. Furthermore, due to the variability of the patients, the ideal and successful treatment strategy for an individual cannot be anticipated at this time, forcing "trials and mistakes" that raise expenses and delay clinical response. As a result, developing novel treatment options for RA remains a top goal.

Nonetheless, with a greater understanding of the pathophysiology of RA, new therapeutic methods are emerging to provide individuals with precision therapy. Adverse effects caused by the non-selective activity of currently accessible RA therapeutics can be whittled down by enclosing these active substances in nanocarriers for a more targeted approach to administering the drugs at the desired site of action (i.e., the joints) by avoiding frequent or high dosing, resulting in an effective drug concentration locally. The most important strategy used by leading companies in the global rheumatoid arthritis treatment market to keep ahead of the competition is research and development. Nanotechnology is such a multi-dimensional method that employs a wide range of tools and techniques aimed at disease diagnosis and therapeutic agent delivery through the use of submicrometric size carriers, or nanocarriers.

7.3 NANOTECHNOLOGY FOR INFLAMMATION CONTROL

Today's treatment options include the use of steroidal or nonsteroidal anti-inflammatory medications. However, these treatments are not always enough to provide maximal pharmacological activity. Non-specific biodistribution, limited bioavailability, and/or a short half-life in the body are all examples of drug limitations. Furthermore, considerable doses must be delivered to patients, resulting in off-target adverse effects and only little efficacy in treating inflammatory disease symptoms. To overcome some of these constraints, the usage of nanoparticles (NPs) ranging in size from several tenths to a few hundred nanometers has grown in popularity. Biocompatible nanomedicines (NPs loaded with active components) with highly regulated shape, size, and surface charge are now possible.

Nanoparticles can concentrate efficiently in inflammatory microenvironments of arthritic joints characterized by angiogenic arteries and an aberrant peripheral lymphatic system, the development of nanomedicine in RA has recently acceler-ated. Indeed, nanoparticles (NPs) can be deliberately tailored to travel selectively to the target tissue from the site of administration, solving traditional therapy concerns such as off-target organ adverse effects and systemic toxicity, which are increased by frequent and long-term dosage. Considerable emphasis has been paid to the development of more potent anti-inflammatory nanomedicines in order to overcome the negative effects found with traditional therapy.

7.4 NANOMEDICINES FOR RA

The development of all nanosized instruments for clinical diagnosis, prevention, and therapy falls under the purview of "nanomedicine." A significant amount of previous research has produced strategies for adding therapeutic compounds to biocompatible nanodevices, such as polymer nanoparticles, liposomes, micellar systems, inorganic nanoparticles, nanotubes, and dendrimers. The research on nanomedicine in RA has significantly increased since nanoparticles can concentrate effectively in inflammatory microenvironments of arthritic joints marked by angiogenic arteries and an abnormal peripheral lymphatic system. Nanoparticles (NPs) have the potential for drug delivery applications due to their high surface-area-to-volume ratio, surface functionalization with targeting ligands, compact scale (as various proteins can be attached to their surface), high drug loading efficiency, multi-modality imaging capability, passive and/or active targeting effects. Therapeutic or imaging agents can be delivered selectively and continuously to the targeted inflammation sites using nanoscale drug carriers. By doing so, it is possible to significantly improve the therapeutic effects of conventional anti-RA medications while obviating the side effects that are brought on by their short biological half-life and low bioavailability. Notably, nanomaterials give synergistic multifunctional nanomedicine a strong framework into which numerous therapeutic and/or imaging agents can be incorporated. Delivery methods based on nanomedicine have great opportunities to enhance and maximize current therapeutic alternatives while avoiding the frequent side effects of immunosuppressives and biologics. The clinical utility of novel nanomedicine technologies for inducing immunosuppression and immunological tolerance in autoimmune illnesses to correct immune malfunction is being recognized[24]. With improved anti-inflammatory and analgesic properties, nanoparticles have also overcome selenium's poor bioavailability and toxicity as reported by El-Ghazaly et al.[25]

In RA, utilizing nanocarriers capable of simultaneously serving as a diagnostic imaging agent and a targeted drug delivery system, also known as nanotheranostics, may allow for an increased effectiveness and safety pharmacologic profile, rapid diagnosis, and disease tracking. When medications or bioactive molecules are delivered specifically to cells or tissues that display a tissue-specific molecular signature that distinguishes them from healthy tissues in the body, it is known as a targeted drug delivery system. The release and activity of anti-rheumatic drugs can thus be increased and maintained successfully without causing injury to healthy tissues and organs, while also providing a non-invasive and precise imaging tool for RA. Due to its excellent specificity, nanomedicine has also played a significant role in the diagnosis of inflammatory arthritis with increased sensitivity, cost-effectiveness, and reduced overdiagnosis. Nanomaterial drug delivery is superior to traditional therapy due to its improved targeted specificity via controlled drug release, higher ability to solubilize hydrophobic medicines, additive combinatorial chemistry, and superior drug delivery ability. Several nanostructures nourished with improved drug delivery in treating inflammatory arthritis include NSAID-based metallic and polymeric NP conjugates (chitosan-dexamethasone NPs), surface-engineered liposomes, human serum albumin NPs (arginine-glycine aspartic acid attached with gold nano half-shells conjugated with methotrexate).

The primary use of traditional nanoparticles in the management of rheumatoid arthritis is the administration of anti-inflammatory drugs. Nanomaterials have enhanced the targeting specificity of drugs used in drug delivery systems, as well as the drugs' biodistribution, permeability, intracellular delivery, and capacity to cross biological membranes. By modifying the carrier's surface in different ways, drugs can be transported to the joint site, boosting drug accumulation there and augmenting pharmacological effects. There are now drug-release nanocarriers on the market (nanomedicines collectively), including liposomes, micelles, polymeric and solid lipid nanoparticles, inorganic nanoparticles, and sub-micrometric emulsions. Moreover, antibodies, polymer-protein conjugates, and polymer-drug conjugates are categorized as nanomedicines[26].

Nanomedicines may indeed be produced to: shield the therapeutic agent from deterioration, prolong blood circulation, and be customized for macrophage absorption or directed at specific receptors as inter endothelial cell gaps are typically 1–2 nm, in healthy tissues but can reach 600 nm in diseased tissues or sick tissues, such as swollen joints[27]. However, when building nanomedicine, it is important to take into account the characteristics of the active chemical to be administered, the biological site, the atmosphere before and around the the target sites.

7.5 PASSIVE AND ACTIVE DELIVERY OF NANOMEDICINES

Nanomedicines, a hybrid of nanotechnology and medicine, use nanotechnology to deliver pharmaceuticals passively or actively to specific tissues, cells, or subcellular domains. These techniques are ideally intended to optimize medication uptake, therapeutic concentration, and longevity, resulting in successful drug targeting. Because of the widespread systemic nature of inflammation, the most crucial aspect for the management of RA and other inflammatory process illnesses is increased permeability and retention. Synthesis of properly sized (10-1000 nm) nanoparticles and surface modification with appropriate functional groups might improve their circulation duration, thereby giving optimum advantage in executing their targeted activity[28]. The nanomedicine concentrates in the affected joints either actively or passively due to improved permeability and retention effect.

Typically, active targeting makes use of both selective and high-affinity binding to increase therapeutic efficacy. Nanomedicines with active targeting capability must first surmount three obstacles in order to be effective in alleviating RA[29]: (a) reticuloendothelial system, (b) inflamed vascular endothelium, and (c) appropriate ligands coupled to the nanoplatforms. Thus, when constructing nanocarriers, appropriate ligands, a sufficient size (10–100 nm), and surface charge should be considered. Through many processes, including adsorption, covalent coupling, ligand-receptor attachment[30], and internalization, nanoparticles can enter the systemic circulation.

Numerous in vivo biodistribution studies have validated the passive targeting of these[31,32] nanocarriers to inflamed tissues based on increased permeability. The primary element influencing the passive targeting method is particle size. Ishihara et al. investigated the size of nanoparticles ranging from 45 to 115 nm and discovered that 115 nm nanoparticles have the greatest anti-inflammatory capacity[33]. The second element is the surface chemistry. The most popular technique, known as PEGylation, involves coating the surface of the nanomedicine with polyethylene glycol (PEG). PEGylated nanomedicine is shown to collect more on inflamed synovium but to be less removed by the spleen and liver[34]. Similar to size, shape is a key characteristic of NPs that is important for the biological tasks for which they are intended. In general, NPs are spherical in form. Recent years have seen the emergence of many NP shapes and forms with novel geometrical, physical, and chemical properties thanks to enhanced nanofabrication techniques. It affects the biodistribution and the pace of a nanoparticle's uptake by macrophages. Margination can also be improved by changing a nanoparticle's shape. Non-spherical particles are shown to marginate and exit the blood flow more easily[35]. Because the microenvironment of RA and tumors is comparable, it is plausible to assume that the form of nanocarriers influences passive targeting efficacy in RA, despite the fact that research on particle shape tends to concentrate on tumors (Figure 7.5).

Studies of nanomedicines for potential treatment of RA are summarized in Table 7.1. These include in vitro, in vivo, and clinical investigations utilizing nanomedicines for targeted drug delivery to diseased tissues in RA animal models or patients.

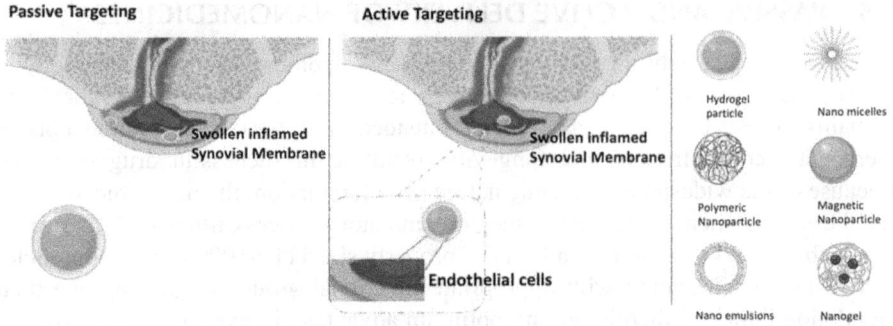

FIGURE 7.5 Schematic illustration of the passive and active targeting delivery system of nanocarriers for treatment of rheumatoid arthritis and different types of nanocarriers.

TABLE 7.1

Studies of Nanomedicines for Potential Treatment of RA

Therapy Type	Drug	Nano-Drug Delivery System	Targeting Mechanism	Phase	Ref.
NSAID	Piroxicam	Liposomes	Macrophage uptake	Preclinical, *In vitro*	36
Gold salts	Gold salts	Nanoparticles	Macrophage uptake	Preclinical, *In vitro*	37
Corticosteroid	Betamethasone	PEGylated polymersomes	Passive	Preclinical, *In vivo*	33
Corticosteroid	Dexamethasone	PEGylated liposomes; liposomes	Passive	Preclinical, *In vivo*	38

Nonsteroidal anti-inflammatory drugs (NSAIDs) are typically prescribed to manage pain, stiffness, and inflammation while also improving patient physical function; corticosteroids, which also have anti-inflammatory, anti-angiogenic, and immunoregulatory properties, allow for the promotion of a reduction in the expression of cellular adhesion molecules and cytokines on endothelial cells and thereby prevent joint erosions.

7.6 POLYMERIC NANOPARTICLES

The active ingredient in polymeric nanoparticles ranges in size from 1 to 1000 nm and is either trapped inside the polymeric core or has been adsorbed onto the surface of the polymeric core. These have been used for RA treatment recently because the leaky nature of the vasculature enables them to passively accumulate into inflamed synovial tissues[39].

Zheng et al.[40] created nanoparticles using triptolide that were grafted with poly—glutamic acid and di-tert-butyl L-aspartate hydrochloride (PAT). These particles had an average diameter of 79 nm, a narrow polydispersity index of 0.18, a strong zeta potential of -32 mV, and high drug encapsulation efficiency (EE1) and loading. In vivo, research revealed that tumor necrosis factor transgenic mice had a higher survival rate than TP animals and fewer adverse effects. The effective development of new nanoparticles decreased toxicity and boosted efficacy. When mice were injected with 2 mg/kg of free triptolide, all of the mice died on day two, and when mice were injected with 1 mg/kg of free triptolide, all of the mice died on day seven. These findings clearly demonstrated that triptolide's toxicity was reduced when encapsulated in a nanoparticulate system. However, when mice were given 0.5 mg/kg of TP injections, the livability was 70%.

Micelles encapsulating Cy7-dodecylamine accumulated within the inflamed joints of mice model of antibody-induced arthritis, according to Ishihara et al.[41] The glucocorticoid betamethasone was then enclosed within these micelles and administered intravenously. After one day, a single dose resulted in a 35% reduction in paw inflammation, which lasted for nine days. Even at three times the dose, this reaction outperformed a free betamethasone injection.

Polymers, lipids, and inorganic nanostructures can all be used to create nanomedicines. Liposomes, PEGylated liposomes, polymersomes, micelles, dendrimers, and hydrogel nanoparticles are examples of lipid-, polymer-, and hybrid lipid-polymer-based nanomedicines that are often used for intravenous (IV) delivery.

7.7 INORGANIC NANOPARTICLES

The study of therapeutic inorganic nanoparticles (INPs) has had a significant influence on medical sciences. INPs have been applied in biomedicine for both therapeutic and diagnostic purposes. As an illustration, gold nanoparticles (AuNPs) have attracted a lot of attention because of their biocompatibility and the simplicity with which their size distribution and structure (spheres, nanorods, and cubes) can be controlled. Additionally, conjugating different polymers, antibodies, small-molecule drugs, and molecular probes with AuNPs makes it simple to change their surface chemistry. AuNPs may be prepared using wet chemistry, and their form and size can be precisely regulated to satisfy specific requirements. Other than shape, the surface AuNP may be readily changed, resulting in biomolecule conjugations with improved biocompatibility. Because of AuNPs' flexible chemistry, it is simpler to conjugate medicinal and/or contrast chemicals onto AuNPs. Lee et al.[42] synthesized an HA-AuNP/TCZ (hyaluronate gold nanoparticle/Tocilizumab) combination for the treatment of RA. They used the immunosuppressive tocilizumab as a monoclonal antibody to target the interleukin-6 (IL-6) receptor. The citrate technique was used to synthesize gold nanoparticles. They achieved a particle diameter of 64.83 nm and a polydispersity index of 0.18 for the HA-AuNP/TCZ combination. They discovered that TCZ was steadily released from the HA-AuNP/TCZ complex for up to 8 days following incubation in bovine serum albumin. They also discovered that the generated HA-AuNP/TCZ combination had an anti-angiogenic effect on the growth of HUVEC cells by binding to the VEGF receptor[42]. Recent[43] research has linked the downregulation of inflammatory mediators like TNF-, IL-1, COX-2, and transcription factor to nanogold's anti-inflammatory properties. NF-kB (Nuclear factor-kB) (Nuclear factor-kB).

Iron oxide nanoparticles (IONPs) are another type of INP that has been widely used for diagnostic therapeutic and imaging reasons since the 1960s. The generation of superparamagnetic iron oxide nanoparticles with potential effects on human immune cell survival, activity, and as a theranostics in rheumatic disorders has been achieved[44]. The intra-articular adsorption rate of superparamagnetic iron oxide nanoparticles (SPIONs) coated with poly-vinyl-alcohol (PVA-SPIONS) via the synovial membrane in an animal model was investigated by another group of researchers[45]. The NPs were identified in the synovium for nearly a week, indicating that such systems could provide a viable platform for intra-articular medication delivery, particularly for the treatment of acute or chronic joint disorders.

Many studies have reported the use of nanoparticles differently than discussed here. However, only a few nanoparticles have been approved for therapeutic usage, with the majority remaining in the clinical testing stage. At present, iron, gold, and cerium NPs are extensively employed in the treatment of RA.

7.8 NANOMICELLES

Nanomicelles are ultramicroscopically small globular formations with hydrophilic polar heads on the outside and a hydrophobic fatty acyl chain on the inside. Nanomicelles are well-organized supramolecular structures produced by amphiphilic molecules self-assembling in aqueous conditions. Among the drug-delivery systems, nanomicelles have piqued the interest of nanomedicine researchers due to their inexpensive cost, high biocompatibility, simple fabrication methods, and effectiveness. Fan et al.[46] devised a new formulation for RA that included curcumin and hyaluronic acid [HA/Cur] spherical nanomicelles with a diameter of 164 nm. When fed to RA-induced rats, the expression of associated cytokines and vascular endothelial growth factor was observed to be reduced. The HA/ Cur sample had the lowest frictional coefficient of 0.027 0.006, demonstrating that micro micelles can greatly reduce frictional coefficient between joints. Paw edema investigations also revealed that inflammation was reduced from 100 to 60%. Furthermore, friction between the surfaces of cartilage around the joints was shown to be significantly reduced, indicating the potential of nanomicelle for RA treatment. The newly discovered nanomicelles has the potential to be used in clinical practise of RA therapy, considerably reducing pain and enhancing patients' quality of life.

7.9 LIPOSOMES

Nowadays, a number of rheumatoid arthritis medications use the liposome system to increase their effectiveness. These nanocarriers were first to achieve the market recognition in 1995. Liposomes are administered intravenously, accumulating in the synovial tissue of RA patients. When cholesterol and phosphatidylcholine liposomes encapsulated with clodronate are delivered to arthritic rats, bone resorption is reduced due to anti-inflammatory effects. Though several innovative drug delivery technologies have appeared during the last two decades for the targeted administration of anti-rheumatoid medicines to synovial fluid, liposomes provide a convenient and effective drug delivery capable of decreasing side effects due to the following advantages[47,48]: (1) they are adaptable, non-toxic, biodegradable, biocompatible, and nonimmunogenic; (2) they provide both a lipophilic and an aqueous environment "milieu interne" in one system, making them useful for the administration of pharmaceuticals with different solubility profiles, such as hydrophobic, amphipathic, and hydrophilic compounds.

Polyethylene glycol (PEG) is a powerful hydrophilic polymer that can decrease liposome localization and absorption by the reticuloendothelial system (RES), extending the time liposomes spend in the systemic circulation. Wang et al.[49] demonstrated that polymerized stealth liposomes are stable in blood arteries and have a long circulation period. To increase the impact of dexamethasone in the treatment of arthritis, Wang et al. employed polymeric stealth liposomes as a carrier. They prepared the liposome by thin film hydration using 1,2-bis(10, 12-tricosadiynoyl)-sn-glycero-3-phosphocholine (DC89PC) and 1,2-distearoylsn-glycero-3-phospho-ethanolamine-poly(ethyleneglycol) (DSPE-PEG2000), and the PEG chains supplied a stealth layer. After being injected into arthritic rats, the liposomes preferentially aggregate in inflamed joints, limit the amount of pro-inflammatory factors in joint tissues, and diminish the swelling of inflamed joints. This work demonstrates that polymeric stealth liposomes may be exploited as a novel drug delivery vehicle for a variety of therapeutic applications.

Ulmansky et al.[50] investigated the anti-inflammatory impact of sterically stabilized nanoliposomes of methylprednisolone hemisuccinate and betamethasone hemisuccinate in adjuvant arthritis. Both nano-liposome formulations substantially inhibited arthritis when compared to larger dosages of free medication or TNF-antagonists (infliximab, etanercept).

Glucocorticoids are commonly used to treat RA patients and are regarded as powerful anti-inflammatory medicines; however, the specific mechanism of action of this family of pharmaceuticals is unknown. Because of the EPR effect, encapsulating them in liposomes enables for more local distribution and accumulation at inflammation sites, decreasing systemic adverse effects and improving therapeutic efficiency.

However, despite being the most often utilized nanocarriers for RA therapy, the impact of liposomes' physical and chemical features, such as sizes, surface charges, polyethylene glycol (PEG) chain length, and PEG concentrations, on their passive RA targeting effect are not well known. Further research will open paths for more effective targeted delivery.

7.10   CONCLUSION

The goal of therapeutic delivery is to improve patient care by allowing the administration of new complex medications, increasing the bioavailability of existing treatments, and offering spatial and temporal targeting of drugs to reduce adverse effects and increase efficiency.[51-57] Over the past few decades, there have been many developments in drug delivery, and it is now more important than ever to link the published findings in order to acquire deeper knowledge and establish a solid foundation for future research on novel ideas. NPs might be a viable method for improving rheumatoid arthritis diagnosis and therapy options. NPs can perform imaging, efficient transport, and medication delivery to specific target sites. As a result, nanoparticles can be employed to increase the therapeutic and pharmacological qualities of RA-fighting medications. The inclusion of NPs into therapeutic molecules aids in the preservation of the drug while also assuring constant targeting and release.

However, resolving the issue of how nanotechnology may be employed industrially while still protecting health, safety, and the environment remains a major difficulty. It should be noted that gold, even though it is well tolerated by the body, is not a biodegradable material and may remain for a long time inside the body, as previously demonstrated in a mouse model, despite systemic administration of these nanoparticles producing a significant anti-inflammatory activity in vivo on various mouse models.

Attempts have been made to develop strategies that will enable various industrial processes to scale up, with new methods becoming safer and easier to maintain.

REFERENCES

1. McGonagle, D., Hermann, K.G.A. and Tan, A.L., 2015. Differentiation between osteoarthritis and psoriatic arthritis: implications for pathogenesis and treatment in the biologic therapy era. *Rheumatology 54*(1): 29–38.
2. Piyarulli, D. and Koolaee, R.M., 2016. A 22-year-old female with joint pain. *Medicine Morning Report: Beyond the Pearls*. Philadelphia: Elsevier: 65–77.
3. Landré-Beauvais, A.J., 2001. The first description of rheumatoid arthritis. Unabridged text of the doctoral dissertation presented in 1800. *Joint Bone Spine 68*(2): 130–143.
4. McInnes, I.B. and O'Dell, J.R., 2010. State-of-the-art: rheumatoid arthritis. *Annals of the Rheumatic Diseases 69*(11): 1898–1906.
5. Edwards, J.C. and Cambridge, G., 2006. B-cell targeting in rheumatoid arthritis and other autoimmune diseases. *Nature Reviews Immunology 6*(5): 394–403.
6. Birch, J.T. and Bhattacharya, S., 2010. Emerging trends in diagnosis and treatment of rheumatoid arthritis. *Primary Care: Clinics in Office Practice 37*(4): 779–792.
7. Kim, K., Bang, S.Y., Lee, H.S. and Bae, S.C., 2017. Update on the genetic architecture of rheumatoid arthritis. *Nature Reviews Rheumatology 13*(1): 13–24.
8. van der Linden, M.P., Le Cessie, S., Raza, K., van der Woude, D., Knevel, R., Huizinga, T.W. and van der Helm-van Mil, A.H., 2010. Long-term impact of delay in assessment of patients with early arthritis. *Arthritis & Rheumatism 62*(12): 3537–3546.
9. Cho, S.K., Kim, D., Won, S., Lee, J., Choi, C.B., Choe, J.Y., Hong, S.J., Jun, J.B., Kim, T.H. and Koh, E., 2019. Factors associated with time to diagnosis from symptom onset in patients with early rheumatoid arthritis. *The Korean Journal of Internal Medicine 34*(4): 910.
10. Visser, H., 2005. Early diagnosis of rheumatoid arthritis. *Best Practice & Research Clinical Rheumatology 19*(1): 55–72.
11. Arnett, F.C., Edworthy, S.M., Bloch, D.A., Mcshane, D.J., Fries, J.F., Cooper, N.S., Healey, L.A., Kaplan, S.R., Liang, M.H., Luthra, H.S. and Medsger Jr, T.A., 1988. The American Rheumatism Association 1987 revised criteria for the classification of rheumatoid arthritis. *Arthritis & Rheumatism: Official Journal of the American College of Rheumatology 31*(3): 315–324.
12. Majithia, V. and Geraci, S.A., 2007. Rheumatoid arthritis: diagnosis and management. *The American Journal of Medicine 120*(11): 936–939.

13. Staikova, N.D., Kuzmanova, S.I. and Solakov, P.T., 2003. Serologic markers of early rheumatoid arthritis. *Folia Medica 45*(3): 35–42.
14. https://www.arthritis-health.com/types/rheumatoid/rheumatoid-arthritis-ra-diagnosis.
15. https://www.uptodate.com/contents/diagnosis-and-differential-diagnosis-of-rheumatoid-arthritis/print.
16. Monti, S., Montecucco, C., Bugatti, S. and Caporali, R., 2015. Rheumatoid arthritis treatment: the earlier the better to prevent joint damage. *RMD Open 1*(Suppl 1): e000057.
17. Norn, S., Permin, H., Kruse, P.R. and Kruse, E., 2011. History of gold–with Danish contribution to tuberculosis and rheumatoid arthritis. *Dansk Medicinhistorisk Arbog 39*: 59–80.
18. Suarez-Almazor, M.E., Belseck, E. Spooner, C., and Cochrane Musculoskeletal Group. 1996. Penicillamine for treating rheumatoid arthritis. *Cochrane Database of Systematic Reviews* 2011(10):1–43.
19. Smolen, J.S., Landewé, R., Breedveld, F.C., Dougados, M., Emery, P., Gaujoux-Viala, C., Gorter, S., Knevel, R., Nam, J., Schoels, M. and Aletaha, D., 2010. EULAR recommendations for the management of rheumatoid arthritis with synthetic and biological disease-modifying antirheumatic drugs. *Annals of the Rheumatic Diseases 69*(6): 964–975.
20. Zhang, N., Li, M., Hou, Z., Ma, L., Younas, A., Wang, Z., Jiang, X. and Gao, J., 2022. From vaccines to nanovaccines: a promising strategy to revolutionize rheumatoid arthritis treatment. *Journal of Controlled Release 350*: 107–121.
21. Crofford, L.J., 2013. Use of NSAIDs in treating patients with arthritis. *Arthritis Research & Therapy 15*(3): 1–10.
22. Jeske, W., Walenga, J.M., Hoppensteadt, D. and Fareed, J., 2013. Update on the safety and bioequivalence of biosimilars–focus on enoxaparin. *Drug, Healthcare and Patient Safety 5*: 133.
23. Li, S., Su, J., Cai, W. and Liu, J.X., 2021. Nanomaterials manipulate macrophages for rheumatoid arthritis treatment. *Frontiers in Pharmacology 12*: 699245.
24. Gharagozloo, M., Majewski, S. and Foldvari, M., 2015. Therapeutic applications of nanomedicine in autoimmune diseases: from immunosuppression to tolerance induction. *Nanomedicine: Nanotechnology, Biology and Medicine 11*(4): 1003–1018.
25. El-Ghazaly, M.A., Fadel, N., Rashed, E., El-Batal, A. and Kenawy, S.A., 2017. Anti-inflammatory effect of selenium nanoparticles on the inflammation induced in irradiated rats. *Canadian Journal of Physiology and Pharmacology, 95*(2): 101–110.
26. Canal, F., Sanchis, J. and Vicent, M.J., 2011. Polymer–drug conjugates as nano-sized medicines. *Current Opinion in Biotechnology 22*(6): 894–900.
27. Revel, J.P. and Karnovsky, M., 1967. Hexagonal array of subunits in intercellular junctions of the mouse heart and liver. *The Journal of Cell Biology 33*(3): C7.
28. Katsuki, S., Matoba, T., Koga, J.I., Nakano, K. and Egashira, K., 2017. Anti-inflammatory nanomedicine for cardiovascular disease. *Frontiers in Cardiovascular Medicine 4*: 87.
29. Chen, M., Daddy JC, K.A., Xiao, Y., Ping, Q. and Zong, L., 2017. Advanced nanomedicine for rheumatoid arthritis treatment: focus on active targeting. *Expert Opinion on Drug Delivery 14*(10): 1141–1144.
30. Behzadi, S., Serpooshan, V., Tao, W., Hamaly, M.A., Alkawareek, M.Y., Dreaden, E.C., Brown, D., Alkilany, A.M., Farokhzad, O.C. and Mahmoudi, M., 2017. Cellular uptake of nanoparticles: journey inside the cell. *Chemical Society Reviews 46*(14): 4218–4244.
31. Hofkens, W., Schelbergen, R., Storm, G., van den Berg, W.B. and van Lent, P.L., 2013. Liposomal targeting of prednisolone phosphate to synovial lining macrophages during experimental arthritis inhibits M1 activation but does not favor M2 differentiation. *PLoS One, 8*(2): e54016.

32. Mello, S.B., Tavares, E.R., Bulgarelli, A., Bonfá, E. and Maranhão, R.C., 2013. Intra-articular methotrexate associated to lipid nanoemulsions: anti-inflammatory effect upon antigen-induced arthritis. *International Journal of Nanomedicine 8*: 443.

33. Ishihara, T., Takahashi, M., Higaki, M., Mizushima, Y. and Mizushima, T., 2010. Preparation and characterization of a nanoparticulate formulation composed of PEG-PLA and PLA as anti-inflammatory agents. *International Journal of Pharmaceutics 385*(1-2): 170–175.

34. Mitragotri, S. and Yoo, J.W., 2011. Designing micro-and nano-particles for treating rheumatoid arthritis. *Archives of Pharmacal Research 34*(11): 1887–1897.

35. Truong, N.P., Whittaker, M.R., Mak, C.W. and Davis, T.P., 2015. The importance of nanoparticle shape in cancer drug delivery. *Expert Opinion on Drug Delivery, 12*(1): 129–142.

36. Chiong, H.S., Yong, Y.K., Ahmad, Z., Sulaiman, M.R., Zakaria, Z.A., Yuen, K.H. and Hakim, M.N., 2013. Cytoprotective and enhanced anti-inflammatory activities of liposomal piroxicam formulation in lipopolysaccharide-stimulated RAW 264.7 macrophages. *International Journal of Nanomedicine 8*: 1245.

37. Turk, C.T.S., Oz, U.C., Serim, T.M. and Hascicek, C., 2014. Formulation and optimization of nonionic surfactants emulsified nimesulide-loaded PLGA-based nanoparticles by design of experiments. *Aaps Pharmscitech 15*(1): 161–176.

38. Rauchhaus, U., Schwaiger, F.W. and Panzner, S., 2009. Separating therapeutic efficacy from glucocorticoid side-effects in rodent arthritis using novel, liposomal delivery of dexamethasone phosphate: long-term suppression of arthritis facilitates interval treatment. *Arthritis Research & Therapy 11*(6): 1–9.

39. Heo, R., You, D.G., Um, W., Choi, K.Y., Jeon, S., Park, J.S., Choi, Y., Kwon, S., Kim, K., Kwon, I.C. and Jo, D.G., 2017. Dextran sulfate nanoparticles as a theranostic nanomedicine for rheumatoid arthritis. *Biomaterials 131*: 15–26.

40. Zhang, L., Chang, J., Zhao, Y., Xu, H., Wang, T., Li, Q., Xing, L., Huang, J., Wang, Y. and Liang, Q., 2018. Fabrication of a triptolide-loaded and poly-γ-glutamic acid-based amphiphilic nanoparticle for the treatment of rheumatoid arthritis. *International Journal of Nanomedicine 13*: 2051.

41. Ishihara, T., Kubota, T., Choi, T. and Higaki, M., 2009. Treatment of experimental arthritis with stealth-type polymeric nanoparticles encapsulating betamethasone phosphate. *Journal of Pharmacology and Experimental Therapeutics 329*(2): 412–417.

42. Lee, S.M., Kim, H.J., Ha, Y.J., Park, Y.N., Lee, S.K., Park, Y.B. and Yoo, K.H., 2013. Targeted chemo-photothermal treatments of rheumatoid arthritis using gold half-shell multifunctional nanoparticles. *ACS Nano 7*(1): 50–57.

43. Khan, M.A. and Khan, M.J., 2018. Nano-gold displayed anti-inflammatory property via NF-kB pathways by suppressing COX-2 activity. *Artificial Cells, Nanomedicine, and Biotechnology 46*(suppl 1): 1149–1158.

44. Strehl, C., 2016. SP0049 nanoparticles and the immune system. *Annals of the Rheumatic Diseases 75*(2): 13.

45. Oliveira, I.M., Gonçalves, C., Reis, R.L. and Oliveira, J.M., 2018. Engineering nanoparticles for targeting rheumatoid arthritis: past, present, and future trends. *Nano Research 11*(9): 4489–4506.

46. Fan, Z., Li, J., Liu, J., Jiao, H. and Liu, B., 2018. Anti-inflammation and joint lubrication dual effects of a novel hyaluronic acid/curcumin nanomicelle improve the efficacy of rheumatoid arthritis therapy. *ACS Applied Materials & Interfaces 10*(28): 23595–23604.

47. Mufamadi, M.S., Pillay, V., Choonara, Y.E., Du Toit, L.C., Modi, G., Naidoo, D. and Ndesendo, V.M., 2011. A review on composite liposomal technologies for specialized drug delivery. *Journal of Drug Delivery* Vol 2011: Article ID 939851.

48. Gangwar, M., Singh, R., Goel, R.K. and Nath, G., 2012. Recent advances in various emerging vesicular systems: an overview. *Asian Pacific Journal of Tropical Biomedicine 2*(2): S1176–S1188.

49. Wang, Q., He, L., Fan, D., Liang, W. and Fang, J., 2020. Improving the anti-inflammatory efficacy of dexamethasone in the treatment of rheumatoid arthritis with polymerized stealth liposomes as a delivery vehicle. *Journal of Materials Chemistry B 8*(9): 1841–1851.

50. Ulmansky, R., Turjeman, K., Baru, M., Katzavian, G., Harel, M., Sigal, A., Naparstek, Y. and Barenholz, Y., 2012. Glucocorticoids in nano-liposomes administered intravenously and subcutaneously to adjuvant arthritis rats are superior to the free drugs in suppressing arthritis and inflammatory cytokines. *Journal of Controlled Release, 160*(2): 299–305.

51. Yadav, N., Mudgal, D., Anand, R., Jindal, S., & Mishra, V., 2022. Recent development in nanoencapsulation and delivery of natural bioactives through chitosan scaffolds for various biological applications. *International Journal of Biological Macromolecules, 220*: 537–572. 10.1016/j.ijbiomac.2022.08.098.

52. Narang, G., Bansal, D., Joarder, S., Singh, P., Kumar, L., Mishra, V., Singh, S., Tumba, K. and Kumari, K., 2023. A review on the synthesis, properties, and applications of graphynes. *FlatChem, 40*: 100517. 10.1016/j.flatc.2023.100517.

53. Yadav, N. and Mishra, V., 2024. Organic–inorganic hybrid materials as potential antimicrobial nanocoatings for medical device and implants. *Next-Generation Antimicrobial Nanocoatings for Medical Devices and Implants* (pp. 125–159). 10.1016/b978-0-323-95756-4.00011-7.

54. Yadav, N., Mudgal, D., Mishra, S., Sehrawat, H., Singh, N. K., Sharma, K., Sharma, P. C., Singh, J. and Mishra, V., 2023. Development of ionic liquid-capped carbon dots derived from Tecoma stans (L.) Juss. ex Kunth: combatting bacterial pathogens in diabetic foot ulcer pus swabs, targeting both standard and multi-drug resistant strains. *South African Journal of Botany, 163*: 412–426. 10.1016/j.sajb.2023.10.063.

55. Yadav, N., Mudgal, D. and Mishra, V., 2023. In-situ synthesis of ionic liquid-based-carbon quantum dots as fluorescence probe for hemoglobin detection. *Analytica Chimica Acta, 1272*: 341502. 10.1016/j.aca.2023.341502.

56. Yadav, N., Gaikwad, R. P., Mishra, V., & Gawande, M. B. (2022). Synthesis and photocatalytic applications of functionalized carbon quantum dots. *Bulletin of the Chemical Society of Japan*, 95, 1638–1679. 10.1246/bcsj.20220250.

57. Kumar, A., Yadav, A. K., Kumar, D. and Mishra, V., 2023. Recent advancements in triazole-based click chemistry in cancer drug discovery and development. *SynOpen, 07*: 186–208. 10.1055/s-0042-1751452.

8 The Discovery of Personalized Nanomedicine and Nanoparticulate Delivery System

Anil Kumar Mavi, Sonal Gaur, Dheeresh Kumar, Avanish Kumar Shrivastav, Srijita Chowdhury, Vivekanand Bahuguna, and Manoj Kumar

8.1 INTRODUCTION

The fusion of nanotechnology and medicine has given rise to the relatively new emerging field of nanomedicine (Yadav et al., 2023). Its foundation is the manipulation of matter at the nanoscale for uses in the area of human health (Yadav et al., 2022). By altering essential drug properties like solubility, diffusivity, bloodstream half-life, and drug release and distribution profiles, the usage of materials in this range has considerably advanced pharmacology (Zhang et al., 2008; van der Meel et al., 2019; Jain and Triantafyllos, 2010; Schaming et al., 2015). Although the creation and application of nanoparticle matter extend back hundreds of years (Reibold et al., 2006), the field of nanomedicine as we know it now just emerged at the end of the previous century. There is plenty of space below: An Invitation to Enter a New Field of Physics, Richard P. Feynman's 1959 address to the American Physical Society, is regarded by many authors as the fundamental text on nanotechnology (Feynman, 1961).

Feynman described a vision of technology in the future that advances toward the atomic scale and the ultimate restrictions imposed by physical laws. There were some novel suggestions, such as making computer-integrated circuits between 10 and 100 atoms in size (Figure 8.1). It is enough to keep in mind that a computer at the time he presented his ideas probably took up a complete room, if not several. This will help you comprehend the breadth of his forecasts. Feynman stuck to discussing the shrinking of devices and their potential uses; he didn't use the word (or the prefix) nano in his speech. In his speech titled "On the Basic Concept of Nanotechnology," Norio Taniguchi first used the word "nano" in 1974 (Taniguchi, 1974).

DOI: 10.1201/9781003348672-8

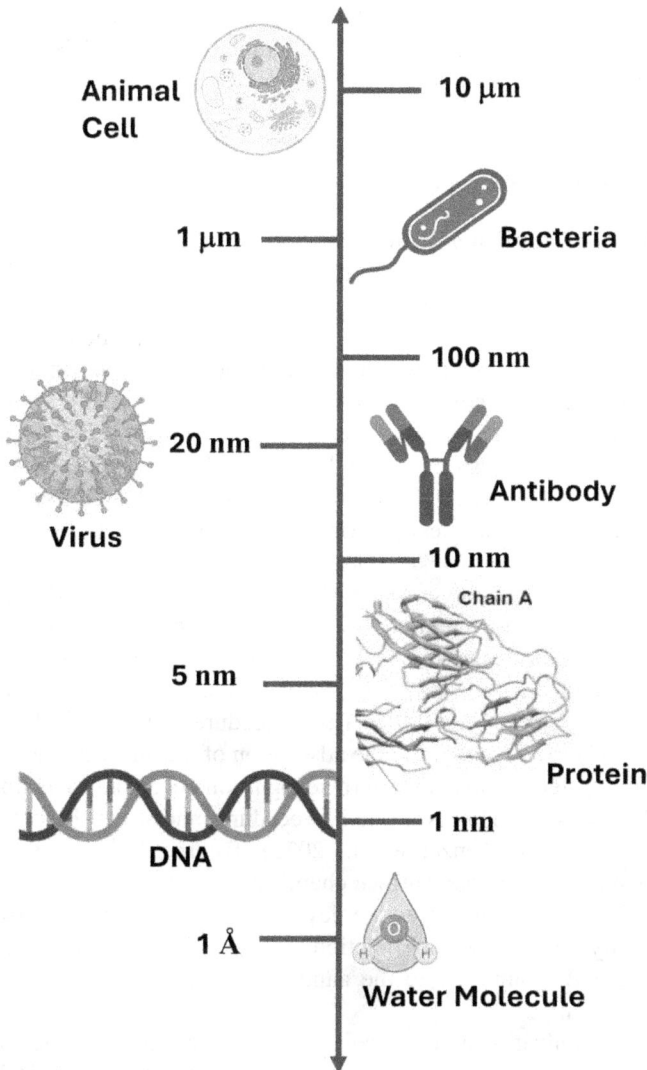

FIGURE 8.1 A scale bar is shown diagrammatically to relate the range of nanomaterials and nanosystems to biological components.

It must be made clear that when the term "nanotechnology" is used to study nanoparticles, it just designates the study of colloidal dispersions (Jindal et al., 2022). Michael Faraday made a significant contribution to this field in 1857 by publishing the first method for synthesizing metal nanoparticles, including gold (Faraday, 1857). Faraday is surprised by the modifications in the metallic colloidal dispersions' optical characteristics that were observed during the study. Gustav Mie finally solved the equations given by Maxwell for particles with a finite volume in 1908, explaining these characteristics (Mie, 1976).

Richard Zsigmondy received the Chemistry Nobel Prize in 1925 for proving the heterogeneity of colloidal dispersions (Zsigmondy, 1926). His methodological innovations have been essential for the study of contemporary colloidal chemistry and nanotechnology.

8.2   NANOPARTICLE DESIGN

Nanoparticles confront many difficulties from the application point to the site of action. The circulatory system is about 106 km long and circulates blood at a rate of 5 L/min, with a range of blood vessel velocities between 1.5 and 33 cm/s (Jones, 1969). This dilutes the nanoparticles and prevents them from interacting with the target tissue. Only a few m/s is the speed of interstitial fluids, where interactions would be encouraged. However, getting to them requires getting through biological a barrier, which is a difficult effort. Finally, it should be noted that the immune system responds negatively to nanoparticles when they enter the body. For these reasons, depending on their intended use, nanoparticles are designed using various design principles in an effort to overcome various barriers.

The mononuclear phagocyte system, a network of phagocytic cells, mostly macrophages present in the liver, spleen, and lymph nodes, is where the nanoparticles first come into touch with the body, as was previously noted. As soon as the nanoparticles are administered, the macrophages sequester the nanoparticles (Moghimi et al., 1998). This procedure begins with the opsonization of the nanoparticles and is based on the adsorption of plasma proteins such albumin, complimentary system proteins, pattern recognition receptors, and immunoglobulins, and uses enzymes. This is a quick procedure, and it can be completed in as little as thirty seconds (Tenzer et al., 2020). By interfering with a variety of attributes, such as size, charge, surface chemistry, and hydrophobicity, this "natural functionalization"—also known as the development of the protein crown—clearly has the capacity to change the function or destiny of nanoparticles. Even the receptors or ligands connected to the nanoparticles can be hidden by this protein crown (Salvati et al., 2013).

To prevent opsonization and consequent immune system clearance, many design techniques have been created. In order to increase the nanoparticles' chances of hitting the target tissue as they circulate through the bloodstream, this immune system evasion tries to prolong their stay in the body. PEGylation forms a steric barrier and hydration layer to opsonization by functionalizing nanoparticle surfaces with polyethylene glycol (PEG) molecules in which the polymer units form very strong connections with the water molecules (Totten et al., 2019). An alternative strategy would involve functionalizing the nanoparticles with endogenous signals commonly present in healthy cells. Rodriguez et al. (2013) functionalized viral particles with the CD47 membrane protein, which serves as a "non-phagocytizing" signal, to prolong circulation (Wernig et al., 2017). To protect the particles from the immune system, a comparable tactic is to encase them in biomimetic polymers like cell membranes (Hu et al., 2011; Parodi et al., 2013). In 2020, a strategy proposal by Nikitin and his colleagues temporarily suppressed the mononuclear phagocyte system with the addition of anti-erythrocyte antibodies as another method to prolong the duration of circulation. By suppressing about 5% of hematocrits, they were able to multiply the circulation half-life of various nanosystems by a factor of up to 32 (Nikitin et al., 2020).

Due to its very low immune response characteristics, silk fibroin can bypass the immune system. The work by Catto et al. (2015) illustrates this and implanted silk fibroin-based tubular matrices in mice. Few macrophages were observed to be stained with anti-ED1 antibodies, which is a sign of a weak inflammatory response. Anti-CD4 antibodies, which are absent in T-cells, showed that a cell-mediated immune response was absent. By utilizing cutting-edge design, Tan and colleagues (Tan et al., 2019) have developed a doxorubicin delivery nanosystem that uses silk fibroin as a Trojan horse. The scientists produced amorphous calcium carbonate nanoparticles that were covered in silk fibroin and contained drugs. It helps the immune system elude detection and inhibits the early release of doxorubicin. Nanoparticles accumulate in malignant tissues as a result of the EPR process before being eventually absorbed by lysosomes. The latter's acidic pH encourages the production of CO_2 from calcium carbonate, which causes the lysosome to burst from the gas's expansion and releases doxorubicin into the target cell. Results in mice showed that silk fibroin-coated nanoparticles were superior to free doxorubicin or uncoated calcium carbonate nanoparticles in terms of lowering tumor volume and minimizing its negative effects. Because the nanoparticles did not produce more CD^{4+} and CD^{8+} T-cells, IgM, IgG, or IgA in contrast to the control group, the immunological toxicity tests also demonstrated that nanoparticles didn't elicit an immune reaction.

8.3 PERSONALIZED MEDICINES

According to one definition of personalized nanoparticles, it is a personalized, individually managed method of getting the appropriate treatment to the right patient at the right dose (Verma, 2012). The strategy was motivated by a number of considerations, such as the widespread occurrence of unjustified pharmacological side effects and the wide variation in treatment efficacy among therapeutic classes, which can range from 25 to 80%.

Proteomic, genomic, and epigenetic research are all part of personalized medicine, along with particular patient health issues and environmental factors (Spear et al., 2001). In contrast, the word "nanotechnology" is broad and covers systems with a diameter between 10 and 100 nm (Auffan et al., 2009). The phrase also suggests the capacity to direct structures at this nanoscale toward a desired result. Nanoscale compounds can interact with cells at the molecular levels and subcellular, which is not conceivable at larger sizes, due to their small size (such that greater than 1 m). Nanomedicine has produced a number of innovations that have improved disease prevention, monitoring, diagnosis, and therapy (Greish, 2012).

There are several points where personalized medicine and nanotechnology converge. The first is diagnostics, where nanotechnology has much to offer in terms of pharmacogenetic testing, the capacity to conduct both *in vitro* and *in vivo* testing, and the examination of the condition of particular drug targets. The second is the therapeutic area, as nanomedicine allows for treatment to be customized to a specific target found for an ailment in a specific patient (Ventola, 2012).

Additionally, due to its targeting powers, nanomedicine enables much elevated dosages than the highest tolerable quantity for an unformulated drug. As a result, the dose can be modified in accordance with the particulars of each patient (Maeda, 2001). And finally, two important factors in individualized drug response related to the variation in cytochrome-P enzymes (CYP) and drug transporters in various populations can be avoided by using nanomedicine (Figure 8.2). Nanomedicine drug formulations could effectively produce pharmaceuticals inside of cells during the endocytic process, which does not rely on a transporter and is imperceptible to enzymes that catalyze metabolism.

In order to give tailored treatments for each patient or group of patients while taking into account environmental factors, genetic and phenotypic that could affect the treatment's safety and efficacy, healthcare practitioners use an approach

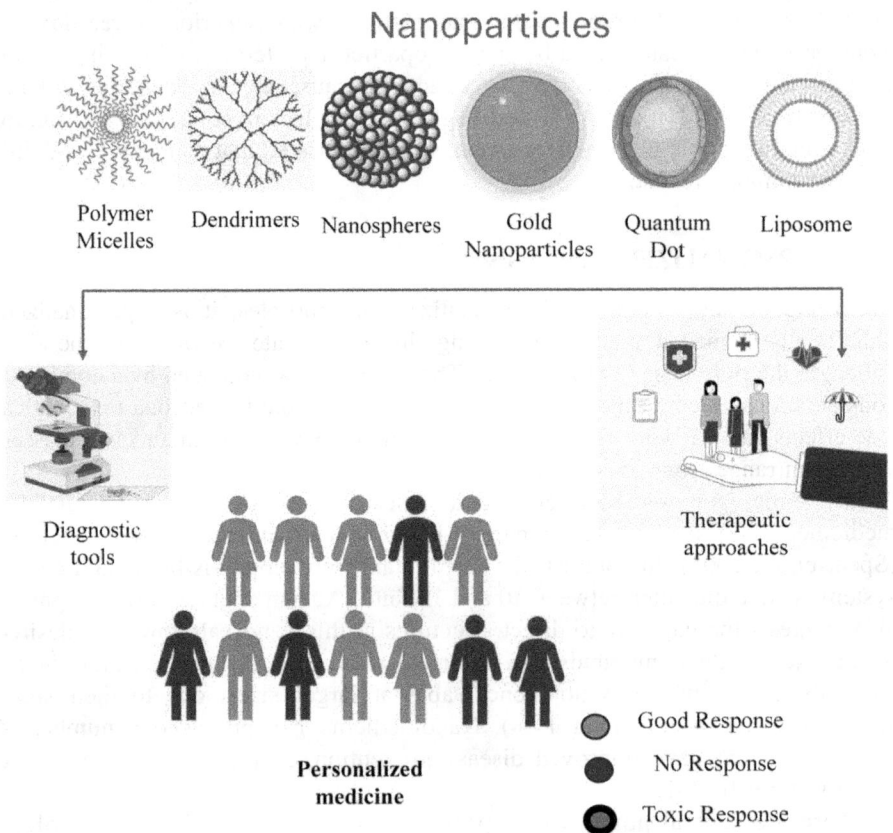

FIGURE 8.2   An illustration of how nanotechnology is applied in personalized medicine.

known as "personalized medicine" (Greish, 2012). The usage of nanomedicines in this sector has also increased exponentially since they offer the chance to treat each person or each cohort of individuals by taking into account the unique requirements specified in each individual's DNA (Ge et al., 2014; Zhang et al., 2012). This review will discuss how nanomedicines are used as therapeutic agents, particularly for the development of personalized treatments, and how the pharmaceutical industry has adopted them as cutting-edge medical procedures. Although there are many different types of nanomedicines, including magnetic nanoparticles, liposomes, polymeric nanosystems, and nanoparticles, in that they typically change the pharmacodynamics and pharmacokinetics (pD/pK) of the active components, they all offer advantages over conventional treatments (Arachchige et al., 2015).

These benefits can be categorized more specifically as follows:

1. Because of their extremely tiny sizes, nanomaterials have a high surface-to-volume ratio that is useful for fine-tuning their surfaces.
2. Any sort of nano-system can have different types of activity (hydrophilic or lipophilic), enabling higher dosages than are possible with conventional treatments because of solubility problems.
3. They block environmental factors like light and nucleases from affecting the confined activity (e.g., light, nucleases).
4. They change the active components' pharmacokinetics, permitting a controlled active release that benefits extending therapeutic action and reducing dose frequency (Figure 8.3).

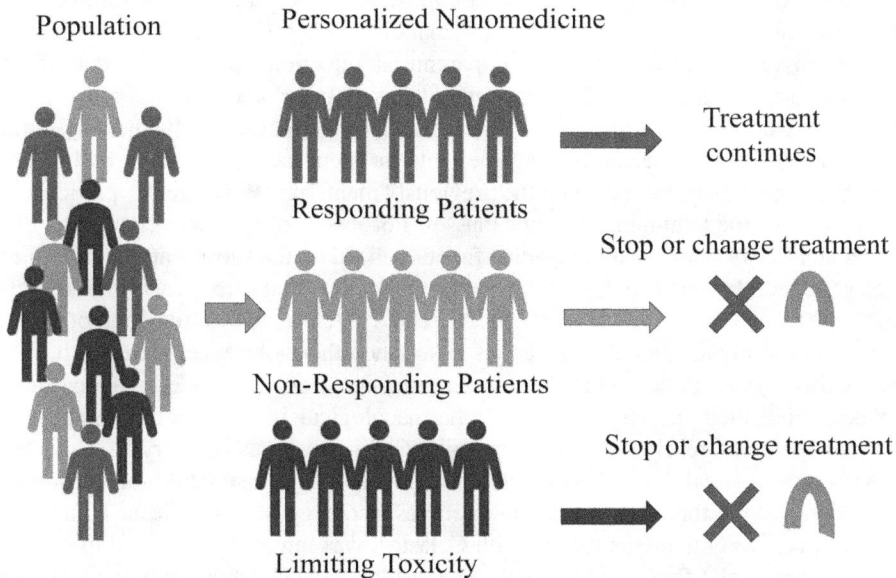

FIGURE 8.3 Personalized nanomedicine can be a great option to differentiate the patients.

5. They can actively be directed at the intended organ, enabling local therapeutic benefits, boosting therapeutic efficacy, and minimizing adverse effects (Figure 8.3).
6. The ability to select from several types of nanosystems offers nanomedicine the necessary flexibility to develop the proper particular treatment to obtain a tailored therapy.

8.4 ADMINISTRATION METHODS FOR CUSTOMIZED NANOPARTICLES

For the transportation of medicinal substances including tiny medicines, proteins, and DNA molecules, silk fibroin nanoparticles (SFN) have proved to be incredibly adaptable (Zhao et al., 2015). The route of administration of these chemicals has a direct impact on their functioning. For instance, nanoparticles can be circulated and passively accumulate in metastatic malignancies using the EPR effect, or they can be injected directly into the tumor mass (Jordan et al., 1997). However, they can also be used topically to treat skin cancer (Dianzani et al., 2014) and similarly to treat lung conditions (Kim et al., 2015; Paranjpe et al., 2014). SFNs are used in a variety of administration techniques (Pham and Tiyaboonchai, 2020). In order to keep things simple, just the transdermal, oral, and pulmonary routes of administration will be discussed. Some research that addresses the application of SFN for these various routes of administration will be provided as examples.

8.4.1 PARENTERAL

Injections administered via parenteral administration are projected for intravenous, intramuscular, subcutaneous, and intradermal distribution (into the skin). Compared to topical or enteral administration, parenteral injection operates more quickly, and the commencement of effect frequently takes place between a few seconds and a few minutes. In essence, the injected drug has a 100% bioavailability and a systemic distribution, which means it may be able to penetrate the entire body. The combination of this final idea with the previously mentioned EPR effect is particularly intriguing for the treatment of tumor masses. For instance, SFN was created by Zhu Ge et al. in 2019 with proanthocyanins functionalized on the surface and indocyanine green added. In vitro and in vivo, indocyanine may absorb near-infrared light (650–900 nm) and have a heat impact. The FDA has given this photothermic substance approval, and it may be used to photothermolyze cells to death. The researchers gave mice with C6 glioma injections of the loaded nanoparticles to determine their effectiveness. The pharmacological investigation revealed that the nanoparticles reached the gliomas following intravenous delivery in vivo, and the pharmacological study revealed that near-infrared light treatment inhibited tumor development. On the other hand, nanoparticles also suggest brief release control. In recent times, SFN that was loaded with Celastrol was intravenously administered to rats by Zhan et al. (ZhuGe et al., 2019). The results showed that prolonging the drug's residence duration and slowing down its metabolism could lessen the effects of an extension of the drug's total exposure period.

8.4.2 ORAL

When getting medication, oral administration is the most typical and likely the patient's preference. The environment of the gastrointestinal system can cause pharmaceuticals to degrade and change when taken using traditional drug delivery systems like capsules and tablets, which discharge drugs fast and with little control (variations in pH and the presence of microbiota and digestive enzymes). Passive diffusion is another typical method of medication absorption through the gastro-intestinal system. As a result, the majority of the first dosage is digested and expelled rather than absorbed. SFN offers the advantages of avoiding the aforementioned problems and could emerge as a candidate for the oral administration of pharmaceuticals. Due to its mucoadhesive properties, SFN may firmly adhere to intestinal epithelial cells (Peyer's lymphatic M cells). Next, endocytosis is used to internalize the cell (Brooks, 2015). SFN has the advantages needed to get over the aforementioned issues and emerge as potential candidates for oral delivery of medicinal substances. SFN's mucoadhesive properties may allow it to strongly adhere to intestinal epithelial cells (Peyer's lymphatic M cells). The internalization of cells through endocytosis follows (Brooks, 2015).

8.4.3 PULMONARY

Both local and systemic therapies may be able to deliver drugs to the lung. In comparison to standard dosage forms, lung and respiratory disorders including TB and lung cancer can be treated locally with a lower dose and fewer adverse effects. Because of the lung's vast surface area, the medication can be absorbed quickly and effectively without first going through first-pass metabolism like it would when administered orally (Gaul et al., 2018). In order to treat lung cancer, Kim (Kim et al., 2015) created SFN that was loaded with cisplatin. The particles and the A549 human lung epithelial cell line were compatible. The findings showed that when cisplatin is incorporated into particles, it enhances cytotoxicity in comparison to when the chemical is administered alone. The particles demonstrated a high aerosolization performance by in vitro lung deposition measurement, which is at the level of commercially available dry powder inhalers, according to the researchers' findings.

8.4.4 TRANSDERMAL

Transdermal medication delivery increases bioavailability and is beneficial for both local and systemic therapy, including pulmonary use. In a study of the in vivo skin permeability of 40 nm SFN on mice, Takeuchi (Takeuchi et al., 2019) discovered that the particles may pass through the stratum corneum, hair follicles, and surrounding epidermis before reaching the dermis within the six hours.

8.5 CURRENT PERSONALIZED THERAPEUTICS IN CLINICAL PRACTICE

The American Food and Drug Administration (FDA) has recognized 486 medications as requiring pharmacogenetic testing. Every medicine has a distinct biomarker that

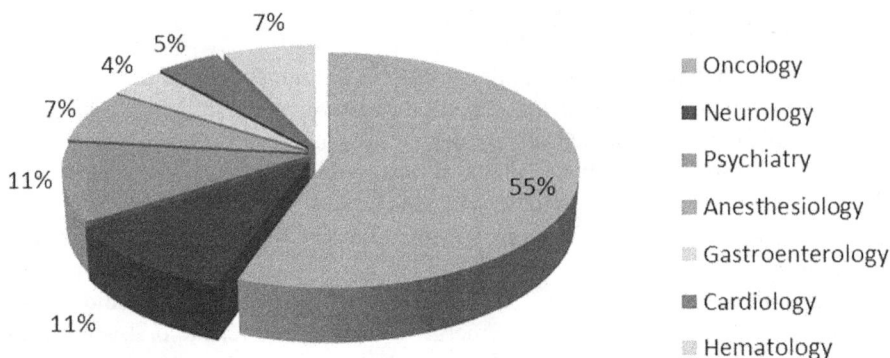

FIGURE 8.4   Personalized medicine system percentage in different clinical areas.

predicts the response based on the genetic profile, and which frequently specifies the usage and/or dosage of the drug in relation to the results of the biomarker (www.fda.gov). Numerous clinical specialties, including oncology, neurology, psychiatry, anesthesia, hematology, cardiology, and gastrointestinal, are included in personalized medicine in Figure 8.4.

8.6   CHALLENGES IN PERSONALIZED MEDICINE

Individualized illness prediction, therapy, and prevention are all a part of personalized nanomedicine. It involves modifying therapy for precise patients in order to achieve the desired outcome (Bobo et al., 2016). Personalized medicine began with the introduction of "omics" (i.e., pharmacoproteomic, pharmacogenomics, and pharmacometabolomic) in the early 2000s, which enabled the study of each person's particular genetic makeup (Zhang et al., 2012). Although there are many nanomedicine products available, none of them are individualized medicines, as was said in the previous section. This is because there are so few publications on the topic. The use of nanomedicines to provide individualized therapeutics is supported by a theoretical framework. The present lack of personalized medicine-related nanomedicine products can be attributed to a number of factors. There are problems with the formulation of nanomedicine, on the one hand. Modern nanotherapeutics, as was already said, do not actively target the goal organ. An example of this is first-generation medications like Doxil, which is projected to reach tumors via the EPR effect.

This formulation is not focused on a particular cell type or organ because it lacks an active targeting moiety. One could argue that this lack of active targeting is an issue with formulation that needs to be fixed. Despite this, Doxil has been used to treat a number of tumors throughout the years. But it's important to remember that every tumor, and even each spot inside a tumor, has its own unique combination of environmental factors (e.g., hypoxic gradient, stromal cells, extracellular matrix, and fenestration). Therefore, a targeted moiety should be a component of innovative second-generation nano-therapies.

Monoclonal antibodies have been the most widely utilized targeting molecules because they specifically target molecules expressed by a single kind of cell (for example, OX26 to target the transferrin receptor, which is overexpressed in blood-brain barrier cells; Beduneau et al., 2008). Bacteriophages and viruses are also tunable nano-systems that can be genetically altered to express or silence a desired gene. These viruses and bacteriophages may be useful for developing novel therapies to treat pancreatic adenocarcinoma by using adenoviral vectors (Mato-Berciano et al., 2017), which is a common cancer.

It's also crucial to keep in mind that, as opposed to pharmacological therapies that use drugs, it is advised to customize therapies using gene material as the active principle. Because gene therapies are being employed more commonly in nanomedicines, research should concentrate on them rather than pharmacological treatments.

Before individualized nanomedicine's success can be assured, economic difficulties must also be resolved. According to estimates, it takes more than ten to fifteen years and costs about one billion dollars to commercialize a novel nano-drug (Bobo et al., 2016); the price is higher for personalized medication. With current technology, it is reasonable to assume that designing personalized treatments for a single patient is neither feasible nor effective; therefore, a major goal of research should be to identify patient groups with shared traits in order to develop personalized therapies for multiple patients.

Modern research on personalized nanomedicine should start with the creation of molecular profiles that reveal the features of each patient's gene expression as well as, more crucially, the patterns that are seen over time and as a result of a disease's progression. With the help of this fundamental knowledge, medical professionals might explain the disease's stage and progression and create nano therapies tailored to each gene sequence (Ge et al., 2014). It has been shown that this defense is effective in stopping metastasis from a local tumor. This strategy was used by the Golub group to show that the tumor response to therapy was dependent on the tumor stroma (Straussman et al., 2012; Stegh, 2013). These results led to the conclusion that stromal and inflammatory variables were crucial for metastasis as well (Ge et al., 2014). Before using or even developing nanotherapy, the genetic and molecular components of a cancer patient must be thoroughly investigated in order to achieve effectiveness (Jiang et al., 2017).

8.7   NANO-BASED DELIVERY SYSTEMS

Recent years have seen significant advancements in delivery techniques that deliver therapeutic medications or naturally occurring active molecules to their intended site for the treatment of various illnesses (Obeid et al., 2017; Miele et al., 2012). Although many drug delivery techniques have been employed successfully in recent years, some problems still need to be fixed and cutting-edge technology still has to be created in order for pharmaceuticals to be successfully delivered to their target places. The enhanced system of medication delivery will therefore be made possible by the nano-based drug delivery systems, which are now being explored.

The importance of delivery systems has increased during the past few years. Such systems are simple to create and have the potential to encourage the body's customized release of active substances. As an illustration, Chen (Chen et al., 2016) talked about the therapeutic effects of their system that utilized nanocarriers for imaging and sensory applications. Additionally, Pelaz et al. (Pelaz et al., 2017) explored new prospects and difficulties for this industry while providing a current evaluation of many usages of nanocarriers in nanomedicine.

8.8 ADVANTAGES OF NANOPARTICLES DELIVERY SYSTEM

Nanoparticles have the ability to alter a drug's diffusivity, solubility, toxicity, half-life, biodistribution, and pharmacokinetics, adding a new point of engineering and control to the field of medicine. Nanoparticles have a wide range of uses, and as technology develops, this list is projected to grow. Numerous investigations conducted recently have shown that they can function as sensors (El-AnsaryandFaddah, 2010), medication carriers (Etheridge et al., 2013; Pham and Tiyaboonchai, 2020; Lammers and Ferrari, 2020), and diagnostic agents (Chen et al., 2013). The term "theragnostic" refers to the processes that have developed as a result of recent efforts to combine therapies and diagnoses in a single application.

At least three mechanisms support the use of nanoparticles as delivery systems, including the potential to deliver insoluble drugs through stable colloidal systems to the bloodstream, the capacity to deliver such drugs through controlled release, and enhanced penetration and retention (EPR) of nanoparticles in solid tumors. The potential benefits of each of these topics will be addressed in this section.

At least three processes support the delivery systems: (i)EPR of nanoparticles in solid tumors; (ii) the potential for stable colloidal systems to carry insoluble pharmaceuticals in the blood; and (iii) the controlled release of such drugs. The potential benefits of each of these topics will be addressed in this section.

8.8.1 IMPROVED RETENTION AND PERMEABILITY (EPR)

Matsumura and Maeda first used the term EPR in 1986 (Drexler, 1981). Neocarzinostatin, an anticancer protein, was shown to accumulate more in tumor tissues when it was coupled to a polymeric matrix, according to the research team's findings. They noticed that up to five times more tagged macromolecules were present in tumor sites than in blood during the course of 19 to 72 hours after being administered to tumor-bearing animals (Drexler, 1981). According to the authors, the fenestrated hypervascularization of tumor masses, which has higher permeability to macromolecules (or nanoparticles), and poor recovery through blood arteries or lymphatic vessels, is what causes the passive accumulation of these macromolecules in tumors (Maeda et al., 1989). Since then, it has been demonstrated that other plasma proteins larger than 40 kDa may both unintentionally and intentionally concentrate at tumor sites (Maeda et al., 2009). The Evans Blue marker, which binds to plasma albumin to create a complex and demonstrates differential accumulation in cancer sites, can be intravenously injected into mice to illustrate the EPR effect.

8.8.2 Insoluble Drug Transport

The majority of medications taken by mouth that are soluble in water and have the ability to pass through biological membranes while traveling through the digestive system will eventually become accessible to the body. When taken orally, water-insoluble medications, however, will typically not be accessible since they cannot dissolve and cross the gastrointestinal barrier. In a similar vein, they cannot be delivered intravenously due to their limited solubility, and parenteral administration does not necessarily boost bioavailability (Wong et al., 2008). In total, 90% of medications thought to be in development are thought to be water-insoluble, compared to only 40% of drugs currently on the market (Loftsson and Brewster, 2010).

These findings might suggest that many medications still in development are not administered to patients because of their poor solubility in water. This results in a decrease in funding for research and development as well as missed opportunities for therapy. In 2011, it was anticipated that the cost of developing a medicine would range from 92 million to 1.8 billion dollars (Morgan et al., 2011), taking an average of between 11.4 and 13.5 years (Paul et al., 2010). Taking all of this into account, it is obvious that poor water solubility presents nanotechnology with both a substantial difficulty and a great opportunity.

8.8.3 Controlled Release

The controlled release of drugs over time using nanoparticles as drug reservoirs has many benefits over the traditional delivery of various dosages. The increase in efficacy, decrease in toxicity, and patient cooperation might be noted among them (Uhrich et al., 1999). While the latter has the benefit of requiring fewer administrations during therapy, the former could be interpreted as an increase in treatment activity when compared to how severe the side effects are. Drugs with relatively short half-lives in the blood because of the body's rapid rate of metabolism and elimination benefit most from controlled release.

As observed, the medication used in traditional dosages spends very little time in the therapeutic range and alternates between sub-therapeutic concentrations and levels exceeding the upper limit of tolerability. The therapeutic concentration window is more slowly reached by the controlled release mechanism, but it does so while maintaining stability. In the therapeutic concentration zone, the system aims to balance the rates of clearance and release. This translates into a variety of advantages in the clinic, such as preventing the concentration from dropping to sub-therapeutic levels and the patient feeling pain during the administration of analgesics. This applies to a wide range of medications, such as anti-inflammatories, antibiotics, anesthetic, hormones, and chemotherapeutics (Kost et al., 1985).

8.9 FUTURE OF DELIVERY SYSTEMS AND NANOMEDICINES

Nanomedicine is one of the most fascinating areas of research today. 1500 patents have already been filed as a result of the completion of several clinical investigations and extensive research in this subject over the preceding 20 years

(Pandit and Zeugolis, 2016). Cancer seems to be the best example of a disease for which non-medical technology has helped with both diagnosis and treatment, as discussed in the several sections above.

Examples of nanoparticles are included in this message: however, their sizes vary, with some actually measuring in nanometers and others in sub-micrometers (over 100 nm). The next line of investigation should focus on materials that have more constant homogeneity and the capacity to load and release drugs. This paper also discusses important advancements in the usage of metals-based nanoparticles for diagnostic purposes. The usage of these metals, such as silver and gold, in both diagnosis and therapy, may lead to an increase in the use of nanomedicines in the future. One major area of interest in this study is gold nanoparticles, which seem to be well absorbed in soft tumor tissues and make the tumor susceptible to radiation-based heat treatment (for example, in the near-infrared range).

Despite the fact that nanomedicine and nano-drug delivery technologies are well known, their real influence on the healthcare system, notably in the treatment and detection of cancer, is still fairly limited. This is because the industry has just recently undergone two decades of serious research and is still mostly undiscovered. Many important, fundamental characteristics are still unknown. Future research will focus heavily on the fundamental indicators of diseased tissues, such as key biological markers that permit absolute targeting without impairing normal cellular function.

In the end, the application of nanomedicine will develop with our growing understanding of diseases at the molecular level or demonstrate marker identification at a nanomaterial-subcellular size equivalent to open up new pathways for diagnosis and therapy. Therefore, the development of future nanomedicine applications will require an understanding of the molecular fingerprints of disease. More research is needed in order to use well-known nanoprobes and nano theragnostic devices to broaden the usage of nanomedicine beyond what has been covered in this review.

The potential of theoretical mathematical models for prediction, technology for the evaluation of these events, medication action in tissues/cellular level, and the concept of controlled release of certain medications at the disturbed regions has not yet been fully realized. Formulation and biomaterial investigations, which seem to be the nascent stages of biomedicine applications, are the subject of many studies in the field of nanomedicine. Important information will be produced by animal studies and trans-disciplinary research, both of which need a large time and financial commitment. This information can then be used for pharmacological therapeutic and diagnostic investigations. An expanding global trend is the hunt for more precise diagnoses and treatments, and nanomedicine and nano-drug delivery technology seem to have a bright future.

8.10 CONCLUSION

The development of customized medicine is aided by nanobiotechnologies because they expand the capabilities of diagnostics and make it easier to combine them with therapies. Targeted treatment using nanoparticles boosts safety by lowering side effects, further improving therapeutic specificity. Researchers have been merging various features of nanotechnology for use in customized medicine during the past few years. A new area of study in precision medicine/personalized is emerging with the use of a precise, tailored diagnosis of a patient's genetic profile and focused therapy of that medical problem.

Nanomedicine has opened up new possibilities for molecular and genetic diagnosis in addition to drug delivery. In personalized medicine, it can be used to enhance bioavailability and compatibility, boost binding affinity, and have maximum therapeutic efficacy with a controlled drug release profile so the drug can reach the correct target, in the right patient, at the right time. As a result, targeted techniques for diagnosis and treatment can be developed. It can also help us comprehend a person's DNA. Nanomedicine may soon be employed on a much larger scale in customized medicine since laboratory-produced nanoparticles have demonstrated promising effects. A combination of personalized and nanomedicine may represent the future of medicine.

REFERENCES

Arachchige M. C. M., Reshetnyak Y. K., Andreev O. A. 2015. Advanced targeted nanomedicine. *J Biotechnol.* 202:88–97. doi: 10.1016/j.jbiotec.2015.01.009.

Auffan M., Rose J., Bottero J-Y., Lowry G. V., Jolivet J.-P., Wiesner M. R. 2009. Towards a definition of inorganic nanoparticles from an environmental, health and safety perspective. *Nature Nanotechnol.* 4(10):634–641.

Bobo D., Robinson K. J., Islam J., Thurecht K. J., Corrie S. R. 2016. Nanoparticle-based medicines: A review of FDA-approved materials and clinical trials to date. *Pharm Res.* 33:2373–2387. doi: 10.1007/s11095-016-1958-5.

Brooks A. E. 2015. The potential of silk and silk-like proteins as natural mucoadhesive biopolymers for controlled drug delivery. *Front Chem.* 3(Nov):1–8.

Béduneau A., Hindré F., Clavreul A., Leroux J. C., Saulnier P., Benoit J. P. 2008. Brain targeting using novel lipid nanovectors. *J Control Release.* 126:44–49. doi: 10.1016/j.jconrel.2007.11.001.

Catto V., Farè S., Cattaneo I., Figliuzzi M., Alessandrino A., Freddi G., Remuzzi A., Tanzi M. C. 2015. Small diameter electrospun silk fibroin vascular grafts: Mechanical properties, in vitro biodegradability, and in vivo biocompatibility. *Mat Sci Eng: C.* 54:101–111.

Chen G., Roy I., Yang C., Prasad P. N. 2016. Nanochemistry and nano-medicine for nanoparticle-based diagnostics and therapy. *Chem Rev.* 116:2826–2885.

Chen H., Zhen Z., Todd T., Chu P. K., Xie J. 2013. Nanoparticles for improving cancer diagnosis. *Mater Sci Eng: Reports.* 74(3):35–69.

Dianzani C., Zara G. P., Maina G., Pettazzoni P., Pizzimenti S., Rossi F., et al. 2014. Drug delivery nanoparticles in skin cancers. *Biomed Res Int.*

Drexler K. E. 1981. Molecular engineering: An approach to the development of general capabilities for molecular manipulation. *Proc Nat Acad Sci* 78(9):5275–5278.

El-Ansary A., Faddah L. M. 2010. Nanoparticles as biochemical sensors. *Nanotechnol Sci Appl.* 3(1):65–76.

Etheridge M. L., Campbell S. A., Erdman A. G., Haynes C. L., Wolf S. M., McCullough J. 2013. The big picture on nanomedicine: The state of investigational and approved nanomedicine products. *Nanomedicine Nanotechnology, Biol Med.* 9(1):1–14.

Faraday M. 1857. LIX. Experimental relations of gold (and other metals) to light.—The Bakerian lecture. *The London, Edinburgh, and Dublin Philosophical Magazine and Journal of Science.* 14(96):512–539.

Feynman R. P. 1961. There's plenty of room at the bottom: An invitation to enter a new field of physics. Miniaturization, Reinhold.

Gaul R., Ramsey J. M., Heise A., Cryan S. A., Greene C. M. 2018. Nanotechnology approaches to pulmonary drug delivery: Targeted delivery of small molecule and gene-based therapeutics to the lung. *Design of Nanostructures for Versatile Therapeutic Applications.Elsevier Inc.* pp. 221–253.

Ge Y., Li S., Wang S., Moore R. 2014. Nanomedicine. *Springer*; Ottawa, ON, Canada. *Nanostruct.*

Greish K. 2012. Enhanced permeability and retention effect for selective targeting of anticancer nanomedicine: Are we there yet? *Drug Discovery Today: Technologies.* 9(2):e161–e166.

Hu C-M. J., Zhang L., Aryal S., Cheung C., Fang R. H., Zhang L. 2011. Erythrocyte membrane-camouflaged polymeric nanoparticles as a biomimetic delivery platform. *Proc Nat Acad Sci.* 108(27):10980–10985.

Jain R. K., and Stylianopoulos T. 2010. Delivering nanomedicine to solid tumors. *Nature Reviews Clinical Oncology.* 7(11):653–664.

Jiang W., von Roemeling C. A., Chen Y., Qie Y., Liu X., Chen J., Kim B. Y. S. 2017. Designing nanomedicine for immuno-oncology. *Nat Biomed Eng.* 29. doi: 10.1038/s41551-017-0029.

Jindal, S., Anand, R., Sharma, N., Yadav, N., Mudgal, D., Mishra, R., Mishra, V. 2022. Sustainable approach for developing graphene-based materials from natural resources and biowastes for electronic applications. *ACS Applied Electronic Materials*, 4:2146–2174. doi: 10.1021/acsaelm.2c00097.

Jones R. T. 1969. Blood flow. *Ann Rev Fluid Mech.* 1(1):223–244.

Jordan A., Scholz R., Wust P., Fähling H., Krause J., Wlodarczyk W., et al. 1997. Effects of magnetic fluid hyperthermia (MFH) on C3H mammary carcinoma in vivo. *Int J Hyperth.* 13(6):587–605.

Kim S. Y., Naskar D., Kundu S. C., Bishop D. P., Doble P. A., Boddy A. V., et al. 2015. Formulation of biologically-inspired silk-based drug carriers for pulmonary delivery targeted for lung cancer. *Sci Rep.* 5(April):1–13.

Kost J., Horbett T. A., Ratner B. D., Singh M. 1985. Glucose-sensitive membranes containing glucose oxidase: Activity, swelling, and permeability studies. *J Biomed Mater Res.* 19(9):1117–1133.

Lammers T., Ferrari M. 2020. The success of nanomedicine. *Nano Today.* 31:100853.

Loftsson T., Brewster M. E. 2010. Pharmaceutical applications of cyclodextrins: Basic science and product development. *J Pharm Pharmacol.* 62(11):1607–1621.

Maeda H. 2001. SMANCS and polymer-conjugated macromolecular drugs: Advantages in cancer chemotherapy. *Adv Drug Del Rev.* 46(1-3):169–185.

Maeda H., Matsumura Y. 1989. Tumoritropic and lymphotropic principles of macro-molecular drugs. *Crit Rev Ther Drug Carrier Syst.* 6(3):193–210.

Maeda H., Bharate G. Y., Daruwalla J. 2009. Polymeric drugs for efficient tumor-targeted drug delivery based on EPR-effect. *EurJ Pharm Biopharm.* 71(3):409–419.

Mato-Berciano A., Raimondi G., Maliandi M. V., Alemany R., Montoliu L., Fillat C. 2017. A NOTCH-sensitive uPAR-regulated oncolytic adenovirus effectively sup-presses pancreatic tumor growth and triggers synergistic anticancer effects with gemcitabine and nab-paclitaxel. *Oncotarget.* 8:22700–22715. doi: 10.18632/oncotarget.15169.

Matsumura Y., Maeda H. 1986. A new concept for macromolecular therapeutics in cancer chemotherapy: Mechanism of tumoritropic accumulation of proteins and the antitumor agent smancs. *Cancer Res.* 46(8):6387–6392.

Mie G. 1976. Contributions to the optics of turbid media, particularly of colloidal metal solutions. *Contributions to the Optics of Turbid Media.* 25(3):377–445.

Miele E., Spinelli G. P., Miele E., Di Fabrizio E., Ferretti E., Tomao S., Gulino A. 2012. Nanoparticle-based delivery of small interfering RNA: Challenges for cancer therapy. *Int J Nanomedicine.* 7:3637.

Moghimi S. M., Patel H. M. 1998. Serum-mediated recognition of liposomes by phagocytic cells of the reticuloendothelial system–the concept of tissue specificity. *Advanced Drug Del Rev.* 32(1-2):45–60.

Morgan S., Grootendorst P., Lexchin J., Cunningham C., Greyson D. 2011. The cost of drug development: A systematic review. *Health Policy (New York).* 100(1):4–17.

Nikitin M. P., Zelepukin I. V., Shipunova V. O., Sokolov I. L., Deyev S. M., Nikitin P. I. 2020. Enhancement of the blood-circulation time and performance of nanomedicines via the forced clearance of erythrocytes. *Nature Biomedical Eng.* 4(7):717–731.

Obeid M. A., Al Qaraghuli M. M., Alsaadi M., Alzahrani A. R., Niwasabutra K., Ferro V. A. 2017. Delivering natural products and biotherapeutics to improve drug efficacy. *Therapeutic Del.* 8(11):947–956.

Pandit A., Zeugolis D. I. 2016. Twenty-five years of nano-bio-materials: Have we revolutionized healthcare? *Fut Med.* 11(9):985–987.

Paranjpe M., Müller-Goymann C. C. 2014. Nanoparticle-mediated pulmonary drug delivery: A review. *Int J Mol Sci.* 15(4):5852–5873.

Parodi A., Quattrocchi N., Van De Ven A. L., Chiappini C., Evangelopoulos M., Martinez J. O., Brown B. S. et al. 2013. Synthetic nanoparticles functionalized with biomimetic leukocyte membranes possess cell-like functions. *Nature Nanotechnol.* 8(1):61–68.

Paul S. M., Mytelka D. S., Dunwiddie C. T., Persinger C. C., Munos B. H., Lindborg S. R., et al. 2010. How to improve RD productivity: The pharmaceutical industry's grand challenge. *Nat Rev Drug Discov.* 9(3):203–214.

Pelaz B., Alexiou C., Alvarez-Puebla R. A., Alves F., Andrews A. M., Ashraf S., Balogh L. P., Ballerini L., Bestetti A., Brendel C., Bosi S. 2017. Diverse applications of nanomedicine. *AcsNano.* 11:2313–2381.

Pham D. T., Tiyaboonchai W. 2020. Fibroin nanoparticles: A promising drug delivery system. *Drug Deliv.* 27(1):431–448.

Reibold M., Paufler P., Levin A. A., Kochmann W., Pätzke N., Meyer D. C. 2006. Carbon nanotubes in an ancient Damascus sabre. *Nature.* 444(7117):286–286.

Rodriguez P. L., Harada T., Christian D. A., Pantano D. A., Tsai R. K., Discher D. E. 2013. Minimal "Self" peptides that inhibit phagocytic clearance and enhance delivery of nanoparticles. *Science.* 339(6122):971–975.

Salvati A., Pitek A. S., Monopoli M. P., Prapainop K., Bombelli F. B., Hristov D. R., Kelly P. M., Åberg C., Mahon E., Dawson K. A. 2013. Transferrin-functionalized nanoparticles lose their targeting capabilities when a biomolecule corona adsorbs on the surface. *Nature Nanotechnol.* 8(2):137–143.

Schaming D., Remita H. 2015. Nanotechnology: From the ancient time to nowadays. *Found Chemistry.* 17(3):187–205.

Spear B. B., Heath-Chiozzi M., Huff J. 2001. Clinical application of pharmacogenetics. *Trends Molecular Med.* 7(5):201–204.

Stegh A. H. 2013. Toward personalized cancer nanomedicine—past, present, and future. *Integr Biol.* 5:48–65. doi: 10.1039/C2IB20104F.

Straussman R., Morikawa T., Shee K., Barzily-Rokni M., Qian Z. R., Du J., Davis A., Mongare M. M., Gould J., Frederick D. T., et al. 2012. Tumour micro-environment elicits innate resistance to RAF inhibitors through HGF secretion. *Nature.* 487:500–504. doi: 10.1038/nature11183.

Takeuchi I., Shimamura Y., Kakami Y., Kameda T., Hattori K., Miura S., et al. 2019. Transdermal delivery of 40-nm silk fibroin nanoparticles. *Colloids Surfaces B Biointerfaces.* 175: 564–568.

Tan M., Liu W., Liu F., Zhang W., Gao H., Cheng J., Chen Y., Wang Z., Cao Y., Ran H. 2019. Silk fibroin-coated nanoagents for acidic lysosome targeting by a functional preservation strategy in cancer chemotherapy. *Theranostics*. 9(4):961.

Taniguchi N. 1974. On the basic concept of nanotechnology. Proceeding of the ICPE.

Tenzer S., Docter D., Kuharev J., Musyanovych A., Fetz V., Hecht R., Schlenk F. et al. 2020. Rapid formation of plasma protein corona critically affects nanoparticle pathophysiology. In *Nano-Enabled Medical Applications*, pp. 251–278. Jenny Stanford Publishing.

Totten J. D., Wongpinyochit T., Carrola J., Duarte I. F., Seib F. P. 2019. PEGylation-dependent metabolic rewiring of macrophages with silk fibroin nanoparticles. *ACS Appl Mater Interfaces*. 11(16):14515–14525.

Uhrich K. E., Cannizzaro S. M., Langer R. S., Shakesheff K. M. 1999. Polymeric systems for controlled drug release. *Chem Rev*. 99(11):3181–3198.

Van der Meel R., Sulheim E., Shi Y., Kiessling F., Mulder W. J. M., Lammers T. 2019. Smart cancer nanomedicine. *Nature Nanotechnol*. 14(11):1007–1017.

Ventola C. L. 2012. The nanomedicine revolution: part 1: Emerging concepts. *Pharmacy Therapeutics*. 37(9):512.

Verma M. 2012. Personalized medicine and cancer. *J Personalized Med*. 2(1):1–14.

Wernig G., Chen S-Y., Cui L., Neste C. V., Tsai J. M., Kambham N., Vogel H., et al. 2017. Unifying mechanism for different fibrotic diseases. *Proc Nat Acad Sci*. 114(18): 4757–4762.

Wong J., Brugger A., Khare A., Chaubal M., Papadopoulos P., Rabinow B., et al. 2008. Suspensions for intravenous (IV) injection: A review of development, preclinical and clinical aspects. *Adv Drug Deliv Rev*. 60(8):939–954.

Zhang L., Gu F. X., Chan J. M., Wang A. Z., Langer R. S., Farokhzad O. C. 2008. Nanoparticles in medicine: Therapeutic applications and developments. *Clinical Pharmacology Therapeutics*. 83(5):761–769.

Yadav, N., Mudgal, D., Anand, R., Jindal, S., Mishra, V. 2022. Recent development in nanoencapsulation and delivery of natural bioactives through chitosan scaffolds for various biological applications. *International Journal of Biological Macromolecules*, 220:537–572. doi: 10.1016/j.ijbiomac.2022.08.098.

Yadav, N., Mudgal, D., Mishra, S., Sehrawat, H., Singh, N. K., Sharma, K., Sharma, P. C., Singh, J., Mishra, V. 2023. Development of ionic liquid-capped carbon dots derived from Tecoma stans (L.) Juss. ex Kunth: Combatting bacterial pathogens in diabetic foot ulcer pus swabs, targeting both standard and multi-drug resistant strains. *South African Journal of Botany*, 163:412–426. doi: 10.1016/j.sajb.2023.10.063.

Zhang X. Q., Xu X., Bertrand N., Pridgen E., Swami A., Farokhzad O. C. 2012. Interactions of nanomaterials and biological systems: Implications to personalized nanomedicine. *Adv Drug Deliv Rev*. 64:1363–1384. doi: 10.1016/j.addr.2012.08.005.

Zhao Z., Li Y., Xie M. B. 2015. Silk fibroin-based nanoparticles for drug delivery. *Int J Mol Sci*. 16(3):4880–4903.

ZhuGe D. L., Wang L. F., Chen R., Li X. Z., Huang Z. W., Yao Q., et al. 2019. Cross-linked nanoparticles of silk fibroin with proanthocyanidins as a promising vehicle of indocyanine green for photo-thermal therapy of glioma. *Artif Cells, Nanomedicine Biotechnol*. 47(1):4293–4304.

Zsigmondy R. A. 1926. Properties of colloids. *Nobel lecture*. 11.

9 Role of Bioinformatics in the Development of Nanomedicines

Gunjan, Himanshu, Archana Gupta, and Manoj K. Yadav

9.1 INTRODUCTION

Over the past few decades, nanotechnology has shown promise in many fields of science and technology advancement. Nanomedicine in medicine is expected to bring up new techniques for diagnosis, prognosis, and treatment. With the increasing severity of diseases in the human population, the demand for data related to biological information is also increasing. To meet the increased demand for data and knowledge management, new biomedical informatics systems must be created as the amount of information available is expanding quickly. Hence the newly emerging field "The field of nanoinformatics," which is connected to nanotechnology, biomedicine, and Informatics, has come (Figure 9.1). The goal of nanoinformatics is to connect information technology and nanomedicine and manage the information generated in the nanomedical field using computational methods (Maojo et al., 2012). Nanoinformatics has the potential to enhance existing accomplishments in Biomedical Informatics by introducing new elements required to investigate various scientific biological and physical aspects at varying levels of complexity (Maojo et al., 2012; Maojo et al., 2010).

Numerous techniques in computing-based applications have been tested over the past ten years in the context of biomedicine to unveil interdisciplinary research in fields like bioinformatics, medical informatics, and others. The translation of findings from the bench side to the bedside for nanomedicine will be accelerated through the integration of biology, nanotechnology, and informatics. In short "Bioinformatics is a branch of the life sciences which integrates biology and information technology" (Bayat, 2002). The goal of bioinformatics, which combines several life sciences disciplines, is to provide methodology and tools to investigate massive amounts of biological data in order to store, organize, systematize, visualize, annotate, query, comprehend, and interpret that data (Li, de Vries, & Peng, 2021). Modern computer science, such as cloud computing, statistics, mathematics, pattern recognition, reconstruction, machine learning, simulation and literature techniques, and molecular modeling/algorithms, are all used to organize massive amounts of biological data ("Action GRID: Assessing the Impact of Nanotechnology on Biomedical

DOI: 10.1201/9781003348672-9

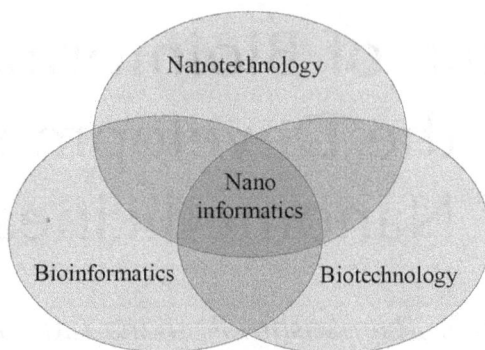

FIGURE 9.1 Nanoinformatics, a relatively new field of informatics combination of nanotechnology, bioinformatics, and biotechnology.

Informatics - PubMed," n.d.-a). Concepts from fields like informatics (computer science and information technologies), nanotechnology, medicine, and other conventional sciences like biology, chemistry, and physics are all included under its umbrella (Breu, Guggenbichler, & Wollmann, 2008).

9.2 BIOINFORMATICS IN NANOMEDICINE: "THE NANOINFORMATICS"

The numerous obstacles of nanotechnology for nanomedicine point to the necessity for a new informatics field (Thomas, Klaessig, et al., 2011). An emerging field called nanomedicine informatics seeks to overcome problems with information management in this field ("Action GRID: Assessing the Impact of Nanotechnology on Biomedical Informatics - PubMed," n.d.-b; Maojo, Martin-Sanchez, Kulikowski, Rodriguez-Paton, & Fritts, 2010a). The term "nanoinformatics" in this biomedical context describes the "use of informatics tools for evaluating and processing information on the structure and physicochemical features of nanoparticles and nanomaterials, their interaction with their surroundings, and their applications for nanomedicine" (Maojo et al., 2010). Nanomedicine is generally understood to be the application of nanotechnology to the medical field. The development of efficient methods for obtaining, exchanging, analyzing, modeling, and analyzing data and information pertinent to the community of nanoscale scientists and engineers. This information covers any information that might be pertinent, such as literature, physical-chemical characteristics, biological, clinical, and toxicological impacts (Khan, Saeed, & Khan, 2019).

Presently, nanomedicine has taken hundreds of various paths, and each one is developing the capacity to alter molecules and devices at the molecular level, which has the potential to have a huge and immediate positive impact on medicine (Freitas, 2005). These applications are concentrated on biological system control, drug administration, treatment, monitoring, and diagnostics (Farokhzad & Langer, 2006). In this, nanoparticles play a major role typically ranging in size from 1 to 100 nm (Zhou, Yu, Qin, & Zheng, 2012). Drug carriers made of nanoparticles may

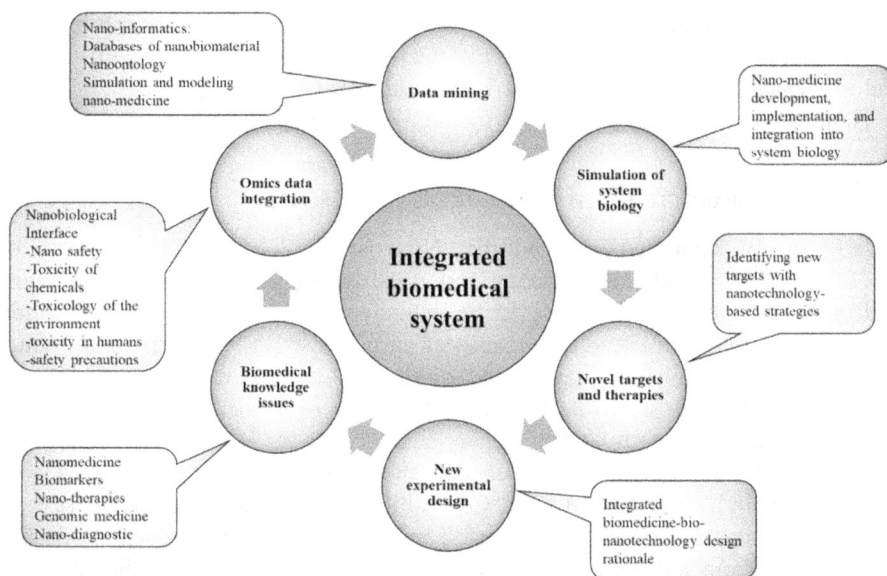

FIGURE 9.2   Strategy for the integration of several research areas, including nanomedicine and nanobiotechnology, around the sophisticated biomedical system.

change a drug's reactivity, potency, and ultimately how it behaves in vivo. Delivery of drugs to a specified tissue, drug release at a regulated rate, and drug detoxification treatments are all made possible by advances in nanotechnology design and delivery. There are a number of nanotechnological study areas in the field of health that can offer new perspectives on pathogenic causes and new directions for therapeutic approaches for example nanomedicine; nano-bio interaction and nano-safety; bioinformatics tools in combination with nanoparticles (nanoinformatics); development, implementation and integration of nanosystem too biological system; new target strategies; rational design of nanosystem integrated into biomedicine nano-biotechnology (Figure 9.2).

9.3   NANOPARTICLES IN NANOMEDICINE

Nanoparticles and nanomaterials are developed as DNA and protein bio detectors. Additionally, automated platforms for nano detection can be created by combining nanodevices like nanowires and nanotubes with nanoarrays. The term "nanoparticle" is equivalent to the term "nanostructure," which is superior to a number of terms: Metal nanoparticles, dendrimers, nanospheres, nanocapsules, quantum dots, and many more (Jeevanandam, Barhoum, Chan, Dufresne, & Danquah, 2018). These many types of nanoparticles can be applied in nanomedicine in various ways including cure, treatment diagnostic, and monitoring purposes in the biomedical field. The safety of patients and other potential side effects of using nanoparticles raise additional concerns for the scientific community. Studies on potential dangers to human health associated with the usage of nanoparticles are becoming more and more popular. Nanotoxicology, a recent field, centered on such problems. Nanoinformatics may be important in this area, assisting in the processing of data obtained from tests and well-planned clinical studies (De La Iglesia et al., 2009).

Nanomaterials are mostly used in medicine for the following purposes.

9.3.1 NANOPARTICLE-BASED GENE AND DRUG DELIVERY

It has already been demonstrated that NPs can be loaded with a variety of medications using both encapsulation and covalent coupling. Genes, medications, and other specialized substances can be delivered using nanoparticles to specific organs, cells, molecules, and other areas of an organism. The surprising introduction of a focused, biologically protected, on-demand tool has resulted in significant advances in scientific study. Furthermore, the range of medications brought is not limited to cancer therapy (Chen, Zhu, Zhang, Liu, & Huang, 2010; Gvili & Machluf, 2006). If specific requirements are met, medications can be released from nanoparticles in a controlled manner. Controlling medicine distribution has several obvious advantages in delivery systems. Targeted delivery protects healthy tissues and systems from any potentially damaging side effects of the medicine. Drug accumulation at target areas reduces the overall dose required. Loading medications into shielding nano structures protects them from physiologically dynamic variables such as pH and permits drugs to reach target tissues with their potency and effectiveness intact (Lee Ventola, 2012). The use of nanoparticles in medication and gene delivery is predicted to continue to gain attention. Many different particles can be used, and each one has unique properties, such as dendrimers, liposomes, buckyballs, Dendrimer-entrapped GNPs (Au DENPs), etc. (Shan et al., 2012).

9.3.2 TREATMENT (NANO THERAPY)

With the use of nanotechnology, patients can receive therapies that are less intrusive and typically require lower dosages than traditional medications. They can aid in lowering the harmful effects of medications by increasing therapeutic efficacy. Additionally, nanoparticles can be created with specific therapeutic capabilities, such as antibacterial (Thomas, Yallapu, Sreedhar, & Bajpai, 2009) or antimicrobial (Chamundeeswari et al., 2010) ones. It is necessary to develop new models of nano-clinical trials to evaluate their effectiveness and any potential side effects. Nanomedicine can benefit from new computerized clinical practice guideline models.

9.3.3 DIAGNOSIS (NANO DIAGNOSIS)

Molecules in living things can directly interact with nanoparticles. They are therefore precise and useful diagnostic instruments for a few clinical disorders and diseases. As previously said, NPs can assist in providing useful information at all stages of the therapeutic process. While improved imaging capabilities provide more gross anatomical and cellular information, sensitive and precise detection of disease-related substances is also vital. To that purpose, NPs have been used to aid in the diagnostic process with a variety of innovative tests. One of the most significant advantages of NPs is the ability to attach any number of proteins to their surface. As a result, GNPs serve as a useful starting point for a variety of biomolecule detection tests. They have swiftly established themselves as important biomarkers and tumor labelers (Yohan & Chithrani, 2014).

9.3.4 Nanomedical Devices and Regenerative Medicine

To aid in the development of new nanomedical devices, research into the biological interactions with particular nanostructures (such as dendrimers) and cell physiology is required techniques. Additionally, new biocompatible materials can be employed to create implants for regenerative medicine and replacement therapy (Maojo et al., 2012).

9.4 A COLLABORATIVE NETWORK PLATFORMS DEVELOPMENT FOR NANOBIOTECHNOLOGY AND NANOMEDICINE

9.4.1 Generate Web Portals

To accelerate and validate the use of nanoparticles, nanomaterials, and nanosystems in nanomedicine by facilitating data sharing (current literature, lectures, publications, websites, and access points to nanomedicine databases (Perez-Acle & Sandoval, n.d.)) in the scientific community such as:

1. **NanoLink** (http://www.nano-link.net): This portal provides links to websites focusing on life quality through technological innovation (LINK=Life Quality through Innovation by a Knowledge Network). Hence it will be a consolidated network of nanotechnology-focused networks (nanoLINKnet) (Nanowerk Nanotechnology Portal).
2. **Nanowerk Nanotechnology Portal** (http://www.nanowerk.com): This portal contains a wide range of connections to and directories related to nano research, daily news, and nanotechnology feature pieces, reports, an events calendar, and a nanomaterial database centered on nanomedicine (NanoLink is a web portal).
3. **CaNanoLab** (http://cananolab.abcc.ncifcrf.gov): This portal also has a web page dedicated to disseminating nanobiological information throughout the scientific community (The Cancer Nanotechnology Laboratory (caNanoLab) Portal).

These are all clear examples of portals dedicated to promoting nanomedicine and nanotechnology information.

9.4.2 Building Storage Systems and Exchanging Data

Certain tools useful for a significant increase of data and information are:

1. Visual analysis of nanoimages (Mauger, Hunter, Drennan, Wright, & O'hagan, 2007),

2. Data-mining (Zweigenbaum, Demner-fushman, Yu, & Cohen, 2007),
3. The cancer Nanotechnology Laboratory (caNanoLab) Portal,
4. Mathematical models from clinical nanomedicine (Bewick, Yang, & Zhang, 2009),
5. Taxonomy of nanomedical application (Neil Gordon et al., 2003),
6. Nano-ontologies (The cancer Biomedical Informatics Grid [caBIG]), and
7. High-throughput experimentation/discovery (Ironi & Tentoni, 2003).

The multidisciplinary development of nanomedicine depends on the establishment of databases (Perez-Acle & Sandoval, n.d.) or repositories that will permit the exchange of data regarding the 3-D structural and data of the physical and chemical properties of nanoparticles with biomedical applications, such as dendrimers, nanotubes and metal nanoparticles, and quantum dots, and others. In this field, numerous initiatives have been created (Mauger, Hunter, Drennan, Wright, & O'Hagan, 2007). Such as

1. **Cancer Nanotechnology Laboratory (caNanoLab)** (https://gforge.nci. nih.gov/projects/canano/): It contains all the technologies and a toolset necessary to model targeted drug delivery and diagnostics using nanoparticles as transport platforms. The third project is a database that includes summaries (abstracts) and references for studies on the effects of nanoscale materials on human health and safety (The ICON EHS Database).
2. **ICON EHS Database** (http://icon.rice.edu/research.cfm), **and Collaboratory for Structural Nanobiology (CSN)** (http://nanobiology. utalca.cl): It is the structural database of different nanoparticles that might be used in nanomedicine. This website provides resources for the viewing of various nanoparticles, including dendrimers, nanotubes, and metallic particles, as well as downloadable nanopdb files, associated research information, and data (CSN).

9.5   APPLICATION OF BIOINFORMATICS IN NANOMEDICINE

Nanoinformatics is a promising discipline that has yet to be fully defined due to its novelty. Although computers have been used in many parts of nanotechnological research, the subject still requires a better articulation of goals, subdisciplines, concepts, and educational requirements, which might lead to more defined research and development agendas. We can think of nanoinformatics as the best technique to integrate multiple areas of study and translation in a fair amount of time as it provides the opportunity to design and test these systems immediately, allowing us to devise a sensible means of growing them as our understanding improves.

There are the following specific nanoinformatics research areas as shown in Figure 9.3.

9.5.1   DATA TERMINOLOGIES, ONTOLOGIES, AND EXCHANGE OF INFORMATION

The need for updated data, information, and digital libraries, as well as for mechanisms of information transmission, is expanding quickly in the field of

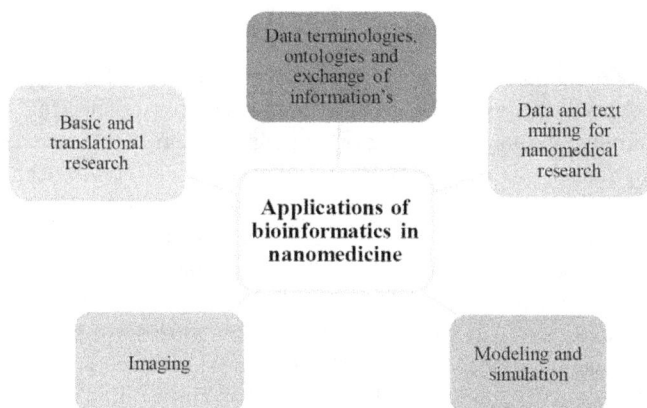

FIGURE 9.3   Application of bioinformatics in nanomedicine.

nanomedicine. A current strategy for easing data transmission through shared terminological references is the development of biomedical ontologies, which are crucial to the semantic web (Bizer, 2009). The following are described in biomedical ontologies: concepts or classes, such as those for flora and fauna life forms, cells, molecules, and proteins; and their corresponding properties. Ontologies have proven crucial for organizing and managing knowledge, especially in the biomedical sector. The integration of multilevel data, data mapping, search, storage, and extraction are all made possible by ontologies today (Renear & Palmer, 2009; Spasic, Ananiadou, McNaught, & Kumar, 2005). As previously stated, the development of an informatics gateway with tools similar to those used in conjunction with the Protein Data Bank is highly needed. The main focus of such a site should be the structural models of nanomaterials that must be stored, regulated, validated, and distributed (Council, 2012; Thomas, Pappu, & Baker, 2011).

9.5.2   DATA AND TEXT MINING FOR NANOMEDICAL RESEARCH

Enormous medical and biological databases have typically been used for data mining to create or validate research hypotheses. Data mining issues can be divided into two primary categories from the viewpoint of machine learning: supervised learning and unsupervised learning. Classification and numerical prediction are two further subcategories of supervised learning. The class label is discrete in a classification problem. In contrast, the class label is continuous in a problem of numerical prediction. Predicting the toxicology of nanoparticles is an example of supervised learning (Horev-Azaria et al., 2011). When toxicity is categorically specified (toxic or nontoxic), classification methods are utilized, and quantitative-based models are used when toxicity is described as a numerical feature. In unsupervised learning, clustering is a common issue (Dorney et al., 2012).

9.5.3 Modeling and Simulation

Molecular modeling and simulation approaches are crucial in systems biology research. They will be essential in the nanoworld for connecting aggregation, molecular, cellular, tissue, organ, and organismal system-level impacts with nano-level effects. The fundamental physical, chemical, and biological features of nanoparticles and nanomaterials can be analyzed and understood using methods from quantum mechanics, molecular modeling, and simulation (Varga & Driscoll, 2011). Characterizing the characteristics of nanoparticles is made easier by computationally demanding techniques like hybrid quantum mechanics and molecular dynamic simulations. Additionally, this offers comprehensive details on biological events connected to the interactions between nanoparticles and physiological systems (Archakov & Ivanov, 2007). These simulations allow one to explore the fundamental physicochemical characteristics of nanoparticles and speed up their research.

9.5.4 Imaging

For many biomedical applications, semiconductor luminous Quantum dots (QDs) are used as probes (Gao et al., 2005; Papagiannaros, Levchenko, Hartner, Mongayt, & Torchilin, 2009). Small size (around 10 nm in diameter), greater photostability, specialized adjustable or configurable optical and electrical properties, size-tunable light emission, remarkable signal brightness, barrier properties to photobleaching, and broad absorption spectra for simultaneous excitation of numerous fluorescence colors and multimodality to facilitate in vivo diagnosis are just a few of their many characteristics. For instance, they can be used to diagnose various cancers. They are capable of being joined to specific molecules found inside malignant tumors, aiding early diagnosis and treatment with the goal of enhancing patient outcomes and early tumor development [13, 14, 15]. Controlled gold nanoparticles can improve cancer molecular computed tomography (CT) imaging in a manner similar to this. In order to create CT contrast agents for blood pools, various nanoprobes, such as gold nanoprobes and nanotags, iodine-based emulsions, and tantalum oxide nanoparticles, have been developed (Reuveni, Motiei, Romman, Popovtzer, & Popovtzer, 2011; Sperling, Gil, Zhang, Zanella, & Parak, 2008). Then, using cutting-edge informatics techniques, tissue banks, images of tissues, and histological findings might all be linked together to enable increased image annotation at the nanoscale.

9.5.5 Basic and Translational Research

"Translational nanoinformatics" is a new subfield that aims to translate fundamental nano-level research into clinical applications. In this, research findings as well as adverse effects like nanotoxicity, a significant clinical concern—may aid in the development of new understandings about how in vitro and model results might be applied to clinical settings and practice (Lavik & Von Recum, 2011; Maojo et al., 2010). The goal of translational nanoinformatics is to transform measurements and data taken at the nano or atomic level into new understanding that can help patients receive high-quality diagnoses and treatments. The polymorphic and polydisperse character of nanomaterials is one of the specific problems that face nanoinformatics. For the nanoscale integration of data and knowledge, new strategies are needed. To ensure the accuracy of the data and analysis techniques employed in nanomedicine, expert annotation and curation of the data are required (Maojo et al., 2010).

9.6 OBSTACLES FOR BIOINFORMATICS IN NANOMEDICINE

The following are the main research obstacles and requirements, as previously said, as a result of a lack of information:

1. Enhanced characterization of nanomaterials as reported in databases and literature;
2. Determining the analytical methods' sensitivity to changes in experiments, supplies, and methodological approaches;
3. Evaluating and managing various sorts of risks;
4. Assessing the mistake and uncertainty in the procedures and techniques used to obtain the data (Kuiken, 2011; Sandler, 2009).

Nanoinformatics has to deal with two key problems at the same time:

1. The requirement for system control as a result of the huge and constantly changing sets of variables resulting from nano-scale testing; and
2. The necessity for data analysis.

Furthermore, the intricacy of the research apparatus itself as well as the sophistication of the experiments were greatly boosted by the variables that the researcher intended to alter. All of these need to be managed using computerized models at the atomic, molecular, and nanoscale, which necessitates the processing and analysis of enormous datasets. The following growth of ever-expanding applications of nanotechnology and nanomedicine has revealed a wide range of issues that can be solved with or without the aid of nanoinformatics approaches (Maojo, Fritts, de la Iglesia, et al., 2012).

9.7 FUTURE PROSPECTIVE OF BIOINFORMATICS IN NANOMEDICINE

Nanomedicine derived by using bioinformatics offers a remarkable potential to reduce the devastating impacts of untreatable diseases like cancer and many more, which annually affect millions of people worldwide. There are still many obstacles that nanomedicines in healthcare must overcome. The scientific difficulties of transitioning nanomedicines from the lab scale from initial proof-of-principle phases to verified, dependable, and commercially licensed products with established efficacy and safety will be another significant hurdle. In order to achieve this, academic-pharmaceutical industry partnerships must be strengthened (Ratner, 2011). In a few years, we anticipate that clinicians will be able to select from a vast array of clinically approved nanocarrier building blocks that can be quickly combined with the appropriate therapeutic agent, imaging agent, and targeting molecules in accordance with the patient's unique pharmacological and molecular characteristics derived from multi-level "omics" information and bioinformatics tools in the future will help us to achieve this. Consequently, makes it possible for doctors to realize the full potential of individualized therapy and to produce better therapeutic results at a reasonable cost. Future uses of nanotechnology in healthcare to develop nanomedicine via bioinformatics and how it might propel the sector into a new stage of development are piquing the interest of inventors more and more which will enable them to develop some vital bioinformatics tools that can overcome the obstacles aroused (Jain, 2008).

9.8   CONCLUSION

This chapter summarized key ideas and offered organizational principles for a novel use of informatics that poses major difficulties for both informaticians and experts in nanotechnology and nanomedicine. As we've already indicated, nanoinformatics can offer solutions to many issues that arise in nanomedicine. Physicians and biologists have recently encountered issues in their fields of study and practice that, at least in an abstract sense, are not dissimilar to those that nanotechnologists and experts in the field of nanomedicine are currently dealing with. Data integration, standards, decision support, information storage and access, simulation, and modeling are the main information-related concerns and also the obstacles have arisen. The significance of this area will enable experts to create various computational strategies to deal with the significant problems in nanoinformatics.

REFERENCES

Action GRID: Assessing the Impact of Nanotechnology on Biomedical Informatics - PubMed. (n.d.-a). Retrieved November 23, 2022, from https://pubmed.ncbi.nlm.nih.gov/18998944/

Action GRID: Assessing the Impact of Nanotechnology on Biomedical Informatics - PubMed. (n.d.-b). Retrieved November 28, 2022, from https://pubmed.ncbi.nlm.nih.gov/18998944/

Archakov, A. I., & Ivanov, Y. D. (2007). Analytical nanobiotechnology for medicine diagnostics. *Molecular BioSystems*, *3*, 336–342.

Bayat, A. (2002). Science, medicine, and the future: Bioinformatics. *BMJ: British Medical Journal*, *324*, 1018.

Bewick, S., Yang, R., & Zhang, M. (2009). Complex mathematical models of biology at the nanoscale. *Wiley Interdisciplinary Reviews: Nanomedicine and Nanobiotechnology*, *1*, 650–659.

Bizer, C. (2009). The emerging web of linked data. *IEEE Intelligent Systems*, *24*, 87–92.

Breu, F., Guggenbichler, S., & Wollmann, J. (2008). Intracellular delivery – fundamentals and applications. *Vasa*, 433–456.

Chamundeeswari, M., Sobhana, S. S. L., Jacob, J. P., Kumar, M. G., Devi, M. P., Sastry, T. P., & Mandal, A. B. (2010). Preparation, characterization and evaluation of a biopolymeric gold nanocomposite with antimicrobial activity. *Biotechnology and Applied Biochemistry*, *55*, 29–35.

Chen, Y., Zhu, X., Zhang, X., Liu, B., & Huang, L. (2010). Nanoparticles modified with tumor-targeting scFv deliver siRNA and miRNA for cancer therapy. *Molecular Therapy: The Journal of the American Society of Gene Therapy, 18,* 1650–1656.

Council, N. R. (2012). A research strategy for environmental, health, and safety aspects of engineered nanomaterials. *A Research Strategy for Environmental, Health, and Safety Aspects of Engineered Nanomaterials,* 1–230.

De La Iglesia, D., Chiesa, S., Kern, J., Maojo, V., Martin-Sanchez, F., Potamias, G., ... & Mitchell, J. A. (2009). Nanoinformatics: New challenges for biomedical informatics at the nano level. *Studies in Health Technology and Informatics, 150,* 987–991.

Dorney, J., Bonnier, F., Garcia, A., Casey, A., Chambers, G., & Byrne, H. J. (2012). Identifying and localizing intracellular nanoparticles using Raman spectroscopy. *Analyst, 137,* 1111–1119.

Farokhzad, O. C., & Langer, R. (2006). Nanomedicine: Developing smarter therapeutic and diagnostic modalities. *Advanced Drug Delivery Reviews, 58,* 1456–1459.

Freitas, R. A. (2005). What is nanomedicine? *Nanomedicine: Nanotechnology, Biology and Medicine, 1,* 2–9.

Gao, X., Yang, L., Petros, J. A., Marshall, F. F., Simons, J. W., & Nie, S. (2005). In vivo molecular and cellular imaging with quantum dots. *Current Opinion in Biotechnology, 16,* 63–72.

Gvili, J., & Machluf, M. (2006). 544. PLGA nanoparticles for DNA vaccination–waiving complexity and increasing efficiency. *Molecular Therapy, 13,* S209.

Horev-Azaria, L., Kirkpatrick, C. J., Korenstein, R., Marche, P. N., Maimon, O., Ponti, J., ... & Villiers, C. (2011). Predictive toxicology of cobalt nanoparticles and ions: Comparative in vitro study of different cellular models using methods of knowledge discovery from data. *Toxicological Sciences, 122,* 489–501.

Ironi, L., & Tentoni, S. (2003). A model-based approach to the assessment of physico-chemical properties of drug delivery materials. *Computers & Chemical Engineering, 27,* 803–812.

Jain, K. K. (2008). Nanomedicine. *NanoBioTechnology: BioInspired Devices and Materials of the Future,* 303–327.

Jeevanandam, J., Barhoum, A., Chan, Y. S., Dufresne, A., & Danquah, M. K. (2018). Review on nanoparticles and nanostructured materials: History, sources, toxicity and regulations. *Beilstein Journal of Nanotechnology, 9,* 1050.

Khan, I., Saeed, K., & Khan, I. (2019). Nanoparticles: Properties, applications and toxicities. *Arabian Journal of Chemistry, 12,* 908–931.

Kuiken, T. (2011). Nanomedicine and ethics: Is there anything new or unique? *Wiley Interdisciplinary Reviews: Nanomedicine and Nanobiotechnology, 3,* 111–118.

Lavik, E., & Von Recum, H. (2011). The role of nanomaterials in translational medicine. *ACS Nano, 5,* 3419.

Lee Ventola, C. (2012). The nanomedicine revolution: Part 1: Emerging concepts. *Pharmacy and Therapeutics, 37,* 512.

Li, J., de Vries, R. P., & Peng, M. (2021). Bioinformatics approaches for fungal biotechnology. *Encyclopedia of Mycology,* 536–554.

Maojo, V, Fritts, M., Martin-Sanchez, F., De La Iglesia, D., Cachau, R. E., Garcia-Remesal, M., ... & Kulikowski, C. (2012). Nanoinformatics: Developing new computing applications for nanomedicine. *Computing in Science & Engineering, 94,* 521–539.

Maojo, V., Fritts, M., de la Iglesia, D., Cachau, R. E., Garcia-Remesal, M., Mitchell, J. A., & Kulikowski, C. (2012). Nanoinformatics: A new area of research in nanomedicine. *International Journal of Nanomedicine, 7,* 3867–3890.

Maojo, V., Martin-Sanchez, F., Kulikowski, C., Rodriguez-Paton, A., & Fritts, M. (2010). Nanoinformatics and DNA-based computing: Catalyzing nanomedicine. *Pediatric Research, 67,* 481–489.

Mauger, B., Hunter, J., Drennan, J., Wright, A., & O'Hagan, T. (2007). Building a data grid for the Australian nanostructural analysis network. *Third IEEE International Conference on E-Science and Grid Computing (e-Science 2007)*, 312–319. https://www.10.1109/e-Science.2007.26

Neil Gordon, A., President, M., Sagman, U., Rémi Quirion, S., Warren Chan, A., Professor, A., … NanoBusiness Alliance Nanomedicine Taxonomy, C. (2003). *Canadian NanoBusiness Alliance Nanomedicine Taxonomy*.

Papagiannaros, A., Levchenko, T., Hartner, W., Mongayt, D., & Torchilin, V. (2009). Quantum dots encapsulated in phospholipid micelles for imaging and quantification of tumors in the near-infrared region. *Nanomedicine: Nanotechnology, Biology and Medicine, 5*, 216–224.

Perez-Acle, T., & Sandoval, C. (n.d.). New challenges for bioinformatics and computational chemistry in nanobiotechnology. *Isp.Ncifcrf.Gov*. Retrieved from https://www.academia.edu/22295303/New_challenges_for_Bioinformatics_and_Computational_Chemistry_in_NanoBiotechnology

Ratner, M. (2011). Pfizer reaches out to academia—again. *Nature Biotechnology, 29*, 3–4.

Renear, A. H., & Palmer, C. L. (2009). Strategic reading, ontologies, and the future of scientific publishing. *Science, 325*, 828–832.

Reuveni, T., Motiei, M., Romman, Z., Popovtzer, A., & Popovtzer, R. (2011). Targeted gold nanoparticles enable molecular CT imaging of cancer: An in vivo study. *International Journal of Nanomedicine, 6*, 2859.

Sandler, R. (2009). Nanomedicine and nanomedical ethics, *9*, 16–17. http://Dx.Doi.Org/10.1080/15265160902995117

Shan, Y., Luo, T., Peng, C., Sheng, R., Cao, A., Cao, X., … & Shi, X. (2012). Gene delivery using dendrimer-entrapped gold nanoparticles as nonviral vectors. *Biomaterials, 33*, 3025–3035.

Spasic, I., Ananiadou, S., McNaught, J., & Kumar, A. (2005). Text mining and ontologies in biomedicine: Making sense of raw text. *Briefings in Bioinformatics, 6*, 239–251.

Sperling, R. A., Gil, P. R., Zhang, F., Zanella, M., & Parak, W. J. (2008). Biological applications of gold nanoparticles. *Chemical Society Reviews, 37*, 1896–1908.

Thomas, D. G., Klaessig, F., Harper, S. L., Fritts, M., Hoover, M. D., Gaheen, S., … & Baker, N. A. (2011). Informatics and standards for nanomedicine technology. *Wiley Interdisciplinary Reviews: Nanomedicine and Nanobiotechnology, 3*, 511–532.

Thomas, D. G., Pappu, R. V., & Baker, N. A. (2011). Nanoparticle ontology for cancer nanotechnology research. *Journal of Biomedical Informatics, 44*, 59.

Thomas, V., Yallapu, M. M., Sreedhar, B., & Bajpai, S. K. (2009). Fabrication, characterization of chitosan/nanosilver film and its potential antibacterial application. *Journal of Biomaterials Science. Polymer Edition, 20*, 2129–2144.

Varga, K., & Driscoll, J. A. (2011). Computational nanoscience: Applications for molecules, clusters, and solids. *Computational Nanoscience: Applications for Molecules, Clusters, and Solids, 9781107001701*, 1–431.

Yohan, D., & Chithrani, B. D. (2014). Applications of nanoparticles in nanomedicine. *Journal of Biomedical Nanotechnology, 10*, 2371–2392.

Zhou, C., Yu, J., Qin, Y., & Zheng, J. (2012). Grain size effects in polycrystalline gold nanoparticles. *Nanoscale, 4*, 4228–4233.

Zweigenbaum, P., Demner-fushman, D., Yu, H., & Cohen, K. B. (2007). Frontiers of biomedical text mining: Current progress. *Briefings in Bioinformatics, 8*, 358.

10 Nanotechnology for Diagnosis and Therapy of Rheumatoid Arthritis

Tanya Singh, Anjali Priyadarshini, and V. Samuel Raj

10.1 INTRODUCTION

An arthritic condition is characterized by inflammation of one or more joints (Chow and Chin, 2020). Redness of the joints, swelling of the joints, joint discomfort, and joint warmth are some of the signs and symptoms of this disease (Ng and Azizudin, 2020). Osteoarthritis (OA) and rheumatoid arthritis (RA) are the most common types of arthritis. The OA is a mechanical condition resulting from wear and tear of joints, while the RA is an autoimmune disease (Chua et al., 2019). There are numerous joints in the body that are affected by RA. In the absence of treatment, RA damages bone and cartilage, making it difficult for patients to work or attend social activities. This condition is called chronic RA (Guo et al., 2018). An illustration of arthritis joints is shown in Figure 10.1. It has been demonstrated that inflammation of the tendon (tenosynovitis) can result in both cartilage loss and bone erosion (Lin et al., 2020). In RA, different treatments have heterogeneous clinical effects (Conigliaro et al., 2019).

RA affects approximately 5 in 1,000 people and, tragically, 80% of those affected experience disability within 20 years of initial symptoms. There are several anti-arthritic drugs on the market today, but most of them are relatively expensive, have limited efficacy, and have unavoidable side effects. Inflammatory drugs are one of the most expensive healthcare treatment categories (Fonseca et al., 2019). Nonsteroidal anti-inflammatory drugs (NSAIDs), glucocorticoids (GCs), disease-modifying anti-inflammatory drugs (DMARDs), and biologics are commonly prescribed for the treatment of RA. NSAID-induced nephrotoxicity, liver damage, and heart failure are potential side effects of these treatments but may slow disease progression (Khilfeh et al., 2019). If drugs do not work, surgery is the only option (Ganhewa et al., 2019).

Tumor necrosis factor (TNF-α) plays an important role in the pathogenesis of rheumatoid arthritis and is emerging as a new therapeutic target. TNF-α inhibitors such as adalimumab and etanercept are important biologics in the treatment of rheumatoid arthritis. Ten studies have shown that these clinical drugs can cause

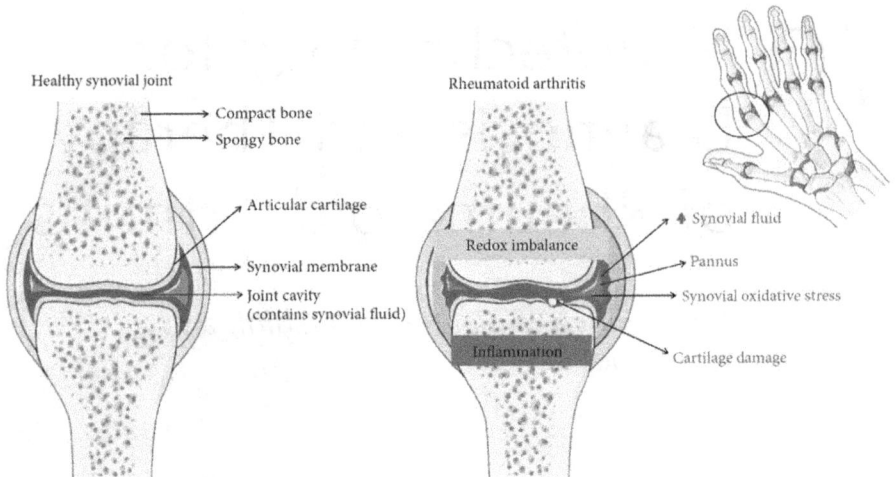

FIGURE 10.1   Normal joint vs RA joint.

serious neurological and hematological side effects and harm the human body (Guidelli et al., 2020). Rheumatoid arthritis Most of the current treatments for HIV are combination therapy with methotrexate and biologics, which are far superior to monotherapies, but expensive biologics can be an unbearable financial burden for many patients and their families. Therefore, developing biocompatible drugs that can treat joint damage is our goal, and nanotechnology promises to improve conventional drug treatments (Peng et al., 2019). This chapter summarizes current progress in the application of various nanomaterials in the treatment of rheumatoid arthritis.

10.2   CURRENT DIAGNOSIS AND TREATMENT STRATEGIES FOR RA

In clinical practice, physicians currently use the American College of Rheumatology (ACR) in 1987 (Arnett et al., 1988) and the ACR/European League Against Rheumatism (EULAR) in 2010 (Aletaha et al., 2010) is recommended. However, such a diagnosis is primarily based on physical examination and observation of characteristic symptoms such as pain, stiffness, and swelling in multiple joints in a symmetrical pattern. This means that a purely clinical diagnosis can only be confirmed from six months to one year after RA onset, making early diagnosis of RA almost impossible. Furthermore, the symptoms and pathological features of RA are usually nonspecific, resulting in low clinical, radiological, or immunological diagnostic efficiency, and lack of a gold-standard approach to RA diagnosis (Visser, 2005). With this in mind, the Chinese College of Rheumatology formulated the 2018 edition of the Chinese Guidelines for the Diagnosis and Treatment of RA. The 2018 guidelines state that physicians should base their diagnosis on a patient's clinical presentation, laboratory, and imaging studies (Figure 10.2) (Jans et al., 2018).

Serological tests are performed to detect various circulating blood factors, such as immune-mediated antibodies (RF, ACPA) and/or acute-phase reactants (C-reactive protein (CRP), erythrocyte sedimentation rate (ESR)), which increase during

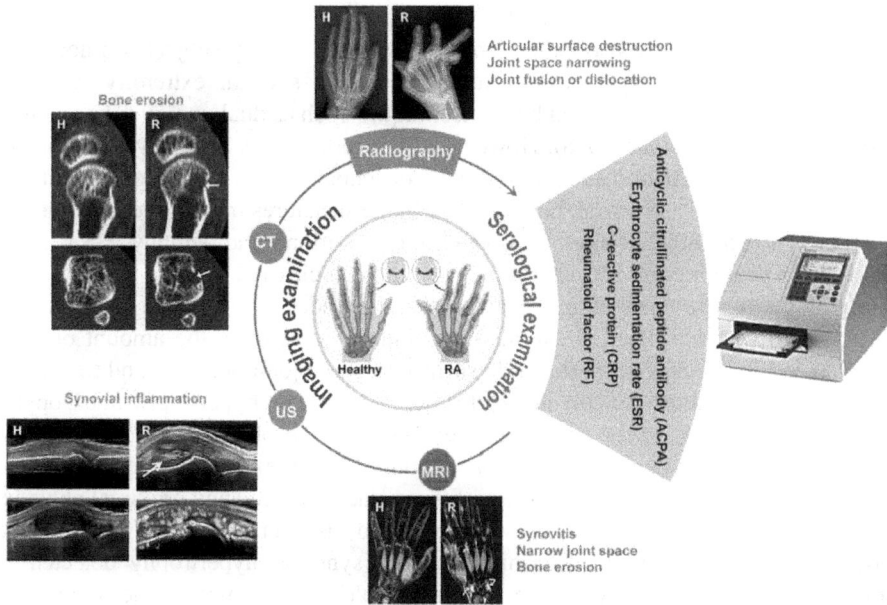

FIGURE 10.2 RA diagnostic techniques used in clinic.

inflammation. Used to detect biomarkers. A patient may be diagnosed with RA if at least one of RF and ACPA has a positive titer and elevated levels of acute-phase reactants (CRP or ESR) are observed (Aletaha et al., 2010). Imaging modalities for RA include conventional radiography, ultrasonography (US), computed tomography (CT), and magnetic resonance imaging (MRI) (Figure 10.2). Imaging criteria for RA are based on the size and number of joints involved and the duration of synovitis. Patients with RA must meet criteria for two or more medium or large joint involvement or one or more small joint involvement. Or the duration of synovitis exceeds her six weeks. Among the various imaging approaches, conventional radiography such as X-ray is the most commonly used imaging tool to assess structural damage in the RA joint. A conventional her radiograph of a healthy subject shows a consolidated baseline joint, with well-defined rims of cortical bone (McQueen, 2013). If erosions are present, joint margins in RA patients may be destroyed or may fit more closely to the adjacent cortex if the joints are narrowed. Her radiographs in early RA showed periarticular soft tissue swelling and periarticular or juxtaarticular osteoporosis. As the disease progresses, joint surface destruction, joint space narrowing, joint fusion, or joint dislocation may occur. X-rays can visualize destruction of joint surfaces, narrowing of the joint space, periarticular osteoporosis, cysts, and, in severe cases, joint fusion or dislocation, but early signs such as soft tissue changes and bone erosions can be visualized. It cannot detect disease symptoms. X-rays, while convenient and inexpensive, suffer from radiation damage and low sensitivity for early diagnosis. CT can detect calcified tissue destruction, such as bone erosion in RA, and achieve 3D visualization of joints (Barile, 2017). This increases the sensitivity of erosion detection, especially in complex areas like the wrist, and aids in the earliest possible diagnosis. The metacarpophalangeal (MCP) joints of RA patients show obvious erosions, whereas healthy subjects do not show erosions in the metacarpal heads. Additionally, the skeletal extremity status of patients with RA can be assessed by CT techniques such as dual-energy CT and high-resolution CT (Jans et al., 2018). However, CT is radioactive, expensive, and cannot detect active inflammation such as synovitis or tenosynovitis. US is convenient and inexpensive to assess synovial, bony, and cartilage structures in multiple joints and to monitor synovial inflammation. Compared to conventional radiography, US is more sensitive to detecting joint structural damage and can clearly show the thickness and morphology of the synovium, synovial sac, joint cavity effusion, and articular cartilage. In addition, the US can also dynamically determine the amount of joint effusion and its distance from the body surface to guide joint puncture and treatment. US imaging of healthy subjects shows that neither synovial hypertrophy nor Doppler activity, independent of the presence of exudate, can be observed (Agostino et al., 2017). If synovial hypertrophy, with or without exudate, extends to the level of the horizontal line joining the bony surface of the metacarpal head and proximal phalanx, but the surface is flat or convex (curved downward), the person may be an RA of the Doppler signal. Severity is determined by the synovial hypertrophy detected in grayscale and the intensity of the power Doppler signal (within the synovium) (Agostino et al., 2017). Doppler ultrasound can be used to confirm the presence of synovitis, monitor disease activity and progression, and assess inflammation (Gaujoux-Viala et al., 2014). However, US is highly dependent on operator skill.

MRI is the most sensitive tool for diagnosing early RA lesions such as synovitis, joint space narrowing, and bone erosion, but has the disadvantage of high cost (Hodkinson et al., 2013). It was detected in early RA by MRI, which is important for early detection of RA. Compared with healthy subjects, MR signal intensity in the synovial compartment was enhanced in RA patients after gadolinium injection, her MR signal intensity in cortical bone increased, but trabecular bone signal decreased. Detection of early inflammation by MRI and US is superior to clinical examination. It can be used not only to predict whether undifferentiated arthritis will progress to RA, but also to predict future joint damage in clinical remission and assess the presence of persistent inflammation. However, early diagnosis of RA remains challenging due to the difficulty of identifying characteristic symptoms in the early stages.

Regarding treatment, the 2018 guidelines prescribe early standardized treatment with regular monitoring and aftercare as the principle of treatment for RA. By inhibiting the production and action of cytokines as early as possible, we can effectively prevent or delay joint synovitis and cartilage lesions, ultimately controlling the disease state, reducing the disability rate, and ultimately improving the patient's health. Treatment of RA has been constantly optimized through years of continuous research. As summarized in Table 10.1, there are currently four basic categories for the treatment of RA: disease-modifying anti-inflammatory drugs (DMARDs), glucocorticoids (GCs), and non-steroidal anti-inflammatory drugs (NSAIDs) and biologics (Umar et al., 2012).

Methotrexate (MTX) is a classic DMARD and has been the first-line treatment for RA since the early 1980s and can be used alone or in combination with other agents. GCs can interfere with macrophage accumulation and impair capillary

TABLE 10.1

Current Therapeutic Agents for RA

Classification	Instance	Mechanism of Action	Side Effects
DMARDS	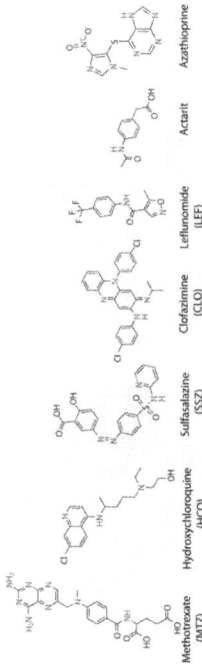 Methotrexate (MTZ), Hydroxychloroquine (HCQ), Sulfasalazine (SSZ), Clofazimine (CLO), Leflunomide (LEF), Actarit, Azathioprine	Immunosuppression, Inhibition of genetic	Hepatic cirrhosis, myelosuppression, interstitial pneumonitis, gastrointestinal disorders, etc.
GCs	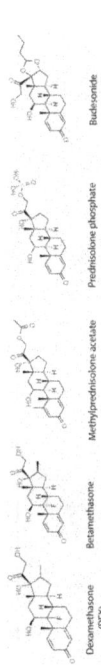 Dexamethasone (DEX), Betamethasone, Methylprednisolone acetate, Prednisolone phosphate, Budesonide	Prevention of phospholipid release, anti-inflammation, immunosuppression	Insulin resistance, infection, hyperadrenocorticism, hypertension and atherosclerosis, osteoporosis and osteonecrosis, skin thinning, obesity, and inhibition of wound repair, etc.
NSAIDs	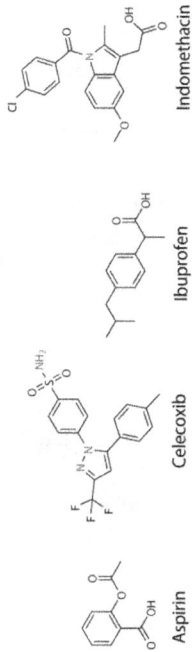 Aspirin, Celecoxib, Ibuprofen, Indomethacin	Inhibition of COXs, reduce acute inflammation, analgesia	Gastrointestinal disturbance, renal malfunction, increase cardiovascular risk, etc.

(Continued)

TABLE 10.1 (Continued)
Current Therapeutic Agents for RA

Classification	Instance	Mechanism of Action	Side Effects
Biological agents	 Etanercept　Infliximab　Adalimumab (ADA)　Golimumab (GOL)　Anakinra (AKR)　Tocilizumab (TCZ)	Antagonism of TNF-α, IL-1 receptor, or IL-6 receptor	Infection, tuberculosis reactivation, gastrointestinal perforation
	 Auranofin　Cyclosporine　Rituximab (RIT)	Reduce the formation of rheumatoid factor and antibody, downregulate T-cell activation, deplete B-cell	Infection, hypersensitivity, hypertension, renal disease, respiratory difficulty, diarrhea

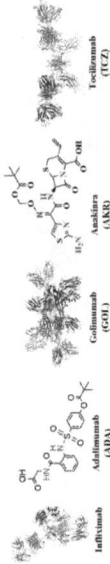

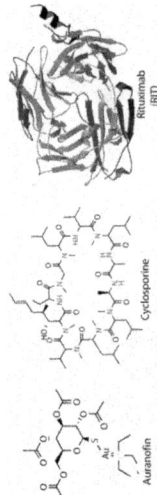

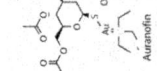

permeability and are therefore primarily used for the initial treatment of aggressive RA. NSAIDs provide relief from symptoms associated with inflammation by suppressing prostaglandin production. Biologic agents such as infliximab (INF), etanercept (ETA), and tocilizumab (TCZ), which can block IL-6 receptors and inhibit TNF-α, have been used in the treatment of RA in the clinic. Although these treatments are effective, their use is limited due to adverse side effects such as cardiac complications, ulcers, gastrointestinal disturbances, and immuno-suppression leading to the development of opportunistic infections (Umar et al., 2012). Therefore, there is an urgent need to propose safer and more effective approaches to RA treatment.

10.3 SUPERIORITIES OF NANOTECHNOLOGY FOR RA DIAGNOSIS AND THERAPY

Nanomaterials are booming today, and their high drug-loading efficiency, multi-modal imaging capabilities, and passive and/or active targeting effects have dramatically increased biomedical applications, including diagnostics and thera-peutics. Therapeutic or imaging agents can be selectively, controllably, or sustainably delivered to the desired site of inflammation by using nanoscale drug carriers. In this way, the therapeutic efficacy of conventional anti-RA drugs can be greatly enhanced, and side effects caused by short biological half-life and low bioavailability can be obviously reduced (Wang et al., 2020). Tao et al. synthesized a respiratory jet to inhale NO produced at the RA site and exhale CO under visible light to improve nitrite levels and inflammatory cytokines at the RA site, leading to more effective treatment of RA (Tao et al., 2020). More importantly, nanomaterials provide a robust framework into which multiple therapeutics and/or contrast agents can be incorporated to provide synergistic multifunctional nanomedicine. Nanoscale genetically engineered biomaterials such as polylactic acid (PLA), poly-L-lysine (PLL), hyaluronic acid (HA), and chitosan are used to encapsulate therapeutic agents to form local drug delivery systems and can create porous scaffolds that Stimulate local immune responses or chemotherapy, radiotherapy, etc. to achieve more effective treatments (Cai et al., 2020). Cai et al. modified his two targeting molecules and his two therapeutic agents on the surface of dendrigraft PLL nanoparticles, making the nanoparticles specific to the blood-brain barrier and damaged neurons. Various mild binding strategies, such as covalent bonding, hydrogen bonding, and electrostatic interactions, are well-established for attaching therapeutic and contrast agents to the surface of nanomaterials (Hermanson, 2008). Indeed, nanomaterials are widely used to combine diagnostic molecules and drugs into a single drug (Chen et al., 2017). The hydrophobic near-infrared dye IR-797 was self-assembled into nanoparticles using a solvent exchange method and surface-modified with an amphiphilic polymer (C18PMH-PEG5000) to improve biocompatibility. The resulting nanoparticles can be aggregated at the lesion site to achieve fluorescence/photoacoustic/photothermal imaging-guided chemotherapy/photothermal therapy.

Nanotheranostics can provide specific targeting, non-invasive imaging, and effective treatment at the lesion site without affecting surrounding healthy cells

(Ma et al., 2020). For example, PLGA nanoparticles encapsulate DOX by emulsion evaporation and bind to the target molecule mAb through aramid bonds, while the outer layer encapsulates a PEI layer to electrostatically absorb siRNA, making the nanoparticles specific for triple-negative breast cancer, which can increase therapeutic efficacy and toxicity and reduce side effects (Liu et al., 2020). Horse et al. synthesized a chimeric peptide composed of a lipophilic palmitate, a photosensitizer, a fluorophore, a cystasparin-3-responsive peptide, and a hydrophilic PEG layer that can self-assemble into nanoparticles (Ma et al., 2020). Affixed to tumor cell membranes, photodynamic (PDT) therapy can be achieved, enhancing therapeutic efficacy while monitoring therapeutic feedback via fluorescence changes. In general, nanotheranostic probes consist of several functional components, such as diagnostic imaging agents, therapeutic moieties, targeting moieties, and some surface modification or coating moieties to improve biocompatibility and water solubility. Figure 10.3 (Shi et al., 2020) shows the functional components commonly used in RA nanotheranostic probes. By combining diagnosis and treatment in a single platform, nanotheranostics have shown significant advantages for RA diagnosis and treatment. On the one hand, nanotheranostics can enable early diagnosis of RA, which in turn facilitates early treatment of RA and improves therapeutic efficacy. Second, in-treatment monitoring can improve prognosis, thereby hastening physician treatment decisions (Wong et al., 2020). Third, the introduction of targeting units will reduce anti-RA drug abuse and treatment costs.

The search for new diagnostics and treatments for RA remains an open and hot research field. Nanotechnology represents a new strategy for the diagnosis and

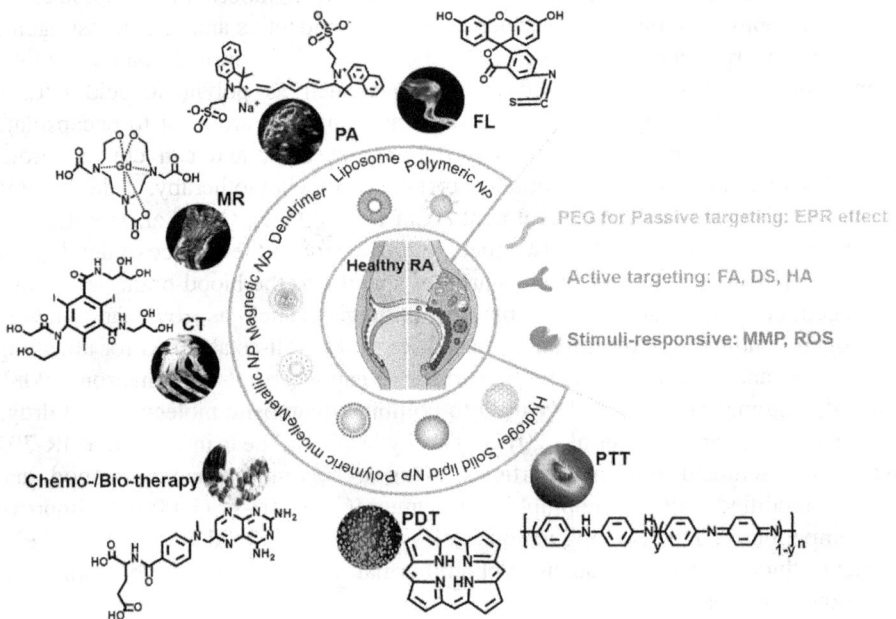

FIGURE 10.3   The summary of the key components for RA theranostics.

treatment of RA. This review summarizes the current development of nanoprobes for the diagnosis and treatment of RA. A particular focus of this chapter is nanotheranostics, which are promising for theranostics approaches in RA.

10.4 NANOMATERIALS FOR THE DIAGNOSIS OF INFLAMMATORY ARTHRITIS

10.4.1 TRADITIONAL APPROACHES

Diagnosis of the disease is difficult because there are over 100 different types of arthritis, and some symptoms are the same among the various diseases that affect the joints (Reginato and Olsen, 2002). The following classes are commonly defined as arthritis: inflammatory arthritis, degenerative arthritis, infectious arthritis, and metabolic arthritis (Furuzawa-Carballeda et al., 2008). The most common form of arthritis is inflammatory arthritis (Cappelli et al., 2017). Historically, several standard laboratory and imaging tests have been used to diagnose inflammatory arthritis. Common laboratory tests include the detection of antinuclear antibodies in blood, joint aspiration (removal and examination of synovial fluid), complement testing, and blood counts (white blood cells, red blood cells, platelets) (Rolle et al., 2019). For example, erythrocyte sedimentation rate (ESR) determines how easily red blood cells sink to the bottom of a test tube. Inflammation in the body increases the amount of ESR (Bray et al., 2016). The amount of red blood cells present in a blood sample is determined by the hematocrit or packed cell volume (PCV). A low red blood cell count (anemia) is common in arthritic patients (de Carvalho Franca et al., 2019). Rheumatoid factor (RF) monitors the presence of antibodies in most RA patients (Bugatti et al., 2016). Interestingly, in inflammatory arthritis, uric acid and CRP are increased in gout (Ghosh et al., 2016). Biomarkers, on the other hand, allow diagnosis of inflammatory arthritis at an early stage of the disease. The ACR/EULAR 2010 criteria for the diagnosis of RA focus on the detection of antibodies to RF and cyclic citrullinated proteins (anti-CCP), but early diagnosis includes antibodies to carbamylated proteins (anti-CarP), and a mutant citrullinated vimentin antibody (anti-CCP) is also included. included-MCV), and cartilage oligomeric matrix protein (anti-COMP).

Imaging, on the other hand, allows us to better understand the processes that occur in inflammatory arthritic joints. X-ray, ultrasound (US) MRI, and arthroscopy are available imaging tests for inflammatory arthritis (Bakewell et al., 2020). X-rays show the joint changes and bone damage seen in inflammatory arthritis. US is based on radiation-free sound waves to see the condition of synovial tissue, ligaments, tendons, and joints. MRI scans are more accurate than X-rays and show damage to joints, including muscles and tendons (Noguerol et al., 2017). An arthroscopy consists of a thin tube (arthroscope) with a flashlight and a camera that allows you to see through your joints. It is used to diagnose joint weakness and/or arthritic changes, classify bone diseases and tumors, and assess the severity of bone inflammation and pain (Memon et al., 2018).

All methods have many drawbacks, such as: despite the widespread use of conventional methods for diagnosing arthritis, they suffer from low accuracy, low image resolution, and high cost. However, important advances in nanomedicine have been made recently, and nanotechnology has the potential to introduce new platforms for high-precision diagnosis of inflammatory arthritis (Rabiei et al., 2020).

10.4.2 NANOIMAGING

Various imaging modalities have contributed to the diagnosis and assessment of inflammatory arthritis, but proper assessment of arthritis, especially in the early stages of the disease, can be problematic (Jo et al., 2018). Therefore, various studies are currently being conducted to improve the sensitivity and accuracy of imaging methods to facilitate the diagnosis of early-stage inflammatory arthritis. The biomedical field is increasingly using the engineering of nanoscale materials to achieve this goal (Cormode et al., 2009). The following sections describe the use of SPIOs, gold, polymeric NPs, and multimodal nanomaterials (cerium and silica NPs). These may offer promising biomedical applications in imaging inflammatory arthritis (Figure 10.4).

In both preclinical animal models and human clinical trials, SPIONs have been used as imaging agents for various diseases, including coronary artery disease, malformations, muscular dystrophies, cancer, inflammation, graft failure, and arthritis. SPION can image many types of infections, such as RA, at the cellular

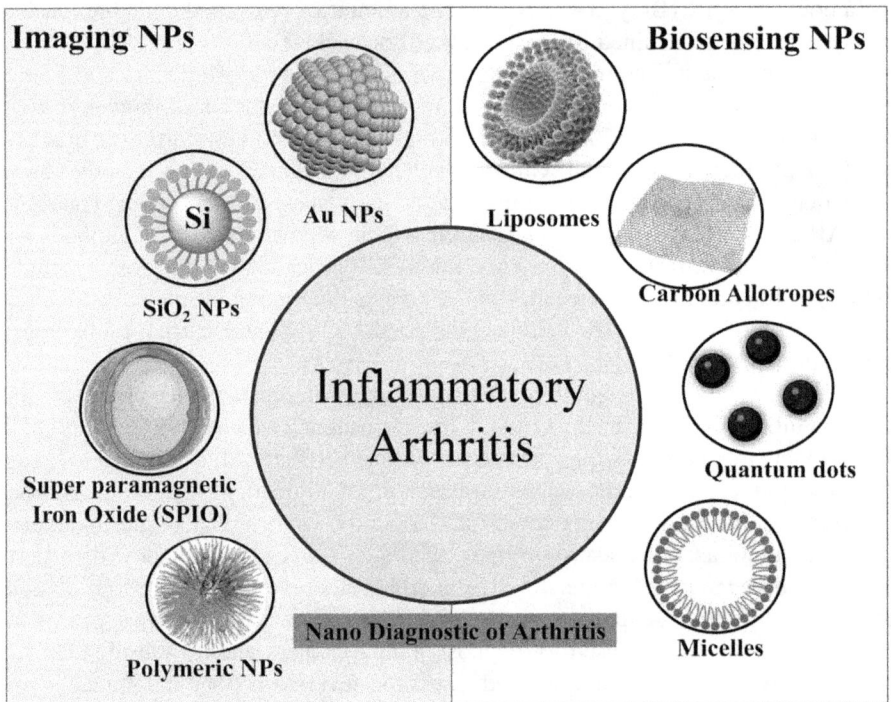

FIGURE 10.4 Different nanoparticles (NPs) for imaging and biosensing of inflammatory arthritis.

level. Chen et al. prepared targeted SPIONs for in vivo MRI of T-cells in RA via conjugation of an anti-CD3 monoclonal antibody to carboxylated polyethylene glycol (PEG)-SPIONs (IOPC-CD3). A series of MRI analyzes showed a selective reduction in the signal-to-noise ratio of her IOPC-CD33-injected femoral growth plates in a rat collagen-induced arthritis (CIA) model of RA. This means that the T-cell and SPION aggregates are in the target area.

Gold nanostructures including injectable auranofin for RA have been used for medicinal purposes for decades. Gold nanostructures have been widely evaluated in a number of imaging techniques, including CT, MRI, Raman spectroscopy, fluorescence, and photoacoustic imaging owing to its unique light scattering abilities and configurable surface plasmon resonance (Ma et al., 2020). The desirable imaging features and simplicity of gold nanomaterial preparation make it a good substrate for selective inflammation and arthritis imaging (Zhao et al., 2018). Using a fast-scanning optoacoustic imaging device based on a pulsed Nd:YAG laser and a single centered US transducer, they demonstrated a longitudinal improvement of optoacoustic signal magnitudes after injection of infliximab- but not certolizumab-modified and PEGylated control particles on arthritic and healthy control mice. Gold nanostructures containing injectable auranofins in RA have been used for medical purposes for decades. Gold nanostructures have been extensively evaluated in various imaging modalities, including CT, MRI, Raman spectroscopy, fluorescence, and photoacoustic imaging, due to their unique light scattering capabilities and configurable surface plasmon resonance (Ma et al., 2020). The favorable imaging properties and ease of fabrication of gold nanomaterials make them excellent substrates for selective imaging of inflammation and arthritis (Zhao et al., 2018). They used a pulsed Nd:YAG laser-based fast-scanning optoacoustic imaging device and a single central US transducer to show longitudinal improvement in optoacoustic signal intensity after injection of infliximab, but Certolizumab-modified and PEGylated control particles did not show any improvement on arthritic and healthy control mice.

Given their superior light-trapping properties, bioactivity, and configurable adsorption capacity, the use of conjugated polymer nanomaterials has solved the limitations of conventional contrast agents as they are superior contrast agents (Sarkar and Levi-Polyachenko, 2020). Tocilizumab-loaded nanopolymers show high-resolution images of swollen and cartilaginous tissue using NIR-II PMI of RA joint tissue, demonstrating the ability to non-invasively track the development of RA disease. In a related study, Vu-Quang et al. (2019) used NIR imaging and 19 F MRI in combination with labeled NP injections in vitro and in CIA mice. NPs were fabricated from poly(lactic glycolic acid) (PLGA)-PEG-folate (folate-NP) or from PEG-Block-PLGA loaded with indocyanine green (ICG) and perfluorooctyl bromide (PFOB). Excessive macrophages have been identified in the inflamed synovium/synovial fluid and in the pannus of inflamed vascular tissue in RA-affected joints. At early time points (two hours), the presence of folate as a targeting ligand strongly enhanced her NIR signal from inflamed tissue. In another study, Xiao et al. designed a cartilage-targeted cationic nanoprobe to enhance photoacoustic imaging (PAI) based on poly-L-lysine-melanin (PLL-M) NPs to track the development of arthritis. In vitro assays demonstrated the ability of PLL-MNPs to discriminate between various sensitive concentrations of anionic glycosaminoglycans (GAGs). By detecting changes in GAG substances using nanoprobe-enhanced PAI, we were able to comfortably and consistently visualize the development of arthritis.

Multimodal imaging modalities, which combine the strengths of multiple imaging modalities, can also be used for NPs. For example, silica-based NPs are attractive as multimodal imaging agents due to their biocompatibility, photostability, multivalent binding capacity, and biodistribution. Nanoceria, a cerium oxide-based NP, is another form of biocompatible NP used for multimodal imaging of arthritis.

10.4.3 NANODIAGNOSIS

The prevalence of arthritis has increased alarmingly since the beginning of the post-industrial era (Gavrila et al., 2016). Historically, traditional medical diagnosis of arthritis has focused on symptoms of pain and decreased function, and computed tomography (joint damage), which often appears late in the course of the disease (Humby et al., 2017). Analyzing biological parameters can be an attractive and realistic alternative. For example, RF and anti-CCP are used for diagnosis of inflammatory arthritis according to EULAR 2010 guidelines. Indeed, the most promising alternative for future diagnosis and treatment of inflammatory arthritis is NP (Rabiei et al., 2020). Nanomaterials such as quantum dots, carbon nanoallotropes, micelles, and liposomes are discussed in subsequent sections (Figure 10.4).

RA is characterized by the development of autoantibodies, synovial inflammation, and bone loss, and RF autoantibodies, as mentioned above, are the most recognized biomarkers of arthritis. To address this issue, Veigas et al. (2019) have developed an inexpensive and simple approach to detect and quantitatively measure HF markers. This colorimetric nanosensor was based on the cross-linking of Au nanoprobes, resulting in strong accumulation near the pentameric IgM RF. Accumulation of the nanoconjugate results in a color change from red to purple that is easily visible to the naked eye. The nanoplatform achieved a limit of detection (LOD) of 4.15 UA/mL IgM RF.

For biological applications, hybrid organic-inorganic nanomaterials have been investigated. This is due to structural and compositional changes in each section. A mixture of these hybrid NPs and metal nanomaterials would be desirable for plasmonic particle pairing for photonics-based biosensing applications. Huang et al. fabricated silver/gold (Ag@Au) core-shell NP) hybrid poly(aniline) nanostructures (CBCPHN) for early diagnosis of RA.

Nanohybrids were used for surface-enhanced Raman scattering (SERS)-based multiplexed detection of autoantibodies (RF IgM and anti-CCP). The LODs of RF IgM and anti-CCP were 0.93 IU/mL and 0.68 IU/mL, respectively. Animal studies have confirmed an association between Mycoplasma pneumoniae (MP) and RA for decades, with an increased risk of RA in patients with Mycoplasma pneumoniae (Chu et al., 2019). Zia et al. prepared Raman-based immunoassay strips to accurately detect MP contamination in blood samples. In this immunoassay, two layers of Raman dye 5,50-dithiobis-(2-nitrobenzoic acid) (DTNB) were loaded onto Au@Ag NPs as SERS tags. The LOD for RF was 0.1 ng/ml. H. 100 times more accurate than the colorimetric assay.

Cardiovascular disease (CVD) and RA are commonly associated with human immunodeficiency virus (HIV) infection, a global public health concern. Islam et al. (2019) developed a unique biosensor based on graphene-based field effect transistors for the detection of HIV and its related diseases (CVD and RA). In this study, amine-functionalized graphene (afG) was integrated with antibodies (anti-CCP for RA, anti-cTn1 for CVD, and anti-p24 for HIV) to detect multiple biomarkers. Antibodies were covalently attached to afG via carbodiimide activation. The nanosensor was highly sensitive and showed linearity to the biomarkers p24, cTn1, and CCP. The LOD was 10 fg/mL for CCP and cTn1 and 100 fg/mL for p24.

10.5   NANOMATERIALS FOR THE TREATMENT OF INFLAMMATORY ARTHRITIS

RA is one of the most common autoimmune and inflammatory progressive diseases and is diagnosed with several main symptoms, including synovial joint damage and dramatic cartilage and bone tissue malformations (Oliveira et al., 2018). Approximately 1.5 million people worldwide suffer from RA. The prevalence of this inflammatory disease in women is nearly three times higher than in men (Paradkar et al., 2018). This inflammation can also occur in other tissues such as the heart, lungs, kidneys, and pleura. Although there are biologic-containing drugs (DMARDs) such as anti-interleukin-6 receptor (anti-IL-6) and anti-TNF-α antibodies (Meka et al., 2019). Although they are considered powerful and effective drugs, long-term use can cause serious side effects. The drug is widely distributed throughout the body, except for the affected joints. For this reason, treatment of chronic arthritis is often associated with several methods of treating RA, none of which are reliably effective. Several groups of anti-arthritic drugs are currently used to treat RA, including NSAIDs and disease-modifying anti-inflammatory drugs that destroy several vital organs such as the liver, kidney, and lungs. Therefore, there is a need to effectively deliver such drugs to inflamed RA sites to enhance their effectiveness in treating arthritis (Meka et al., 2019).

Nanomaterials can provide customized tools to address this issue. Nanomaterials have been extensively used to enhance drug bioavailability, bioactivity, pharmacokinetics, and pharmacodynamics in RA. Therefore, there is a need to expand and explore new and suitable therapeutic modalities for the treatment of RA that precisely and appropriately target diseased joints without damaging other healthy tissues. Various studies have used NPs to treat RA, including liposomes, polymeric NPs, niosomes, metallic NPs, quantum dots, SLNs, and polymeric micelles. The results of these studies support these studies due to specific physicochemical properties such as biocompatibility, lack of toxicity, ability to promote sustained drug release, and selective drug delivery to injured and inflamed tissues in RA animal models. We have demonstrated the performance of the system (Oliveira et al., 2018).

10.5.1   LIPOSOMES

Liposomes are recognized as successful nano-vehicles formed from a lipid bilayer surrounding an aqueous core for drug delivery strategies. They are known nanoscale

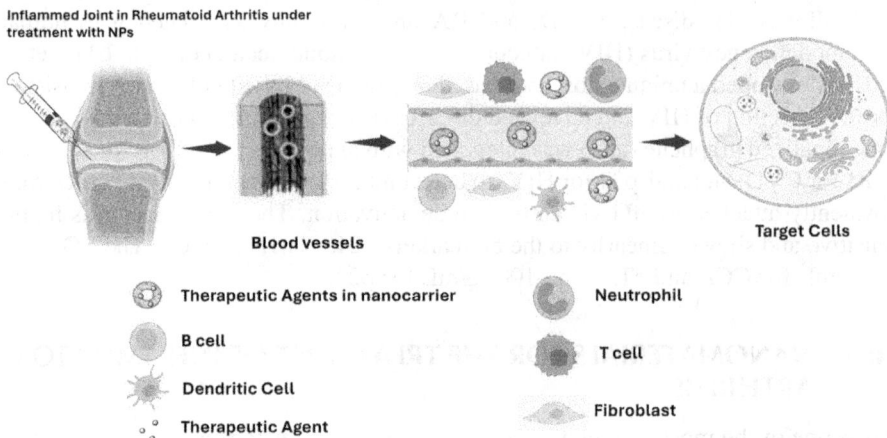

FIGURE 10.5 Liposomes as nanocarriers for the delivery of drugs in the treatment of RA.

systems with low toxicity for therapeutic drug delivery and few side effects. Liposomes as drug-delivery nanocarriers have demonstrated low immunogenicity and high biocompatibility, the ability to load and bind both hydrophilic and lipophilic drugs, and physical properties that enhance drug stability and biological half-life. It has many advantages such as suitable size with chemical properties. Specialized drugs for damaged or inflamed joints (Figure 10.5) (Wang et al., 2020).

Although liposomes have certain advantages, two important challenges remain for the therapeutic application of conventional liposomes. First, the blood circulation time of liposomes is limited as they can be rapidly cleared by hepatic phagocytic cells. Second, under physiological conditions, liposomes generally do not have long-term stability. The presence of these challenges can lead to the release of drugs encapsulated at off-target sites. Several factors can affect liposome instability, including osmotic pressure, lipid hydrolysis, and detergent degradation. The lipid polymerization process in the bilayer has been shown to be a powerful method for maintaining the structural integrity of liposomes (Saper et al., 2019).

MTX is a commonly prescribed drug for the treatment of RA. Due to the inherent side effects of this drug, loading MTX into liposomes may be a suitable delivery method to reduce toxicity while maintaining its properties and efficacy. The encapsulation efficiency (EE) of MTX (or other drug types) in liposomes is controlled by properties such as liposome water content and membrane stiffness. Encapsulation can also be affected by the hydrophilic/hydrophobic portion of the drug, which can affect its ability to interact with the liposomal membrane bilayer. The loading of MTX into liposomes occurs via a passive process controlled by the ability of the liposomes to remove the drug-containing aqueous phase. This method results in low EE as drug retention is limited to the size of the aqueous portion within the liposome and drug solubility. In a recent study, Guimarães et al. (2020) showed that by reducing the initially formed solution (1:1 - v/v - 20% in organic: aqueous phase ratio) using a method based on ethanol injection, the amount of water is outside the liposomes. Improved loading of MTX into liposomes. Ethanol dissolution was reduced, promoting interaction between MTX and lipids, resulting in an appropriate size distribution and larger drug EE. They found a suitable polydispersity index (PDI) with a small size and high MTX loading. The efficiency was over 30% compared to the traditional ethanol injection method. Results obtained by nuclear magnetic resonance (NMR) indicated a bidirectional connection between the drug and the primary phospholipid via hydrogen bonds that increase the EE. Thus, the authors were able to develop a novel pre-concentrated ethanol injection technique to achieve higher MTX encapsulation within liposomes. This is an important advance for the treatment of RA.

The presence of liposomes in the bloodstream for several hours is thought to play a major role in passive targeting, depending on several factors such as hydrophobicity, surface charge, and particle size. Liposome diameter is a fundamental factor affecting perfusion time and biological release after intravenous injection. In addition, liposome diameter affects penetration across leaky synovial vascular spaces and retention in injured joints. Their targeting ability is largely due to the leaky vasculature triggered by inflammatory cytokines such as IL-1β, IL-6, and TNF-α, resulting in enhanced permeability and retention (EPR) in tumors. The size of intercellular endothelial gaps is within a certain range due to adsorption of plasma proteins and phagocytosis by the reticuloendothelial system (RES), but may vary from patient to patient (Wang et al., 2020).

In a recent study, Ren et al. (2019) studied the mechanism of passive targeting of liposomes and demonstrated the effects of their biophysical and biochemical properties on retention time in the bloodstream. The authors prepared liposomes with different sizes and surface charges and different PEG chain lengths (1, 2, and 5 kDa) and concentrations (5%, 10%, and 20% of total fat by lipid film dispersion and extrusion). A NIR fluorescence imaging array was used to assess the targeting ability. We then used the optimal liposome system (loading, size, etc.) to deliver his Dex to CIA rats. Pharmacodynamic studies showed that Dex-liposomes greatly enhanced the anti-arthritic effects of His Dex in this RA model in vivo. In RA, when the walls of blood vessels become inflamed, the blood vessels may become weak, enlarged, or leaky in the inflamed joint. Passive targeting involves the secretion of nano-sized drug delivery vehicles across leaky vasculature, followed by inflammatory cell-mediated sequestration (ELVIS), resulting in increased anti-inflammatory potency, especially at sites of inflamed joints. In another study, Wang et al. prepared 1,2-bis(10,12-tricosadiynoyl)-sn-glycero-3-phosphocholine (DC8,9PC) and 1, 2-distearoyl sn-glycero-3-phosphoethanolamine PEG (DSPE-PEG 2000) using a thin-film hydration process to prepare polymerized stealth liposomes. To enhance liposome integrity and increase perfusion time, the authors used DC8,9PC molecules crosslinked in the liposome bilayer by ultraviolet (UV) radiation and PEG chains to create camouflage layers, respectively. Next, administration of biocompatible liposomes to arthritic rats effectively recruited injured joints. Administration of Dex by encapsulation in such polymerized stealth liposomes suppressed the concentration of pro-inflammatory cytokines such as TNF-α and IL-1β in joint tissue, reduced swelling in inflamed and injured joints, and it completely prevented further progression of RA. In addition, Shen et al. (2020) prepared novel thermosensitive liposomes based on dipalmitoylphosphatidylcholine (DPPC), hydrogenated soybean phosphatidylcholine (SPC), and cholesterol to load the water-soluble drug sinomenine hydrochloride (SIN). A liposomal delivery system with an appropriate particle size possesses excellent compatibility and storage stability, allowing the release of SIN into the bloodstream before reaching the target site in RA rats after complete release by microwave hyperthermia. A thermosensitive liposome delivery system has demonstrated improved controlled release and side effect-free RA, especially when combining SIN therapy with microwave hyperthermia as an optimized combination therapy to potentially treat the clinical manifestations of RA. Reduced symptoms increased drug concentration at the site of inflammation in RA.

10.5.2 POLYMERIC NPS

Polymer NPs are prepared from colloidal particles and a diameter range is considered (1–1000 nm). In fact, polymeric nanoparticles have great potential in the medical field due to their advantageous properties such as biodegradability, biocompatibility, good synthetic flexibility, precise tuning, and suitable mechanical properties (Xie et al., 2020). To prevent uptake by macrophages, the surface of NPs can be coated with a stealth polymer such as PEG. Increasing the density and thickness of the PEG coating increased the circulation time of polymeric NPs in blood. Modification of NPs by PEGylation, a covalent process that prevents their removal from the reticuloendothelial system, or by conjugation with other small molecules (peptides, vitamins, and antibodies), circulates in the blood system. It can significantly increase the time and improve effectiveness. Administered anti-RA drugs such as NSAIDs, corticosteroids, DMARDs, small interfering RNA (siRNA), and therapeutic peptides (Jeong and Park, 2020). Synthetic cationic polymers such as polyethyleneamine (PEI), poly-L-lysine (PLL), and dendrimers are commonly used to deliver nucleic acids such as DNA and interfering RNA (RNAi) (Yu et al., 2020). Among these, PEI is the most commonly used due to its large number of protonated amino functional groups, allowing higher cationic charge densities at physiological pH and facilitating nucleic acid attachment by electrostatic adsorption.

Espinosa-Cano et al. (2020) have shown the advantage of using polymeric NPs conjugated with naproxen and dex to reduce inflammation and prevent IL-12 expression in macrophages. Through either COX-dependent or COX-independent regulatory mechanisms, IL-12 and IL-23 have been identified as therapeutic targets in the treatment of long-lasting inflammatory diseases in which T-cells are the major dysfunctional immune cells. Note the recent emergence. The authors prepared an anti-inflammatory polymeric NP by mixing dex and ketoprofen (Ket) with appropriate chemical and physical properties and properly accumulating and releasing both drugs in injured joints. As a result, these structures have a pronounced anti-inflammatory effect by reducing general nitric oxide (NO) levels and expression of the M1 macrophage marker and increasing levels of the M2 macrophage marker after rapid macrophage uptake, showing an inflammatory effect. This may facilitate their retention at sites of inflammation via extravasation through leaky vessels and subsequent inflammatory cell-mediated sequestration effect (ELVISE).

Tofacitinib (TFC) is another candidate for the treatment of RA as a novel oral non-traditional Janus kinase (JAK) inhibitor with efficacy and safety similar to other DMARDs. However, its clinical use has been hampered by its short plasma half-life. Bashir et al. (2020) designed innovative PLGA-based NPs to facilitate sustained release and target-specific delivery of TFCs. PLGA is one of the most widely used biocompatible and biodegradable polymers used in various drug delivery systems. Hydrolysis of PLGA produces two major monomers in water: polylactic acid (PLA) and polyglycolic acid (PGA). The authors encapsulated TFC into PLGA-NPs by nanoprecipitation as a novel nanocarrier structure targeting the inflamed synovium, and such TFC-PLGA-NPs supported tailored TFC pharmacokinetic profiles.

A study by Howard et al. (2009) demonstrated the effect of CS-siRNA NPs on suppressing inflammatory TNF-α expression in macrophages from CIA mice. Histological examination of joints of anti-TNF-α-treated mice reveals mild cartilage damage and inflammatory cell infiltration, benefiting CS-siRNA NP-mediated TNF-α knockdown approach on local and systemic inflammation was demonstrated (Figure 10.6).

Some investigators have taken a similar approach to control RA progression in mice using nanostructured polymeric siRNAs (poly-siRNAs) targeting TNF-α containing thiolated glycol-CS (TGC) polymers. I'm here. TNF-α expression was downregulated at arthritic sites in the joints of RA mice in vitro by application of these NPs. MD et al. investigated the potential of photothermally organized drug delivery using multifunctional NPs (MNPs) with NIR irradiation sites to improve therapeutic efficacy and reduce side effects in patients suffering from RA. In this approach, a layer of Au film was deposited on the MTX-encapsulated PEG-PLGA NPs, allowing proper encapsulation of her MTX in the MNPs. The synergistic

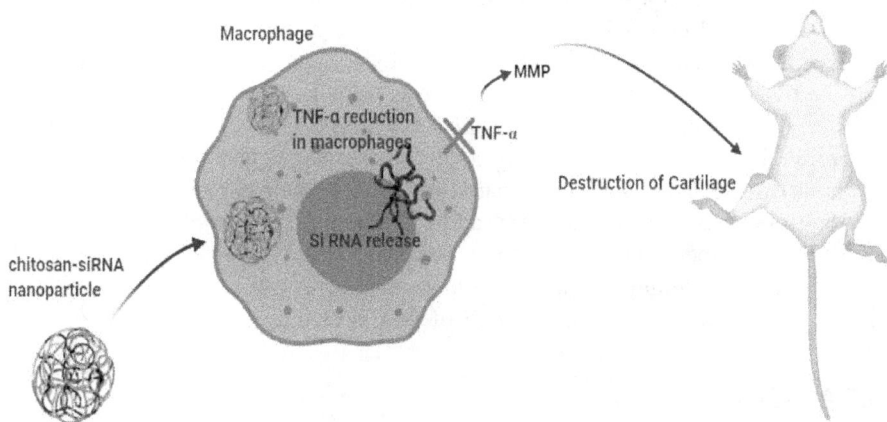

FIGURE 10.6 CS-siRNA NP delivery in macrophages to suppress TNF-α expression. Macrophage elimination by CS-siRNA was established to inhibit local production of IL-1β, IL-6, TNF-α, and matrix metalloproteinases (MMPs) and thus reduce the pathogenesis of inflammatory arthritis.

interaction of MTX-encapsulated MNPs with NIR irradiation was tested in fibroblast-like RA synovial cells (FLS) and CIA mice (Md et al., 2020). An advantage of using the Au-shell NIR resonance is that it accelerates the local release of MTX from the NP. Her NIR images of MNPs loaded with MTX showed proper translocation of MNPs into inflamed joints. Moreover, repeated administration of MNPs encapsulated in a 1/1400 solution of MTX showed a stronger anti-RA effect in CIA mice than the MTX solution itself and was more effective than alone. Overall, MTX-loaded MNP therapy with NIR irradiation represents a suitable treatment for single low-dose MTX-based RA (Md et al., 2020).

10.5.3 NIOSOMES

Niosomes are formed when nonionic surfactant vesicles self-associate. Some factors that influence niosome formation include the type of nonionic detergent used, hydration temperature, and manufacturing method (Bhardwaj et al., 2020). Primary surfactant vesicles are generally composed of ionic surfactants. This study showed that the highest toxicity was associated with cationic surfactants, followed by anionic surfactants, and the lowest toxicity of nonionic surfactants. For these reasons, niosomes made from nonionic surfactants are an ideal choice for transdermal delivery. Hydrophilic-lipophilic balance (HLB) values play an important role in the generation of niosomes, and the range of HLB 4–8 is commonly used. Common detergents used for niosome generation include Span, Brij, and Tween (Lu et al., 2019).

In a recent study, Rajaram et al. (2020) designed a promising system to deliver piroxicam (PC) encapsulated in nonionic surfactant vesicle carriers as a transdermal patch. It is a drug delivery system suitable for enhancing the solubility of poorly soluble drugs and increasing the drug's retention time at the absorption site. This approach may be a useful construct for the treatment of RA. Another report by Paradkar et al. demonstrated the feasibility of preparing a topical niosome thiocorticoside gel consisting of a span 60:cholesterol molar ratio using the thin-film hydration method. This niosome gel extended local retention time and controlled RA-related pain and its side effects with less frequent dosing. Mujibet et al. designed a study of the treatment of RA with the goal of reducing side effects and prolonging the duration of drug action. Topical gel formulations containing niosome-loaded ibuprofen were prepared by varying the ratio of various nonionic surfactants (span20, span60, span80, and cholesterol) by thin-film hydration and ether injection methods. The results indicated that niosome nanocarriers in ibuprofen gel containing carbopol serve as the basis for a suitable local drug delivery system that delays the duration of drug action.

10.5.4 QUANTUM DOTS

Quantum dots (QDs) are inorganic nanomaterials or semiconductor nanocrystals with a size of 1–10 nm, consisting of a central semiconductor core with a shell of inorganic salts (CdS, ZnS) (Nikazar et al., 2020).

QDs are used in several nanotechnology processes, including drug delivery, bioimaging of abnormal cells, and diagnosis and treatment of RA. We tested mercaptopropionic acid (MPA) nanoconjugates coated with Cd-Te-QDs and celecoxib, a potent COX-2 inhibitor, for bioimaging of carrageenan-induced paw inflammation in mice.

10.5.5 POLYMERIC MICELLES

Biocompatible and biodegradable polymers are widely used in pharmaceutical processes as useful components in pharmaceutical formulations and as nanocarriers in drug delivery systems (Hwang et al., 2020). Currently, micelles are based on the use of amphiphilic block copolymers in aqueous solution. They can be used as nanocarriers for poorly soluble drugs that can be covalently attached to polymer chains or non-covalently arranged in micelles (Hwang et al., 2020). In general, they are suitable nano-vehicles for enhancing various biochemical and bio-pharmaceutical properties such as solubility, bioavailability, and targeting of these hydrophobic drugs. They are suitable for use in combination with other therapeutic agents to treat RA. Twenty years ago, a novel micelle-based system was developed for the treatment of RA (Yun et al., 2019).

Glucocorticoids (GLCs) are one of the most important drugs used in RA, but they show serious side effects when used in high doses. We applied GLC in a rat model of arthritis using micellar nanosystems. This enables targeted low-dose drug delivery to injured joints, safely enhancing therapeutic efficacy. Dex-loaded micelles self-assembled from amphipathic PEGblock-poly(caprolactone) (PEG-PCL) polymers by membrane dispersion were successfully treated in rats with adjuvant-induced arthritis using only a single dose of 0.8 mg/kg. Micelles remained in circulation for a long time and accumulated in inflamed joints. Dex delivered by micelles reduced joint pain and swelling and pro-inflammatory cytokine expression in both joint tissue and blood. PEG-PCL micelles not only reduced the adverse effects on body weight, but also lowered lymphocyte counts and blood glucose levels. These results demonstrate that loading Dex into her PEG-PCL micelles enables appropriate and effective low-dose GC therapy targeting inflammatory diseases. We have prepared novel dextran stearate polymer micelles by dialysis method as a means of delivering indomethacin. Indomethacin is an NSAID that can successfully relieve pain and inflammation in RA and reduce otherwise severe side effects. Such micelles provided a more potent and useful drug to reduce inflammation in rat models of arthritis compared to treatment with indomethacin alone.

10.6 CONCLUSIONS, CHALLENGES, AND FUTURE OPPORTUNITIES

RA is a chronic inflammatory disease associated with abnormal functioning of the immune system. In RA, the immune system primarily attacks joints such as knees, wrists, and hands, causing inflammation. This tissue damage can cause long-term pain and inappropriate deformation of the body. In some patients, RA can damage most of our bodies, including the skin, eyes, heart, lungs, and blood vessels. The main goals of RA treatment are to control inflammation and pain, to slow or stop the progression of the disease. Early treatments include MTX and sulfasalazine, which suppress the immune system. These drugs are suitable, but suppressing the immune system increases the risk of infection. It's also important to keep in mind the possible side effects of the drug, such as nausea, abdominal pain, and severe damage to the liver and lungs. The effects of these drugs usually last 6 to 12 weeks, so rheumatologists may also give NSAIDs to treat pain and inflammation. Despite these problems, DMARDs are still used as first-line therapy. In this article, our goal was to describe several types of nanomaterials for therapeutic application in RA. The results of this review demonstrate that all nanocarriers encapsulate anti-RA drugs and possess unique properties to reduce drug side effects. The review also showed that these systems can enhance the bioavailability of hydrophobic drugs and improve their efficacy in RA. Briefly, the current review article describes several useful and successful nanocarriers for the precise delivery of multiple therapeutic agents to target sites in RA treatment (Hosseinikhah et al., 2021).

On the other hand, the growing use of nanomaterials in diverse biomedical applications has also raised questions about their toxicity. Morphological and physicochemical properties of nanomaterials play an important role in determining toxicity in various body organs such as liver, kidney, skin, brain, and heart. It is removed by modifying the surface with various types of natural or synthetic polymers and other compounds. Some studies have investigated the toxicity of nanomaterials for biomedical applications, but to date, there is no detailed information on these aspects (Hosseinikhah et al., 2021).

REFERENCES

Agostino, M.A.D, Terslev, L., Aegerter, P., et al., RMD Open., 3, e000428, 2017.
Aletaha D., Neogi T., Silman A. J., et al., Arthritis Rheumatol., 62, 2569–2581, 2010.
Arnett F. C., Edworthy S. M., Bloch D.A., et al., Arthritis Rheumatol., 31, 315–324, 1988.
Bakewell, C., Aydin, S.Z., Ranganath, V.K., Eder, L., Kaeley, G.S. Imaging techniques: Options for the diagnosis and monitoring of treatment of enthesitis in psoriatic arthritis. J. Rheumatol., 47, 973–982, 2020.
Barile, A., Arrigoni, F., Bruno, F., et al., Radiol. Clin. N. Am., 55, 997–1007, 2017.
Bashir, S., Aamir, M., Sarfaraz, R.M., Hussain, Z., Sarwer, M.U., Mahmood, A., Akram, M.R., Qaisar, M.N. Fabrication, characterization and in vitro release kinetics of tofacitinib-encapsulated polymeric nanoparticles: A promising implication in the treatment of rheumatoid arthritis. Int. J. Polym. Mater. Polym. Biomater., 70, 449–458, 2020.
Bhardwaj, P., Tripathi, P., Gupta, R., Pandey, S. Niosomes: A review on niosomal research in the last decade. J. Drug Deliv. Sci. Technol., 56, 101581, 2020.
Bray, C., Bell, L.N., Liang, H., Haykal, R., Kaiksow, F., Mazza, J.J., Yale, S.H. Erythrocyte sedimentation rate and C-reactive protein measurements and their relevance in clinical medicine. WMJ, 115, 317–321, 2016.
Bugatti, S., Bogliolo, L., Vitolo, B., Manzo, A., Montecucco, C., Caporali, R. Anti-citrullinated protein antibodies and high levels of rheumatoid factor are associated with systemic bone loss in patients with early untreated rheumatoid arthritis. Arthritis Res. Ther., 18, 226, 2016.
Cai, L., Xu, J., Yang, Z., et al., Med. Comm., 1, 35–46, 2020.
Cappelli, L.C., Gutierrez, A.K., Baer, A.N., Albayda, J., Manno, R.L., Haque, U., Lipson, E.J., Bleich, K.B., Shah, A.A., Naidoo, J. Inflammatory arthritis and sicca syndrome induced by nivolumab and ipilimumab. Ann. Rheum. Dis., 76, 43–50, 2017.

Chen, C.-L., Siow, T.Y., Chou, C.-H., Lin, C.-H., Lin, M.-H., Chen, Y.-C., Hsieh, W.-Y., Wang, S.-J., Chang, C. Targeted superparamagnetic iron oxide nanoparticles for in vivo magnetic resonance imaging of T-cells in rheumatoid arthritis. Mol. Imaging Biol., 19, 233–244, 2017.

Chow, Y., Chin, K. The role of inflammation in the pathogenesis of osteoarthritis. Mediators of Inflammation, 2020, 2020, Article ID 8293921.

Chua, J.R., Jamal, S., Riad, M. et al., Disease burden in osteoarthritis is similar to that of rheumatoid arthritis at initial rheumatology visit and significantly greater six months later. Arthritis & Rheumatology, 71(8), 1276–1284, 2019.

Chu, K.-A., Chen,W., Hsu, C.Y., Hung, Y.-M., Wei, J.C.-C. Increased risk of rheumatoid arthritis among patients with mycoplasma pneumonia: A nationwide population-based cohort study in Taiwan. PLoS One, 14, e0210750, 2019.

Conigliaro, P., Triggianese, P., de Martino, E. et al., Challenges in the treatment of rheumatoid arthritis. Autoimmunity Reviews, 18(7), 706–713, 2019.

Cormode, D.P., Skajaa, T., Fayad, Z.A., Mulder, W.J. Nanotechnology in medical imaging: Probe design and applications. Arterioscler. Thromb. Vasc. Biol., 29, 992–1000, 2009.

de Carvalho Franca, L.F., da Silva, F.R.P., di Lenardo, D., Alves, E.H.P., Nascimento, H.M.S., da Silva, I.A.T., Vasconcelos, A.C.C.G., Vasconcelos, D.F.P. Comparative analysis of blood parameters of the erythrocyte lineage between patients with chronic periodontitis and healthy patients: Results obtained from a meta-analysis. Arch. Oral Biol., 97, 144–149, 2019.

Espinosa-Cano, E., Aguilar, M.R., Portilla, Y., Barber, D.F., San Román, J. Anti-inflammatory polymeric nanoparticles based on ketoprofen and dexamethasone. Pharmaceutics, 12, 723, 2020.

Fonseca, L. J. S. da, Nunes-Souza, L., Goulart, J. S. da, M. O. F., Rabelo L. A., Oxidative stress in rheumatoid arthritis: What the future might hold regarding novel biomarkers and add-on therapies. Oxidative Medicine and Cellular Longevity, 2019, 16, 2019, Article ID 7536805.

Furuzawa-Carballeda, J., Macip-Rodriguez, P., Cabral, A. Osteoarthritis and rheumatoid arthritis pannus have similar qualitative metabolic characteristics and pro-inflammatory cytokine response. Clin. Exp. Rheumatol., 26, 554, 2008.

Ganhewa, A., Wu, R., Chae, M., et al., Failure rates of base of thumb arthritis surgery: A systematic review. J. Hand Surg., 44(9), 728–741, 2019.

Gaujoux-Viala, C., Gossec, L., Cantagrel, A., et al., Joint Bone Spine, 81, 287–297, 2014.

Ghosh, B., Baidya, D., Halder, P., Mandal, S. Correlation of serum uric acid with disease activity and C-reactive protein in patients suffering from rheumatoid arthritis. Open J. Rheumatol. Autoimmune Dis., 6, 79–84, 2016.

Gavrila, B., Ciofu, C., Stoica, V. Biomarkers in rheumatoid arthritis, what is new? J. Med. Life, 9, 144, 2016.

Guidelli, G., Viapiana, O., Luciano, N., et al., Clin. Exp. Rheumatol., 38, 2020.

Guimarães, D., Noro, J., Loureiro, A., Lager, F., Renault, G., Cavaco-Paulo, A., Nogueira, E. Increased encapsulation efficiency of methotrexate in liposomes for rheumatoid arthritis therapy. Biomedicines, 8, 630, 2020.

Guo, Q., Wang, Y., Xu, D., Nossent, J., Pavlos, N. J., and Xu J., Rheumatoid arthritis: Pathological mechanisms and modern pharmacologic therapies. Bone Research, 6, 2018.

Hermanson, G.T., Bioconjugate Techniques, 2nd ed., Elsevier Inc., San Diego, 2008.

Hodkinson, B., van Duuren, E., Pettipher, C., et al., S. Afr. Med. J., 103, 576–585, 2013.

Hosseinikhah, S. M., Barani, M., Rahdar, A., Madry, H., Arshad, R., Mohammadzadeh, V., Cucchiarini, M. Nanomaterials for the diagnosis and treatment of inflammatory arthritis. Int. J. Mol. Sci., 22(6), 3092, 2021.

Howard, K.A., Paludan, S.R., Behlke, M.A., Besenbacher, F., Deleuran, B., Kjems, J. Chitosan/siRNA nanoparticle–mediated TNF-α knockdown in peritoneal macrophages for anti-inflammatory treatment in a murine arthritis model. Mol. Ther., 17, 162–168, 2009.

Humby, F.C., Al Balushi, F., Lliso, G., Cauli, A., Pitzalis, C. Can synovial pathobiology integrate with current clinical and imaging prediction models to achieve personalized health care in rheumatoid arthritis? Front. Med., 4, 41, 2017.

Hwang, E.Y., Lee, J.H., Lim, D.W. Compartmentalized bimetal cluster-poly (aniline) hybrid nanostructures for multiplexed detection of autoantibodies in early diagnosis of rheumatoid arthritis. Sens. Actuators B Chem., 321, 128482, 2020.

Islam, S., Shukla, S., Bajpai, V.K., Han, Y.-K., Huh, Y.S., Kumar, A., Ghosh, A., Gandhi, S. A smart nanosensor for the detection of human immunodeficiency virus and associated cardiovascular and arthritis diseases using functionalized graphene-based transistors. Biosens. Bioelectron., 126, 792–799, 2019.

Jans, L., De Kock, I., Herregods, N., et al., Ann. Rheum. Dis., 77, 958–959, 2018.

Jeong, M., Park, J.-H. Nanomedicine for the treatment of rheumatoid arthritis. Mol. Pharm., 18, 539–549, 2020.

Jo, J., Tian, C., Xu, G., Sarazin, J., Schiopu, E., Gandikota, G., Wang, X. Photoacoustic tomography for human musculoskeletal imaging and inflammatory arthritis detection. Photoacoustics, 12, 82–89, 2018.

Khilfeh, I., Guyette, E., Watkins, J., Danielson, D., Gross, D., Yeung, K., Adherence, persistence, and expenditures for high-cost anti-inflammatory drugs in rheumatoid arthritis: An exploratory study. J. Manag Care Spec Pharm, 25(4), 461–467, 2019.

Lin, Y. J., Anzaghe, M., Schülke, S., Update on the pathomechanism, diagnosis, and treatment options for rheumatoid arthritis. Cells, 9(4), 880, 2020.

Liu, Z., Yang, X., Duan, C., et al., ISO: Signal Transduct. Target. Ther., 5, 82, 2020.

Lu, B., Huang, Y., Chen, Z., Ye, J., Xu, H., Chen, W., Long, X. Niosomal nanocarriers for enhanced skin delivery of quercetin with functions of anti-tyrosinase and antioxidant. Molecules, 24, 2322, 2019.

Ma, W., Sha, S. N., Chen, P.L., et al., Adv. Healthc. Mater., 9, 1901100, 2020.

Ma, J., Liu, X., Wang, R., Zhang, J., Jiang, P., Wang, Y., Tu, G. Bimetallic core-shell nanostars with tunable surface plasmon resonance for surface-enhanced Raman scattering. ACS Appl. Nano Mater., 3, 10885–10894, 2020.

McQueen, F. M., Best Pract. Res. Clin. Rheumatol. 27, 499–522, 2013.

Md, S., Alhakamy, N.A., Aldawsari, H.M., Husain, M., Kotta, S., Abdullah, S.T., Fahmy, U., Alfaleh, M.A., Asfour, H.Z. Formulation design, statistical optimization, and in vitro evaluation of a naringenin nanoemulsion to enhance apoptotic activity in a 549 lung cancer cells. Pharmaceuticals, 13, 152, 2020.

Meka, R.R., Venkatesha, S.H., Acharya, B., Moudgil, K.D. Peptide-targeted liposomal delivery of dexamethasone for arthritis therapy. Nanomedicine, 14, 1455–1469, 2019.

Memon, M., Kay, J., Ginsberg, L., de Sa, D., Simunovic, N., Samuelsson, K., Athwal, G.S., Ayeni, O.R. Arthroscopic management of septic arthritis of the native shoulder: A systematic review. Arthrosc. J. Arthrosc. Relat. Surg., 34, 625–646.e1, 2018.

Ng, J. Y., Azizudin, A. M., Rheumatoid arthritis and osteoarthritis clinical practice guidelines provide few complementary and alternative medicine therapy recommendations: A systematic review. Clin Rheumatol, 39(10), 2861–2873, 2020.

Nikazar, S., Sivasankarapillai, V.S., Rahdar, A., Gasmi, S., Anumol, P., Shanavas, M.S. Revisiting the cytotoxicity of quantum dots: An in-depth overview. Biophys. Rev., 12, 703–718, 2020.

Noguerol, T.M., Luna, A., Cabrera, M.G., Riofrio, A.D. Clinical applications of advanced magnetic resonance imaging techniques for arthritis evaluation. World J. Orthop., 8, 660, 2017.

Oliveira, I.M., Gonçalves, C., Reis, R.L., Oliveira, J.M. Engineering nanoparticles for targeting rheumatoid arthritis: Past, present, and future trends. Nano Res., 11, 4489–4506, 2018.

Paradkar, M., Vaghela, S. Thiocolchicoside niosomal gel formulation for the pain management of rheumatoid arthritis through topical drug delivery. Drug Deliv. Lett., 8, 159–168, 2018.

Peng, B., Liang, H., Li, Y., Dong, C., Shen, J., Mao, H. Q., Leong, K. W., Chen Y., Liu L., Angew. Chem., Int. Ed. Engl., 58, 4254–4258, 2019.

Rabiei, M., Kashanian, S., Samavati, S.S., Derakhshankhah, H., Jamasb, S., McInnes, S.J. Nanotechnology application in drug delivery to osteoarthritis (OA), rheumatoid arthritis (RA), and osteoporosis (OSP). J. Drug Deliv. Sci. Technol., 61, 102011, 2020.

Reginato, A.M., Olsen, B.R. The role of structural genes in the pathogenesis of osteoarthritic disorders. Arthritis Res. Ther., 4,1–9, 2002.

Ren, H., He, Y., Liang, J., Cheng, Z., Zhang, M., Zhu, Y., Hong, C., Qin, J., Xu, X., Wang, J. Role of liposome size, surface charge, and PEGylation on rheumatoid arthritis targeting therapy. ACS Appl. Mater. Interfaces, 11, 20304–20315, 2019.

Rolle, N.A., Jan, I., Sibbitt, W.L., Band, P.A., Haseler, L.J., Hayward, W.A., Muruganandam, M., Emil, N.S., Fangtham, M., Bankhurst, A.D. Extractable synovial fluid in inflammatory and non-inflammatory arthritis of the knee. Clin. Rheumatol., 38, 2255–2263, 2019.

Saper, V.E., Chen, G., Deutsch, G.H., Guillerman, R.P., Birgmeier, J., Jagadeesh, K., Canna, S., Schulert, G., Deterding, R., Xu, J. Emergent high fatality lung disease in systemic juvenile arthritis. Ann. Rheum. Dis., 78, 1722–1731, 2019.

Sarkar, S., Levi-Polyachenko, N. Conjugated polymer nano-systems for hyperthermia, imaging and drug delivery. Adv. Drug Deliv. Rev., 163, 40–64, 2020.

Shen, Q., Zhang, X., Qi, J., Shu, G., Du, Y., Ying, X. Sinomenine hydrochloride loaded thermosensitive liposomes combined with microwave hyperthermia for the treatment of rheumatoid arthritis. Int. J. Pharm., 576, 119001, 2020.

Shi, Y.S., Xie, F.F., Rao, P.S., et al., J. Control. Release. 320, 304–313, 2020.

Subashini Rajaram, A.S., Dharmalingam, S.R., Chidambaram, K. Fabrication of non-ionic surfactant vesicular gel for effective treatment of rheumatoid arthritis. JEMDS, 9, 2289–2296, 2020.

Tao, S., Cheng, J., Su, G., et al., Angew. Chem. Int. Ed. 59, 1–7, 2020.

Umar, S., Asif, M., Sajad, M., Ansari, M. M., Hussain, U., Int. J. Drug Dev. Res. 4, 210–219, 2012.

Veigas, B., Matias, A., Calmeiro, T., Fortunato, E., Fernandes, A.R., Baptista, P.V. Antibody modified gold nanoparticles for fast colorimetric screening of rheumatoid arthritis. Analyst, 144, 3613–3619, 2019.

Visser, H., Best Pract, Res. Clin. Rheumatol. 19, 55–72, 2005.

Vu-Quang, H., Vinding, M.S., Jakobsen, M., Song, P., Dagnaes-Hansen, F., Nielsen, N.C., Kjems, J. Imaging rheumatoid arthritis in mice using combined near infrared and 19 F magnetic resonance modalities. Sci. Rep., 9, 14314, 2019.

Wang, S. S., Lv, J., Meng, S. S., Tang, J.X., Nie, L.M., Adv. Healthc. Mater. 9, 1901541, 2020.

Wong, X.Y., Sena-Torralba, A., Alvarez-Diduk, R., Muthoosamy, K., Merkoci, A., ACS Nano. 14, 2585–2627, 2020.

Xie, Y., Tuguntaev, R.G., Mao, C., Chen, H., Tao, Y., Wang, S., Yang, B., Guo, W. Stimuli-responsive polymeric nanomaterials for rheumatoid arthritis therapy. Biophys. Rep., 6, 193–210, 2020.

Yu, Z., Reynaud, F., Lorscheider, M., Tsapis, N., Fattal, E. Nanomedicines for the delivery of glucocorticoids and nucleic acids as potential alternatives in the treatment of rheumatoid arthritis. Wiley Interdiscip. Rev. Nanomed. Nanobiotechnol., 12, e1630, 2020.

Yun, L., Shang, H., Gu, H., Zhang, N. Polymeric micelles for the treatment of rheumatoid arthritis. Crit. Rev. Ther. Drug Carr. Syst., 36, 219–238, 2019.

Zhao, Y., Liu, Y., Li, X., Wang, H., Zhang, Y., Ma, H., Wei, Q. Label-free ECL immunosensor for the early diagnosis of rheumatoid arthritis based on asymmetric heterogeneous polyaniline-gold nanomaterial. Sens. Actuators B Chem., 257, 354–361, 2018.

11 Targeted Drug Delivery in Rheumatoid Arthritis Diagnosis and Treatment

Riya Mukherjee, Vandana Dahiya, Amrita Soni, and Chung-Ming Chang

11.1 INTRODUCTION: DISEASE OVERVIEW

Rheumatoid arthritis (RA) is an autoimmune chronic inflammatory disease in which healthy cells in the body are attacked by the immune system. It is characterized by symmetric synovial joint inflammation, which can harm the cartilage and bone and cause a progressive loss of function. Due to the bone and cartilage degradation brought on by RA over time, radiographs can show anatomical abnormalities in the joints (Figure 11.1). Hand, wrist, and knee joints are frequently affected by RA. The patient's joints are commonly damaged by RA, and the inflammation of the joint lining can affect various tissues throughout the body and negatively impact organs including the lungs, heart, and eyes (1).

Patients with RA may not initially notice any redness or swelling in the joints, although soreness and pain are always possible side effects. It has been observed that many RA patients experience exhaustion or mild fevers. Patients often experience morning stiffness for at least 30 minutes. Small joints (such as the wrists, several joints in the hands, and feet) are typically affected initially (Figure 11.2).

The likelihood that the patient may develop an RA risk depends on a variety of hereditary and environmental factors. The most important element is thought to be age. Adults in their sixties had the highest incidence of RA onset. It is impossible to ignore inherited or genetic qualities. HLA (Human Leukocyte Antigen) class II genotypes are genes that can exacerbate arthritis. Those who possess these genes may also be more susceptible to other environmental variables like smoking and obesity, which increases their risk of developing RA (Figure 11.3). The physical and social effects of rheumatoid arthritis (RA) are extensive, and they can also affect one's quality of life. Premature cardiac disease, obesity, vasculitis, nodules, and Sicca syndrome are the most common RA side effects. A subset of RA patients had higher mortality rates, which have been linked to a high prevalence of cardiovascular disease. Therefore, it is crucial to understand how to diagnose RA early and how to treat it. The chapter will contribute to illuminating targeted medication delivery in RA, as well as its evaluation and management (2).

DOI: 10.1201/9781003348672-11

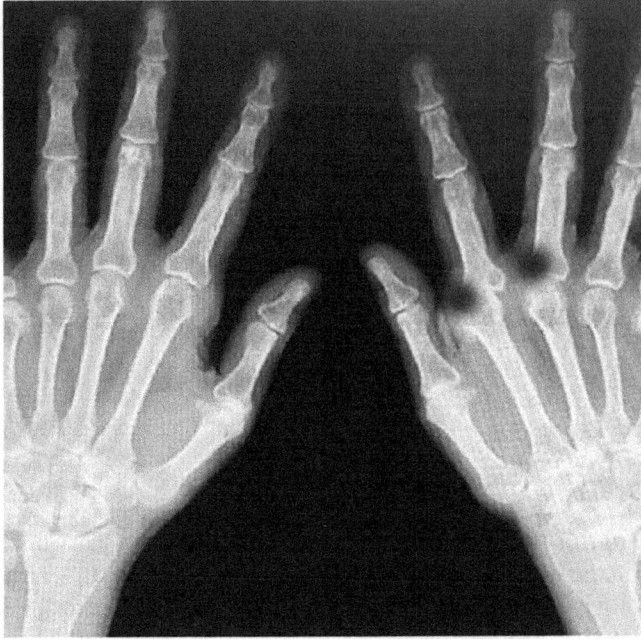

FIGURE 11.1 Hand radiographs of patients exposed to rheumatoid arthritis (RA).

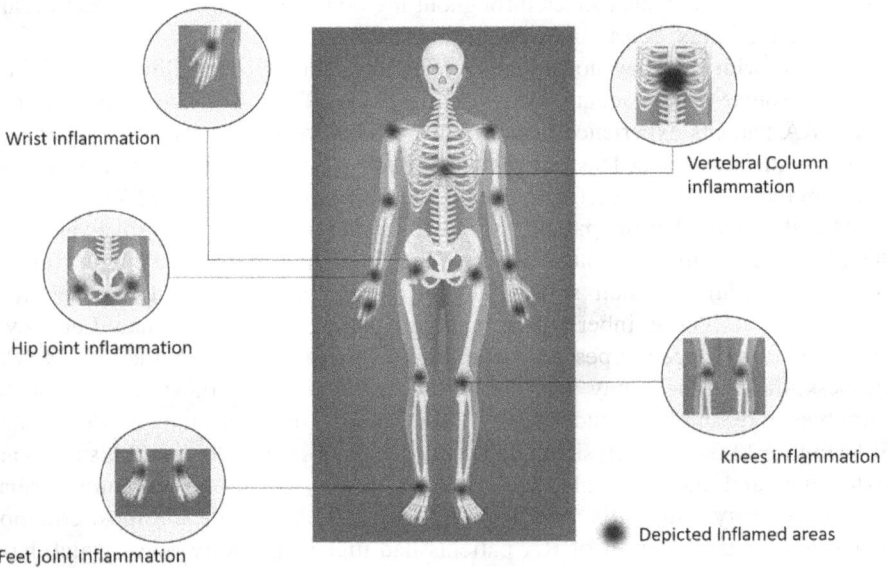

FIGURE 11.2 The common affected areas in a patient suffering from rheumatoid arthritis (RA).

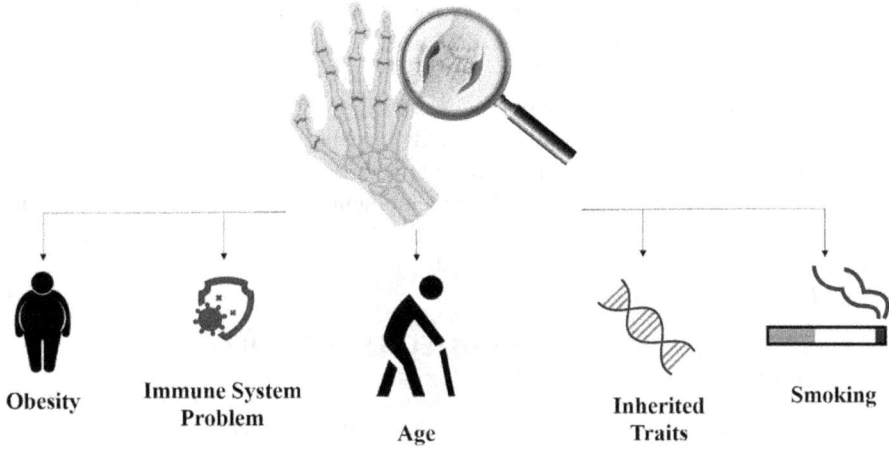

FIGURE 11.3 Causes of rheumatoid arthritis.

11.2 PATHOGENESIS

The majority of the inflammatory process in RA takes place in the synovial membrane, which swells up and releases inflammatory cytokines (Figure 11.4). The synovial membrane, cartilage, and bone are all eventually destroyed as a result of this damage. The majority of the dense cellular infiltrates in the inflammatory rheumatoid synovium are composed of macrophages, T-cells, and B-cells. Synovial lining hyperplasia is a symptom of the accumulation of macrophage-like synoviocytes (MLS) and fibroblast-like synoviocytes (FLS) in the synovial tissue. These macrophages and fibroblast-like cells contribute to inflammation by producing

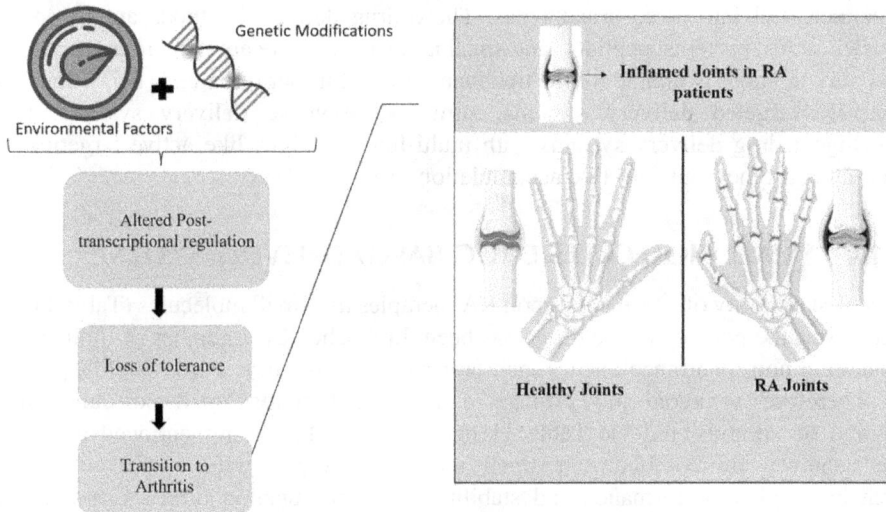

FIGURE 11.4 Pathogenesis of rheumatoid arthritis.

chemical mediators such as pro-inflammatory cytokines like TNF-α and IL-1β. TNF-α and IL-1β both cause the production of tissue-degrading matrix metalloprotease (MMPs) from synovial cells, and TNF-α encourages the growth of osteoclasts, which are responsible for abrasion of the bone. As a result, there is an increase in the number of activated macrophages, lymphocytes, and fibroblasts, and the RA inflammatory process continues. Numerous studies have demonstrated that TNF- and interleukin-17 may work synergistically to enhance the development of IL-1, IL-6, IL-8, MMPs, and granulocyte colony-stimulating factor (G-CSF), all of which are essential for the progression of inflammation and cartilage breakdown (3).

11.3 TARGETED DELIVERY STRATEGIES FOR DIFFERENT NANO-FORMULATIONS

The use of nanotechnology in the biomedical area has been expanding quickly during the past few years. In comparison to traditional formulas or techniques, it has a number of advantages. Nanotechnology has the power to stabilize pharmaceuticals that are encapsulated, control drug release behavior, prolong drug retention, and significantly reduce toxicity. Numerous adjustments can provide the nano delivery system the ability to actively or passively target particular areas, which will both improve the therapeutic efficacy and reduce adverse effects. The synovial in the inflamed joints of RA patients exhibits aberrant enlargement, which is followed by inflammatory cell infiltration and angiogenesis. As a result, the RA microenvironment develops endothelial breaches that may let nanoformulations seep into the afflicted area. Nano-formulations can also be used for imaging and photothermal therapy in addition to chemotherapy. It has been noted that some of the RA therapy's existing agents help reduce inflammation, but in order to increase the effectiveness of these agents for RA, a variety of different drug carriers are being created by focusing on the passive mechanism. The agents utilized in drug-based delivery systems for RA treatment fall into three broad types. These drug delivery methods are based on nucleic acids, proteins, peptides, and small molecules. There are numerous functional delivery methods available for the treatment of RA. Further research is being done on actively targeted delivery systems, stimulus-responsive delivery systems, and intelligent drug delivery systems with multi-functionalities like active targeting to certain cell types and selective accumulation (Table 11.4).

11.4 SMALL MOLECULES DRUG-BASED DELIVERY SYSTEM

The vast majority of current common RA therapies use small molecules (Table 11.1). However, the potency of the drugs has been diminished by a number of limitations, including poor pharmacokinetics, non-targeted distribution, and low solubility.

Therefore, to avoid low efficacy and severe toxicity, small-molecule drugs should be administered via Table 11 nano-carriers. The aforementioned goal can be achieved by combining a small molecule therapy with a macromolecule that has higher performance and stability. Drug conjugation offers a number of advantages for increasing the effects against RA and may result in improved anti-inflammatory actions. Additionally, it is claimed that encapsulating medications

TABLE 11.1

Different Delivery Systems for Small Molecules

Delivery Systems	Agent Name	Nano-Formulations	Ref.
Small Molecules	Dexamethasone	PEG-Dex Conjugates, PCL-PEG micelles, PeGylation Liposomes	(4)
	Methotrexate	Dextran Sulfate-MTX Conjugates, Albumin-MTX Conjugates, Au/Fe half-shell PLGA nanoparticles, SA-Dex-OA/MTX micelles	(4)
	Curcumin	HA-Cur micelles	(4)
	Methylprednisolone	Cyclodextrin-α-methylprednisolone Conjugates	(4)

inside nano-carriers is a successful strategy for protecting the drugs and improving their *in vivo* performance. The well-known nano-carrier known as liposomes increases the bioavailability of medications for the treatment of RA. Since the majority of small molecule medications are hydrophobic by nature, it is also widely used to solubilize and distribute medications in RA therapy by forming micelles with hydrophobic cores. When compared to other traditional treatments, the drug-loaded nanocarriers always offer benefits like improved therapeutic efficacy and fewer adverse effects of RA medication. The two main areas that researchers should concentrate on are further increasing delivery efficacy and reducing negative effects. Numerous changes are made to the cells implicated in the development of RA, which promotes a special binding affinity to the RA-affected cells to support targeted medication delivery in the inflamed areas. In RA, active synovial macrophages express folic acid receptors, which folic acid is known to have a very high affinity for (4). In comparison to other unmodified micelles, the changed FA micelles have a stronger anti-arthritis effect in CIA mice. Similarly, sialic acid (SA), galactosyl, and mannose are utilized to increase the effectiveness of targeted administration to decrease the inflammatory response and promote the bone healing function (Table 11.4).

11.5 NUCLEIC ACID-BASED DELIVERY SYSTEMS

Inflammatory arthritis is frequently treated with gene therapy. Although many medicines are not yet available due to the current clinical trials for gene therapies,

TABLE 11.2

Different Delivery Systems for Nucleic Acid

Delivery Systems	Agent Name	Nano-Formulations	Ref.
Nucleic Acid	IL-1β siRNA	Lipidoid-polymer hybrid nanoparticles	(4)
	P65 siRNA	PCL-PEI and PCL-PEG micelles	(4)
	SiRNA against BTK	PEG-*b*-PLGA nanoparticles	(4)
	TNF-α siRNA	PEGylated solid-lipid nanoparticles	(4)

these treatments have a significant chance of causing the precise knockdown or expression of a variety of genetic targets due to their distinct properties (Table 11.2).

11.6   PROTEIN AND PEPTIDE AGENT-BASED DELIVERY SYSTEMS

However, protein therapies are also attracting a lot of interest due to a number of benefits over small molecules. Drug delivery systems that transfer protein agents to the desired location need to have certain characteristics, such as bioactive peptides that can be utilized to treat chronic inflammatory illnesses and are resistant to protease degradation (Table 11.3).

RGD plays a critical role in improving the effectiveness of how different medicinal drugs are delivered. Numerous other peptides, including RGD, have improved the effectiveness of medicine administration, including macrophage peptide tuftsin and vasoactive intestinal peptide (VIP). Antibodies are frequently used for protein-based targeted delivery. By selectively attaching to the antigens on the surface of cell membranes, antibodies have the capacity to direct precise therapeutic payloads to cells. Albumin can therefore be considered a viable protein drug-based delivery mechanism in inflammatory illnesses like RA. Studies have indicated that joints in active RA have enhanced cell metabolism that has a high need for albumin consumption (Table 11.4).

TABLE 11.3
Different Delivery Systems for Protein and Peptides

Delivery Systems	Agent Name	Nano-Formulations	Ref.
Peptide/Protein	TNF-α siRNA	PEGylated solid-lipid nanoparticles	(4)
	Core peptide	PEGylated liposomes	(4)
	TNF- α antibody	Carboxymethyl cellulose microneedle	(4)
	Etanercept	HA crosslinked microneedle	(4)
	TRAIL	HAS-TRAIL conjugates	(4)
	Tocilizumab	Gold nanoparticles	(4)

TABLE 11.4
Actively Targeted Delivery Systems and Stimulus Responsive Delivery System

Types	Receptor	Drug	Delivery Strategy	Ref.
		Small Molecules		
FA	Folate Receptor β	Etoricoxib	BSA nanoparticles	(4)
		Methotrexate	Dendrimer G5	
		Dexamethosone	FA-PLGA Nps	
		siRNA	FA-PEG-CH-DEAE$_{15}$ Nps	
Mannose	Mannose Receptor	Morin	DSPC/Chol/F-DHPE/Man	(4)
		Withaferin-A	Liposomes	
			DSPC/Chol/Man Liposomes	

TABLE 11.4 *(Continued)*
Actively Targeted Delivery Systems and Stimulus Responsive Delivery System

Types	Receptor	Drug	Delivery Strategy	Ref.
		Small Molecules		
SA	E-Selectin	Methotrexate	SA-Dex-OA micelles	(4)
	L-Selectin	Dexamethasone palmitate	SA-cholesterol conjugated liposomes	
		Protein & Peptides		
Albumin	SPARC	Methotrexate	MTX @ HAS-Nps	(4)
		Tacrolimus	TAC-HAS Nps	
RGD	αvβ3 integrins	Methotrexate	Au/Fe/Au PLGA Nps	(4)
		Methotrexate	Au PLGA Nps	
		Prednisone	RGD-Lip-PRE Liposomes	
VIP	VIP receptor	Camptothecin	DSPE-PEG3400-VIP micelles	(4)
Tuftsin	Fc and Neuropilin-1 receptors	IL-10 DNA	Alginate Nps	(4)

Physiological factors are crucial because they serve as prospective targets when creating bio-responsive drug delivery systems because the characteristics of arthritic tissues and normal tissues are quite different from one another. Drugs may be released by stimulus-responsive drug delivery systems in response to a change in a particular physiological signal or environmental element.

11.7 NOVEL DIAGNOSTIC STRATEGIES

11.7.1 SCREENING TECHNIQUES

11.7.1.1 X-Ray

An X-ray can identify periarticular soft tissue swelling. Early RA manifested primarily periarticular soft tissue inflammation and peri- or juxta-articular osteoporosis on X-rays; when the condition worsens, articular surface degradation, joint space stenosis, joint fusion, or dislocation. Also arthritic surface damage, joint space osteoporosis, juxta-articular osteoporosis, tumors, and, in severe cases, joint fusion or dislocation, and in RA, but it cannot show early disease symptoms such as soft tissue alterations and bone erosion. X-rays are cost-effective and affordable, however, they have low sensitivity for early diagnosis and radiation hazards (5).

11.7.1.2 MRI

The term "MRI" refers to the application of nuclear magnetic resonance and gradient magnetic field principles to produce an interior structural image of an object after detecting the radiation signal given off by the human body. This technique is very helpful in detecting bone and cartilage damage and morphological abnormalities. The amount of hydrogen in the human body is extremely high hence in order to provide the imaging effect in clinical MRI, hydrogen atoms are frequently used (6).

It is the most accurate method for detecting early signs of RA, such as synovitis, joint space narrowing, and bone erosion, is magnetic resonance imaging (MRI), but it is also the most expensive. By using MRI, it is possible to detect early RA's synovial thickening, bone marrow inflammation, and modest degradation of the articular surface (7).

11.7.1.3   CT Imaging

CT imaging involves utilization of software to process X-ray images obtained at various angles, allowing for the generation of 3D imaging of target tissues and organs. Due to its fine spectral resolution, high tissue penetration, and rapid imaging speed, it has been extensively employed in non-invasive cancer and RA diagnosis to see morphological abnormalities (8). This can increase the sensitivity of erosion detection, especially in complicated areas like the wrist, helping with an early diagnosis (9). The metacarpal head of a healthy subject does not show any erosion, however, the MCP joints of an RA patient clearly show erosion. Therefore, CT techniques like dual-energy CT and high-resolution CT can be employed to assess the condition of the appendicular skeleton in RA patients. Although it is costly, radiant, and unable to detect active inflammations such synovitis and tenosynovitis, defects, and other conditions (10).

11.7.1.3.1   Ultrasound (US)

Ultrasound is practical and cost-effective for assessing the synovial, bone, and cartilage structures of numerous joints as well as for keeping track of synovial inflammation (11). As compared to conventional radiographic examination in diagnosing joint structural deterioration US is more sensitive, as it can clearly demonstrate the thickness and morphology of synovium, synovial sac, articular cavity leakage, and articular cartilage either in grayscale or power doppler contrast. In addition, US can also measure the quantity of joint effusion and the distance from the body surface effectively to facilitate joint puncture and treatment (12).

11.7.1.3.2   Photo Acoustic (PA) Imaging

PA imaging is a non-invasive, non-ionizing bioimaging technique that makes use of a pulsed laser as an energy source and ultrasonic waves as inputs (13). The photothermal effect is the basis of PA imaging. When a pulsed laser beam comes into contact with tissues and body components like lipids, melanin, myoglobin, and hemoglobin, the light energy is converted to heat and the temperature of the targeted region rises. This photothermal action causes thermoelastic expansion, which results in ultrasonic waves. PA imaging has lately gained popularity due to its advantages of great penetration depth of ultrasonic imaging and high spatial resolution of optical coherence tomography. Clinically, PA imaging is used to visualize synovial blood vessels with the use of ultrasonic diagnostic tools and shows the possibility of diagnosing RA (14).

11.7.1.3.3   Fluorescence (FL) Imaging

FL imaging monitors the changing level of molecular distortion to give an efficient diagnostic and prognostic evaluation of RA. FL imaging has been used in preclinical studies for a variety of purposes due to its benefits, including its ease of deployment, high sensitivity for real-time identification, and excellent bio-compatibility for biomedical applications. The fundamental drawback of FL imaging is its poor in vivo penetrating capacity. This can be improved by NIR FL imaging which is very similar to MRI and CT scans (15).

11.7.1.3.4   Multimodal Imaging

In order to obtain the effect of complementary advantages and to simultaneously perform several imaging functions, more than two imaging technologies are combined to create multi-modality imaging. This increases the accuracy of diagnostic results. The fusion of various imaging contrast ants is the secret of multimodal imaging. In order to improve the diagnostic outcome for RA, optical imaging and MRI can be used in combination to overcome the weak penetration of optical imaging and the poor sensitivity of MR Multi-modal imaging techniques like FL/PA, FL/MR, and US/PA have also been successfully used to diagnose RA in addition to MR/NIR imaging (7).

11.7.1.3.5   Stimuli-Responsive Imaging

Until now there has been relatively little research on RA stimuli-responsive imaging. Lessons can be drawn from the response imaging of malignancy locations, though, as the milieu of RA and tumors is comparable (16).

11.7.1.3.5.1 Micro RNA   Analysis of miRNA expression may be useful for early diagnosis and for keeping track of medical therapy but there are technical difficulties with extraction and identification brought on by the sample's relatively low miRNA concentration. MiRNAs can be isolated from biological fluids and are Table 11 (blood, plasma, synovial fluid). It is a non-invasive and simplest approach which is estimated by widespread real-time PCR method. The combinations of several miRNAs may improve diagnostic precision and support RA differentiation and for the early rheumatoid arthritis diagnosis certain miRNAs may be helpful in how well a pharmaceutical treatment is working (i.e. DMARDs, biologic therapy, etc.). For the potential and effectiveness, more studies are required (17).

11.7.1.3.5.2 Serological Examination   Blood biomarkers such as antibodies (RF, ACPA) resulting from immune responses and/or acute phase reactants (C-reactive protein (CRP), erythrocyte sedimentation rate (ESR)) that are raised under inflammatory conditions can all be found in serological tests. The patient may be given the diagnosis of RA if at least one of the RF and ACPA tests shows a positive titer and an elevated level of an acute phase reactant (CRP or ESR) is seen (18) (Tables 11.5 and 11.6).

TABLE 11.5

The Contrast Agent's Using in Different Diagnosing Techniques

Imaging Modality	Contrast Agent	Superiority	Limitation	Ref.
FL	FITC	Excellent fluorescence, Good colloidal solubility, High absorptivity quantum yield	Poor colloidal stability	(15)
	ICG	Good biocompatibility, Excellent optical properties	Low cell uptake, Short half-life, Poor colloidal stability	(15)
MR	Gd-EOB-DTPA	High relaxivity	-	(17)
	Gd-DTPA	Weak toxicity	Weak signal in vivo, Short half-life	(17)
CT	Ioversol	Good stability, fewer side effects	Large dose	(8–10)
	Resovisit- Iotrolan	Good colloidal stability, Small dose	High viscosity, Poor colloidal stability	(8–10)
	Iohexol	Good stability, Good colloidal solubility	Large dose	(8–10)
PA	ICG	Good photoacoustic effect, Good biocompatibility	Short half-life Low cell uptake, Poor colloidal stability	(8–10)

TABLE 11.6

Various Current Treatment Strategies with Their Therapeutic Outcome and Side Effects

Class	Drug	Therapeutic Outcome	Side-Effects	Ref.
NSAIDs	aspirin, ibuprofen, naproxen, and Celebrex	Reduce inflammation and pain	Stomatitis, Indigestion, Hemorrhage, Ulceration, Hearing loss, Hepatic abnormalities, Renal abnormalities, etc.	(19–21)
DMARDs	Methotrexate, Leflunomide/ Teriflunomide, Sulfasalazine, Chloroquine/ Hydroxychloroquine.	Inhibit or reduce the immune system's attack on the joints.	Alopeci, Hepatotoxicity, Stomatitis, infrequent myelosuppression, etc.	(22,23)
GCs	Dexamethasone, β-methasone, triamcinolone, prednisone, prednisolone	Reduce pain and swelling,	Depression, hypertension, diabetes sleep disturbance, immunosuppression, weight gain, glaucoma.	(24,25)

TABLE 11.6 *(Continued)*

Various Current Treatment Strategies with Their Therapeutic Outcome and Side Effects

Class	Drug	Therapeutic Outcome	Side-Effects	Ref.
Biological agents	rituximab, certolizumab pegol, golimumab, Infliximab, Etanercept.	biologic response modifiers target immune-related protein molecules	Skin allergy, Pain, Fever, Chills, Nausea, and headache.	(26)

11.8 NOVEL TREATMENT STRATEGIES

11.8.1 CURRENT TREATMENT STRATEGIES

11.8.1.1 Nonsteroidal Anti-Inflammatory Drugs (NSAIDs)

NSAIDs are non-selective cyclooxygenases (COX) enzyme inhibitors. The COX enzyme helps produce prostaglandin (PG), a mediator of the inflammatory process. Therefore, NSAIDs cause remission of pain and inflammation by inhibiting the formation of PG (27). In the early stages of RA, NSAIDs such as indomethacin [1-(4-chlorobenzoyl)-5- methoxy-2-methyl IMCol-3-yl], aspirin, ibuprofen, naproxen, and Celecoxib reduce pain (analgesia) through anti-inflammatory mechanisms without compromising articular function. Due to their short pharmacokinetic half-lives, NSAIDs, like other anti-RA medications, are rapidly metabolized in the body and must be taken often and at large doses, which may result in gastrointestinal issues (like perforations, ulcers, and bleeding) (28) or other symptoms, and they are only moderately effective and unable to block the progression of the disease.

11.8.1.2 Disease-Modifying Antirheumatic Drugs (DMARDs)

DMARDs, such as methotrexate, change RA progress and lessen joint damage. Since DMARD clinical results take 1–6 months to manifest after the first therapy, they are often known as "slowly acting antirheumatic medicines" (29). It mainly includes: Methotrexate, Leflunomide/Teriflunomide, Sulfasalazine, and Chloroquine/Hydroxychloroquine (30). According to studies, compared to other DMARDs, methotrexate may reduce mortality, particularly fatalities from cardiovascular disease, however, it appears to be less successful than newer biological treatments. This medication has a number of benefits, including dependability, potency, long-lasting effects, affordability, and excellent tolerability. Nevertheless, it has several adverse effects also including Hepatic cirrhosis, interstitial pneumonitis, myelosuppression, hypersensitivity and allergic responses, retinopathy, and other conditions (29). Despite these issues, DMARDs are still used as first-line therapy (31).

11.8.1.3   Glucocorticoids (GC)

GCs primarily prevent phospholipid release, anti-inflammation, immuno-suppression (7). It has been shown to lower the activation, proliferation, differentiation, and survival of numerous cells involved in the production of inflammatory mediators in RA patients. Furthermore, the primary benefit of GCs is the relief of arthritis symptoms such as pain and swelling. GCs can inhibit T helper 1 (Th1) cell activity and proliferation, resulting in decreased production of proinflammatory cytokines such as interleukin (IL1, IL2, IL3, IL6) tumor necrosis factor (TNF), interferon, and IL17. Therapeutic techniques aimed at applying GCs RA therapy attempt to relieve symptoms while modifying the course of the disease, such as preventing joint deterioration (32). Despite several properties, it has several side effects also including Insulin resistance, infection, hyperadrenocorticism, hypertension and atherosclerosis, osteoporosis and osteonecrosis, skin thinning, obesity, inhibition of wound repair, etc (33).

11.8.1.4   Biological Agents

Biological agents include TNF-α inhibitors (infliximab, etanercept, adalimumab, golimumab), IL-1 inhibitors (anakinra), IL-6 receptor inhibitor (tocilizumab), Costimulation blockers, Anti-B-cell agents (rituximab), Janus-activated kinase (JAK) inhibitors (tofacitinib), T- cell Inhibitors (abatacept) (34–36) new antibodies (rituximab, certolizumab pegol, golimumab). For targeted immunotherapy, biological therapeutic agents are developed to target key cytokines implicated in the development of RA (37). They are complex proteins synthesized by molecular biology processes in prokaryotic or eukaryotic organisms (38) and have superior therapeutic potential in RA treatment due to their superior targeting activity, but they are accompanied by a number of undesirable properties, including lack of stabilization, poor bioavailability, and a high prevalence of infection and onco-genesis, particularly lymphomas (39).

11.8.1.5   Inflammation-Associated Cells

The inflammation in RA is caused due to various immune cells, which can be B and T lymphocytes, macrophages, and dendritic cells. B-cells produce and respond to cytokines and chemokines which promote leukocyte infiltration in the joints, synovial hyperplasia, formation of ectopic lymphoid structure, and angiogenesis (40). Macrophages help in the progression of RA diseases and are highly active in inflamed areas. It produces large amounts of pro-inflammatory cytokines like IL-1β, IL-6, and TNF-α, which causes aggregation, inflammation, and bone destruction. These cells target a variety of cell surface receptors, which include the folate receptor (FR)(41), scavenger receptor (SR), and vasoactive intestinal peptide (VIP) receptors. On the surface of macrophages and other inflammation cells, folate receptor-beta (FR-β) (42), toll-like receptors, CD44, and other relative receptors are overexpressed. As a result, macrophages and other immune-associated cells may be a key target for anti-rheumatic drugs.

11.8.1.6 Folate Receptor (FR)

It was widely exploited as a therapeutic target for treating oncology before RA because it anchors glycosyl phosphatidylinositol on the cell surface and binds folic acid (FA) with high affinity. The FRs have four subtypes, which include FRβ, FRα, FRγ, and FRδ. Among all the subtypes FRβ is expressed on the CD14+ cells and activated synovial macrophages of Patients with RA and the results indicated that FR high-expression macrophages exhibited a relatively significant absorption of FA conjugated liposomes. (43,44). And meanwhile, FA-targeted nanoparticles are more effective at delivering RA medication. Promoting accumulation in inflamed areas is one benefit. Some scientists used FA as the FR's ligand by conjugating it into a hydrophilic shell. In contrast to other treatments, activated macrophages treated with FA-nanoparticles encapsulated in rhodamine B showed noticeably higher fluorescence intensity (45).

11.8.1.7 SR (Scavenger Receptors)

SR belongs to a family of surface glycoproteins on macrophages by which low-density lipoprotein (LDL) oxidized and acetylated uptake can be efficiently mediated. By using SRs, oxidized LDL, which causes atherogenesis, can be removed by macrophage endocytosis. In recent studies, it has been found that SRs play a major role in inflammatory disease. Inflammation causes the macrophages' surface to become activated, which causes serum albumin, polyanionic macro-molecules, and oxidized LDL to become absorbed. Due to dextran sulfate's excellent biodegradability and biocompatibility, it is intensively explored. It is well known that DS is the ligand for the highly expressed scavenger receptor class A (SR-A) found on activated macrophages. As fewer nanomedicines circulate to other organs, its great selectivity targeting SR is also advantageous for reducing adverse effects (46).

11.8.1.8 CD44

An abundantly found adhesion receptor on epithelial cells, activated lymphocytes, and malignant cells is CD44. Leukocytes and activated macrophages quickly start to express CD44 when exposed to inflammatory stimuli in a variety of inflammatory disorders (47). A common ligand for the CD44 receptor is hyaluronan (HA) a natural polysaccharide, which is employed in drug administration. Using HA for localized RA therapy could improve therapeutic outcomes by increasing accumula-tion while also reducing systemic negative effects (48). Hence, HA binding to CD 44 has the potential to distribute RA treatment medicines.

11.8.1.9 Anti-Angiogenesis

In the early stages of RA, angiogenesis frequently results in inflammatory infiltration and synovial pannus growth, which will eventually cause slow degradation of cartilage and even surrounding bone. In addition to facilitating the movement of oxygen and minerals, Angiogenesis promotes the secretion of inflammatory cytokines, boosts adhesion and recruitment of inflammatory cells to synovitis sites, and promotes the proliferation of excessive synovium. It includes two types of adhesion molecules namely αvβ3-integrin and E-selectin.

11.8.1.10   αvβ3-Integrin

A member of the family of integral proteins, v3-integrin is connected to the stimulation of angiogenesis. According to a study, a v3-integrin antagonist could particularly cause the death of VECs, which would decrease angiogenesis and lessen the severity of arthritis (49). VECs in RA synovium have excessive levels of v3-integrin expression relative to normal tissues. V3-integrin was chosen as another biomarker for an active targeted medication delivery system because of this property. For aiming targets, it has been widely employed in nano-platform (50).

11.8.1.11   E-Selectin

E-selectin, a member of the selectin family of glycoproteins, is often abundantly expressed on endothelial cells in inflammatory and neovascular situations. E-selectin, on the other hand, is hardly detectable (Table 11) in healthy tissues, making it a good candidate for active targeting delivery in inflamed tissues, particularly RA synovium (51). It has been frequently used as a natural target for medical intervention due to its expression in infection, inflammation, and cancer (52).

11.8.1.12   Phototransistor Therapy (PTT)

In recent times, both scientific research and clinical practice have focused a greater emphasis on phototherapy, which comprises photodynamic therapy (PDT) and phototransistor therapy (PTT). It is generally moderate and non-invasive therapy. Photosensitizers are used during PTT to turn light, particularly NIR light, into heat, which kills disease tissues through hyperthermia or overheating because light can successfully enter RA-affected, inflammatory joints (53–55). The precise control of heat release can be accomplished in a dose- and time-dependent way in conjunction with the target administration of photosensitizers. PTT can undeniably cause cell death in the vicinity of inflammatory tissues, but the temperature needs to be carefully managed to prevent unneeded tissue damage when exposed to light. Hence it provides an efficient novel treatment to treat RA.

11.8.1.13   Photodynamic Therapy (PDT)

Photosensitizers in PDT produce reactive oxygen species (ROS) like singlet oxygen, superoxide, and, under the influence of light, hydroxyl radicals, and hydrogen peroxide to eliminate inflammatory or cancerous cells. Likewise, the NIR light is converted by photothermal agents into localized heat for eradicating diseased areas. In order to treat RA, NIR light with a specific depth of penetration can ensure the therapeutic impact of nanoparticles in inflammatory joints both PDT and PTT. In situ ROS production has the ability to kill diseased tissues without invasion or significant side effects. PDT has a lot of potential as a treatment for RA because it can cause cytotoxicity in the synovial membrane when photosensitizers are precisely deposited in the inflammatory areas and triggered by the appropriate light. Moreover, the insufficient oxygen brought on by the hypoxic milieu of the RA site and oxygen consumption during PDT remains a problem for PDT application in RA treatment (56).

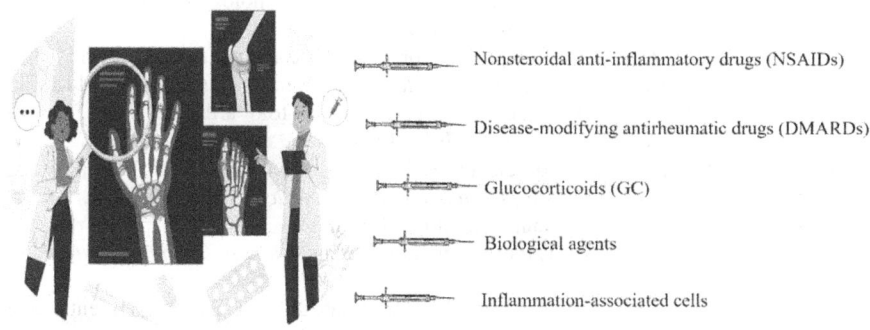

FIGURE 11.5 Treatment strategies currently in use for treating RA.

11.8.1.14 Stimuli-Responsive and Biomimetic Nanoparticles for RA Treatment

The stimuli-responsive nanoplatforms, which may effectively control the pathologic inflammation cascade by targeting specific inflammatory mediators, can reduce the symptoms of RA and prevent further joint damage. Since stimuli-responsive nanoplatforms can only be activated to release drugs at lesion locations, drug leakage can be significantly reduced. Therefore, employing stimuli-responsive nanoplatforms can result in dramatically reduced toxicity and significantly increased therapy efficacy (Figure 11.5).

11.8.1.14.1 Future Treatment Strategies

11.8.1.14.1.1 *Gene Therapy* Although the origin of RA is unknown, there appears to be a substantial link between interaction between genetic and environmental aspects. It entails treating RA without using pharmaceuticals by introducing a gene into a patient's cells. Gene therapy in RA is a local and articular targeted approach to either silence the expression of proinflammatory cytokines genes (TNF-a, IL-1b, and IL-6) or high-expression anti-inflammatory cytokines genes (IL-1ra, IL-4, IL-10, IFN-b), with the hope that long-term expression of these anti-arthritic agents will result in prolonged anti-inflammatory effects while preventing systemic adverse reactions. According to studies, genetic factors contributed between 50 and 60% to the onset of RA. These genes either produced proteins that assisted in inhibiting the generation of inflammatory agents or prevented the production of some inflammatory agents involved in the pathophysiology of RA (57).

REFERENCES

1. Lim, K., Jiang, M. and De Silva, T. (2020). Rheumatoid arthritis. In Rattan, S. (ed.), *Encyclopedia of Biomedical Gerontology*. Academic Press Ltd-Elsevier Science Ltd. **3**: 162–177.
2. Smolen, J.S., Aletaha, D. and McInnes, I.B. (2016). Therapies for bone R. *Lancet*, 30173–30178.

3. Dolati, S., et al. (2016). Utilization of nanoparticle technology in rheumatoid arthritis treatment. *Biomedicine & Pharmacotherapy*, **80**: 30–41.

4. Wang, Q., et al. (2021). Nanomedicines for the treatment of rheumatoid arthritis: State of art and potential therapeutic strategies. *Acta Pharmaceutica Sinica B*, **11**(5): 1158–1174.

5. McQueen, F.M. (2013). Imaging in early rheumatoid arthritis. *Best Practice & Research Clinical Rheumatology*, **27**(4): 499–522.

6. Choi, J.-A. and G.E. Gold (2011). MR imaging of articular cartilage physiology. *Magnetic Resonance Imaging Clinics of North America*, **19**(2): 249–282.

7. Zhao, J., et al. (2021). Nanotechnology for diagnosis and therapy of rheumatoid arthritis: Evolution towards theranostic approaches. *Chinese Chemical Letters*, **32**(1): 66–86.

8. He, W., Ai, K. and Lu, L. (2015). Nanoparticulate X-ray CT contrast agents. *Science China Chemistry*, **58**: 753–760. 10.1007/s11426-015-5351-8.

9. Lee, N., Choi, S.H. and Hyeon, T. (2013). Nano-sized CT contrast agents. *Advanced Materials*, **25**: 2641–2660. 10.1002/adma.201300081.

10. Østergaard, M. and Boesen, M. (2019). Imaging in rheumatoid arthritis: The role of magnetic resonance imaging and computed tomography. *La radiologia medica*, **124**: 1128–1141. 10.1007/s11547-019-01014-y.

11. D'Agostino, M.A. (2015). Ultrasound imaging in rheumatoid arthritis. In Emery, P. (ed.), *Atlas of Rheumatoid Arthritis*. Springer Healthcare. 10.1007/978-1-907673-91-7_7.

12. Gaujoux-Viala, C., et al. (2014). Recommendations of the French Society for Rheumatology for managing rheumatoid arthritis. *Joint Bone Spine*, **81**(4): 287–297.

13. Nie, L. and X. Chen (2014). Structural and functional photoacoustic molecular tomography aided by emerging contrast agents. *Chemical Society Reviews*, **43**(20): 7132–7170.

14. Vonnemann, J., Beziere, N., Böttcher, C., Riese, S.B., Kuehne, C., Dernedde, J., Licha, K., von Schacky, C., Kosanke, Y., Kimm, M., Meier, R., Ntziachristos, V. and Haag, R. (2014). Polyglycerolsulfate functionalized gold nanorods as optoacoustic signal nanoamplifiers for in vivo bioimaging of rheumatoid arthritis. *Theranostics*, **4**(6): 629–641. 10.7150/thno.8518.

15. Schäfer, V.S., Hartung, W., et al. (2013). Quantitative assessment of synovitis in patients with rheumatoid arthritis using fluorescence optical imaging. *Arthritis Research & Therapy*, **15**: R124. 10.1186/ar4304.

16. Han, Q., et al. (2019). A redox-switchable colorimetric probe for "naked-eye" detection of hypochlorous acid and glutathione. *Molecules*, **24**(13): 2455.

17. Filková, M., et al. (2014). Association of circulating miR-223 and miR-16 with disease activity in patients with early rheumatoid arthritis. *Annals of the Rheumatic Diseases*, **73**(10): 1898–1904.

18. Aletaha, D., et al. (2010). Rheumatoid arthritis classification criteria: An American College of Rheumatology/European League against Rheumatism collaborative initiative. *Arthritis & Rheumatism*, **62**: 2569–2581. 10.1002/art.27584.

19. Crofford, L.J. (2013). Use of NSAIDs in treating patients with arthritis. *Arthritis Research & Therapy*, **15** (Suppl 3): S2. 10.1186/ar4174. Epub 2013 Jul 24. PMID: 24267197; PMCID: PMC3891482.

20. Bullock, J., et al. (2018). Rheumatoid arthritis: A brief overview of the treatment. *Medical Principles and Practice*, **27**(6): 501–507.

21. Huang, J., et al. (2021). Promising therapeutic targets for treatment of rheumatoid arthritis. *Frontiers in Immunology*.

22. Benjamin, O., Goyal, A. and Lappin, S.L. (2022 Jan). Disease Modifying Anti-Rheumatic Drugs (DMARD) [Updated 2022 Jul 4]. In *StatPearls [Internet]*. StatPearls Publishing. Available from: https://www.ncbi.nlm.nih.gov/books/NBK507863/.

23. Ragab, O.M., et al. (2017). Effect of early treatment with disease-modifying anti-rheumatic drugs and treatment adherence on disease outcome in rheumatoid arthritis patients. *The Egyptian Rheumatologist*, **39**(2): 69–74.
24. Oray, M., et al. (2016). Long-term side effects of glucocorticoids. *Expert Opinion on Drug Safety*, **15**(4): 457–465.
25. Hua, C., et al. (2020). Glucocorticoids in rheumatoid arthritis: Current status and future studies. *RMD Open*, **6**(1): e000536.
26. Curtis, J.R. and Singh, J.A. (2011 Jun). Use of biologics in rheumatoid arthritis: Current and emerging paradigms of care. *Clinical Therapeutics*, **33**(6): 679–707. 10.1016/j.clinthera.2011.05.044. PMID: 21704234; PMCID: PMC3707489.
27. Yang, M., Feng, X., Ding, J., Chang, F. and Chen, X. (2017 Apr 28). Nanotherapeutics relieve rheumatoid arthritis. *Journal of Controlled Release*, **252**: 108–124. 10.1016/j.jconrel.2017.02.032. Epub 2017 Feb 28. PMID: 28257989.
28. Abbasi, M., et al. (2019). Strategies toward rheumatoid arthritis therapy: The old and the new. *Journal of Cellular Physiology*, **234**: 10018–10031. 10.1002/jcp.27860.
29. van Vollenhoven, R. (2009). Treatment of rheumatoid arthritis: State of the art 2009. *Nature Reviews Rheumatology*, **5**: 531–541. 10.1038/nrrheum.2009.182.
30. Guo, Q., et al. (2018). Rheumatoid arthritis: Pathological mechanisms and modern pharmacologic therapies. *Bone Research*, **6**(15). 10.1038/s41413-018-0016-9.
31. Hosseinikhah, S.M., et al. (2021). Nanomaterials for the diagnosis and treatment of inflammatory arthritis. *International Journal of Molecular Sciences*, **22**(6): 3092.
32. Buttgereit, F., Straub, R.H., Wehling, M. and Burmester, G.-R. (2004). Glucocorticoids in the treatment of rheumatic diseases: An update on the mechanisms of action. *Arthritis & Rheumatism*, **50**: 3408–3417. 10.1002/art.20583.
33. Ban, Q., et al. (2017). Noninvasive photothermal cancer therapy nanoplatforms via integrating nanomaterials and functional polymers. *Biomaterials Science*, **5**(2): 190–210.
34. Mitragotri, S. and Yoo, J.W. (2011). Designing micro- and nano-particles for treating rheumatoid arthritis. *Archives of Pharmacal Research*, **34**: 1887–1897. 10.1007/s12272-011-1109-9.
35. Pham, C.T.N. (2011). Nanotherapeutic approaches for the treatment of rheumatoid arthritis. *WIREs Nanomedicine and Nanobiotechnology*, **3**: 607–619. 10.1002/wnan.157.
36. Meier, F.M., et al. (2013). Current immunotherapy in rheumatoid arthritis. *Immunotherapy*, **5**(9): 955–974.
37. Jung, Y.-S., et al. (2013). Temperature-modulated noncovalent interaction controllable complex for the long-term delivery of etanercept to treat rheumatoid arthritis. *Journal of Controlled Release*, **171**(2): 143–151.
38. Šenolt, L., et al. (2009). Prospective new biological therapies for rheumatoid arthritis. *Autoimmunity Reviews*, **9**(2): 102–107.
39. Scott, D.L., et al. (2010). Rheumatoid arthritis. *The Lancet*, **376**(9746): 1094–1108.
40. Silverman, G.J. and Carson, D.A. (2003). Roles of B cells in rheumatoid arthritis. *Arthritis Research & Therapy* **5**(Suppl 4): S1. 10.1186/ar1010.
41. Yi, Y.S. (2016 Dec). Folate receptor-targeted diagnostics and therapeutics for inflammatory diseases. *Immune Network*, **16**(6): 337–343. 10.4110/in.2016.16.6.337.
42. Chandrupatla, D.M.S.H., et al. (2019). The folate receptor β as a macrophage-mediated imaging and therapeutic target in rheumatoid arthritis. *Drug Delivery and Translational Research*, **9**: 366–378. 10.1007/s13346-018-0589-2.
43. Van Der Heijden, J.W., Oerlemans, R., Dijkmans, B.A.C., Qi, H., Laken, C.J.V.D., Lems, W.F., Jackman, A.L., Kraan, M.C., Tak, P.P., Ratnam, M. and Jansen, G. (2009). Folate receptor β as a potential delivery route for novel folate antagonists to macrophages in the synovial tissue of rheumatoid arthritis patients. *Arthritis & Rheumatism*, **60**: 12–21. 10.1002/art.24219.

44. Xiao, S., et al. (2019). Nanomedicine – advantages for their use in rheumatoid arthritis theranostics. *Journal of Controlled Release*, **316**: 302–316.
45. Wei, J. (2022). Nano-medicine in treating rheumatoid arthritics. *Highlights in Science, Engineering and Technology*, **2**: 186–199. 10.54097/hset.v2i.573.
46. Yu, C., et al. (2022). Dextran sulfate-based MMP-2 enzyme-sensitive SR-A receptor targeting nanomicelles for the treatment of rheumatoid arthritis. *Drug Delivery*, **29**(1): 454–465.
47. Jordan, A.R., et al. (2015). The role of CD44 in disease pathophysiology and targeted treatment. *Frontiers in Immunology*, **6**.
48. Liang, J., et al. (2016). Hyaluronan as a therapeutic target in human diseases. *Advanced Drug Delivery Reviews*, **97**: 186–203.
49. Weis, S.M. and Cheresh, D.A. (2011 Sep). αV integrins in angiogenesis and cancer. *Cold Spring Harbor Perspectives in Medicine*, **1**(1): a006478. 10.1101/cshperspect. a006478. PMID: 22229119; PMCID: PMC3234453.
50. Zhou, H., Chan, H.W., Wickline, S.A., Lanza, G.M. and Pham, C.T.N. (2009). $\alpha_v\beta_3$–Targeted nanotherapy suppresses inflammatory arthritis in mice. *The FASEB Journal*, **23**: 2978–2985. 10.1096/fj.09-129874.
51. Barthel, S.R., et al. (2007). Targeting selectins and selectin ligands in inflammation and cancer. *Expert Opinion on Therapeutic Targets*, **11**(11): 1473–1491.
52. Jiang, M., et al. (2014). Systemic inflammation promotes lung metastasis via E-selectin upregulation in mouse breast cancer model. *Cancer Biology & Therapy*, **15**(6): 789–796.
53. Zhang, S., et al. (2022). Nano-based co-delivery system for treatment of rheumatoid arthritis. *Molecules*, **27**(18): 5973.
54. Kim, H.J., et al. (2015). Drug-loaded gold/iron/gold plasmonic nanoparticles for magnetic targeted chemo-photothermal treatment of rheumatoid arthritis. *Biomaterials*, **61**: 95–102.
55. Lee, S.-M., et al. (2013). Targeted chemo-photothermal treatments of rheumatoid arthritis using gold half-shell multifunctional nanoparticles. *ACS Nano*, **7**(1): 50–57.
56. Wang, S.S., Lv, J., Meng, S.S., Tang, J.X. and Nie, L.M. (2020). Recent advances in nanotheranostics for treat-to-target of rheumatoid arthritis. *Advanced Healthcare Materials*, **9**: 1901541. 10.1002/adhm.201901541.
57. Yamamoto, K., et al. (2015). Genetic studies of rheumatoid arthritis. *Proceedings of the Japan Academy, Series B*, **91**(8): 410–422.

12 Nanobiotechnology in Personalized Oncology

*Umesh Kumar, Mansi Kumari, Bhupendra Sahu,
Daanish Vij, Lakshay Virmani, Neelam Thakur,
and Tanushri Chatterji*

12.1 INTRODUCTION

Personalized medicine refers to prescribing medications that are best suited to an individual. However, other individual patient variations are also considered, including pharmacogenetic, pharmacogenomic, and pharmacoproteomics information. Similarly, cancers of the same histological type behave differently from patient to patient, even when they share the same histological type. Cancer is one of the leading causes of death, and available treatments often merely improve the patient's odds—an unequivocal cure is extremely rare (Kumar et al., 2023). Cancer therapy personalization is based on a better understanding of the disease at the molecular level, and nanotechnology will play a significant role in this area. Nanotechnology is the production and use of materials, technologies, and systems through manipulating matter on a nanometer-length scale, i.e., at the atomic, molecular, and supramolecular levels. Nanobiotechnology uses nanotechnology in life sciences, such as molecular diagnostics, drug discovery, drug delivery, and nanomedicine development. (Yadav et al., 2022; 2023a; 2023b) Several components of individualized cancer therapy are related to nanobiotechnology. The essential component of personalized medicine is molecular diagnostics, and nanobiotechnology will play an important role in refining it and has led to the use of the term nanodiagnostic (Jain, 2005).

Moreover, Personalized oncology is evidence-based, individualized medicine that delivers the proper care to the right cancer patient at the right time and results in measurable improvements in outcomes and a reduction in healthcare costs. This chapter will cover emerging themes in personalized oncology, such as genetic analysis, targeted medications, cancer treatments, and molecular diagnostics. Biomarkers and personalized molecular medicine are displacing traditional "one size fits all" medicine. Cancer treatment will shift from reactive to proactive over the next decade. The use of biomarkers is fundamental to customized oncology. These biomarkers, derived from tissue, serum, urine, or imaging, must be validated. Biomarker-based personalized oncology already has a significant impact. Biomarkers of three sorts are essential: predictive, prognostic, and early response biomarkers. Preventive medicine tools based on genetic and molecular diagnostics

DOI: 10.1201/9781003348672-12

and therapies will increase cancer prevention. Imaging technologies such as computed tomography (CT) and positron emission tomography (PET) are already influencing cancer patient identification and treatment. The application of companion molecular diagnostics is predicted to increase dramatically. It will be integrated into new cancer medicines as a single (bundled) package, providing more efficiency, value, and cost savings. This technique promises a once-in-a-lifetime opportunity for integration and more excellent value in customized oncology (Kalia, 2013). This chapter will first present the notion of personalized cancer therapy and then describe the role of nanobiotechnology in developing personalized cancer therapy.

12.2   SCRUTINIZING NANOBIOTECHNOLOGY FOR DIAGNOSIS

Diagnosis refers to the analysis and interpretation of a particular disease. Diagnosis at the initial stage is crucial for efficient treatment and thereby promotion of public health. precise and early diagnosis of a disease by identification of the nature and cause of the disease and thereby evaluation of relevant laboratory data aids in providing a successful medical response (Nagraik et al., 2021).

Recent years have focused on more diagnosis which helps to develop fast, cheap, accurate and accessible diagnostic devices that can also be used by patient to invigilate their health. Out of various conventional diagnostic bioassays and techniques, some are commonly used assays which include polymerase chain reaction (PCR) based genetic assay, Enzyme-linked immunosorbent assay (ELIZA), etc. Though poor susceptibility, poor sensitivity, and slow pace hinder the process. Therefore, nanotechnology has paved the way for development of the revolutionary diagnostic tools, which have increased functionality, sensitivity, and specificity (Nagraik et al., 2021; Zhang et al., 2019).

The complex, large, and expensive conventional devices have convoluted procedures whereas nanoparticles (NPs) pave the way for manipulation and control of molecules to form nanostructures (1–100 nm) which have high surface area to volume ratio, to aid in highly useful medicinal diagnostic properties. Nanodrugs help Olin's easy regulation of pharmacokinetics with the aid of available interaction sites. The smaller size of NPs helps to transport them easily and distribute them consistently throughout the area. Nanodevices offer possibilities such as nanodrugs, vectors, and underbearing conditions such as pH pressure and bacterial content. Other latest techniques used for cancer diagnosis include Quantum dots (used as fluorescent near-infrared dyes instead of organic dyes), Gold nanoparticles, Dendrimers (polyamidoamines), Carbon nanotubes, Nanoshell, and nanopolymers (chitosan, hyaluronic acid, etc.) (Zhang, 2019; Yadav, 2022).

Genomics and proteomics integrated with nanobiotechnology can help in developing an efficacious, reliable and rapid on-site medical diagnostic tool. Advanced imaging approach integrated with nanotechnology helps in cancer diagnosis which includes Magnetic Resonance Imaging (MRI), Computed Tomography (CT) scan, Positron emission Tomography (PET) scan, Single photon emission CT, and ultrasound (Nagraik et al., 2021).

The applications of nanobiotechnology not only improve current techniques for early diagnosis but can also provide various approaches for cancer treatment (Liang et al., 2022).

12.3 NANOMEDICATED THERANOSTICS

Nanomedicated therapeutic and diagnostic agents have been designed, developed, and approved for clinical applications and commercial markets (Abbasi Kajani et al., 2021). Based on recent reports, the use of nanodrugs and nano-based materials approved by the FDA has increased in the past two decades in pharmaceuticals which have successfully synthesized and used to cure diseases via drug delivery nanosystems (Anselmo & Mitragotri, 2019; McGoron, 2020). Nanomaterial-based particles vary in size, shape and surface chemistry which aids in providing biomedical applications (Abbasi Kajani et al., 2021). Organic (carbon, lipid, etc.), as well as inorganic (metal, Quantum dots, metal oxide) materials, can be synthesized based on the substrate with the aid of methods such (Anselmo & Mitragotri, 2019; McGoron, 2020) as Bottom-up, Top-down, chemical, physical, and biological. The methods are organized because of requisite equipments, efficiency, cost of production, and their potential to synthesize NPs of varied sizes and shapes. However, the potential toxicity of NPs incorporated via different synthesis methods poses a challenge to the production of various biochemical products (Adeel et al., 2020; Karimi-Maleh et al., 2021; Zhao et al., 2015).

According to a recent report, approximately 250 nanodrugs are currently present in the market or in phase, out of which Liposomal nanoformulated drugs are most approved by the FDA which include emulsions, iron polymer complexes, nanocrystals, etc (Martinelli et al., 2019). The Total pharmaceutical global market is anticipated to rise to USD 293.1 billion in 2023 as compared to the year 2019 which was USD 138.8 billion (Martinelli et al., 2019; Zulfiqar et al., 2020).

The approval of Doxil in 1995 by the FDA paved the way for various nanoformulations such as Amphotec, Marqibo, Mepact, Onivyde, ThermoDox, Vyxeous, etc., which are currently in use for drug delivery. (Anselmo AC, 2019; Kajani A.A., 2021). Various Paclitaxel-based liposomal, and albumin-bound polymers have also been synthesized by chemically modifying them into Lipusu and Abraxane (approved in 2006 and 2005 by the FDA) for the treatment of metastatic breast cancer and pancreatic cancers (Abbasi Kajani et al., 2021; McGoron, 2020).

A new Era of nanobiotechnology includes SPIONS which offers high resolution, multi-modal imaging, and high sensitivity for Nanoscale contrast agents. Feraheme and Nanotherm are SPIONS-containing formulations that are used as Therapeutic agents for the treatment of anemia and glioblastoma, respectively (Abbasi Kajani et al., 2021; Smith & Gambhir, 2017). Certain inorganic NP-based therapeutic agents, for ex., NBTXR3 (radiosensitizer hafnium oxide nanoparticle) are also being utilized for radiotherapy of advanced soft tissue carcinoma (Bonvalot et al., 2019).

On the other hand, the development of core-shell NPs targeted three major factors i.e., antigenicity, proliferation, and immunosuppressiveness. A related experiment conducted by a group of researchers includes the incorporation of Gambogic Acid in the outer region of poly(lactic-co-glycolic acid) [PLGA] NPs. Cytosine-phosphate guanine oligonucleotides (CpG-ODNs) were incorporated within nanoparticles. Location-based incorporation of Gambogic acid killed tumor cells and further release of Heparin and CpG-ODNs performed anti-angiogenic and immunostimulatory function, respectively. The upregulation of T-helper 1 type anticancer immune response by CpG-ODN promoted the secretion of antitumor cytokines which further helped in tumor suppression and elimination (Shao et al., 2020). Another experiment showed the blocking of CD-47 and signal regulatory protein-alpha (SIRP-alpha) antibodies of cancer cells with the aid of arginine-coated gold NPs (Ray et al., 2018).

An experiment also provided us with evidence that the use of CRISPR-Cas9 can help to block the expression of PD-L1 and could enhance antitumor immune response. The use of monoclonal antibodies has been approved for PD-L1 blockage but their associated challenges such as immunotoxicity and high cost pose a challenge. Thereby promoting the use of CRISPR-Cas9 components along with paclitaxel, an anti-cancer drug. NPs' inner core consisted of a PEI-PLGA (poly-(ethyleneimine)-poly(lactic-co-glycolic acid)) cationic copolymer. PEI was attached to polyethylene glycol via acid-cleavable linker. The ingression of CRISPR-Cas9 system components in the tumor microenvironment resulted in knocking out the activity of cycling dependent kinase 5 (Cdk5) gene and thereby attenuation of tumor PD-L1 expression. Further, NPs release paclitaxel which stimulates antitumor immunogenic effects, such as dendritic cell activation, macrophage repolarization from type M2 to type M1, etc., which thereby aid in providing theranostic applications in the field of biomedical sciences (Tu et al., 2020).

Therefore, cost-effective, efficacious, and quality control methods help to decide on a capable method and nano-based medicine.

12.4   DRUG DELIVERY

In recent years in the field of biomedicine, nanotechnology has shown an impressive strong impact on early disease diagnosis and helped in the enhancement of various treatment methods. Its major role was seen in the management of cancer, heart disease, and also in brain disorders. For targeting these biomedical challenges nanoparticles (NP) are used, since they have a high surface area/volume ratio, and show high ligand density on targeting (Farokhzad & Langer, 2009a). Stable small molecular compounds or amino acid chains express great stability on targeting (Xiong et al., 2011). Oncology drugs are specific to their target but due to the scattering distribution of anti-cancer drugs, they show toxic side effects on the body. Oral inhalation of anti-cancer drugs shows a high distribution of drugs throughout the body and less in tumor-specific areas as they must pass from various barriers and tissue levels. To deal with this problem, researchers used different drug delivery systems: (i) drug delivered by active targeting; based on ligands affiliation to receptor, (ii) drug delivered by passive targeting based on permeability and microenvironment near onco-regions. Active targeting is considered a smart drug delivery.

12.4.1 ACTIVE TARGETING

Active targeting is a system basically based on the drug-dropping method at a specific site to reduce drug wastage and toxicity that cause side effects on the body. Active targeting was done by using NP as a smart vehicle approved for treatment. NPs are designed by attaching small glycoproteins on their tips, non-antibodies ligands like peptides. Ligand and target-receptor binding are essential for this method and for the pharmacokinetics of the drug. There is a significant difference between oncogenic cells and healthy tissue; receptors are overexpressed on oncogenic cells as they required high energy for their high metabolism (Wang et al., 2016). Receptor-mediated endocytosis occurs to facilitate the entry of nanocarriers which have anti-cancer drugs (Salahpour Anarjan, 2019). Internalization of NP is required for effective delivery of anti-cancer drugs (Huang et al., 2013). Multi-drug resistance (MDR) transporters (integral membrane proteins include P-glycoprotein drug effusion pumps) could be overridden by specialized carriers throughout anti-cancerous drugs. Active targeting methods help in reducing this problem and enhance the bioavailability of anti-cancerous drugs at the sites for action. There are many ligands that bind with specific receptors like Monoclonal antibodies selected as ligands and binds to Breast cancer cells (HER2) and folic acid (FA) as a ligand that binds to folate receptors (FR).

12.5 NANO THERAPIES

12.5.1 POLYMERIC NANOPARTICLES

Due to their distinct characteristics and behaviors brought on by their small size, polymeric nanoparticles (PNPs) have garnered a lot of attention over the past few years (Farokhzad & Langer, 2009b). These nanoparticulate materials, according to many authors, have the potential for a variety of uses, including medication delivery and diagnostics (Crucho, 2015; Lin et al., 2015; Tosi et al., 2008). Controlled release, the possibility to combine therapy with imaging (theranostics), the protection of drug molecules and their precise targeting, and the facilitation of improvements in the therapeutic index are benefits of PNPs as carriers (Kamaly et al., 2012; Krasia-Christoforou & Georgiou, 2013; Zhong et al., 2014).

Nanoparticles are often taken up by cells by endocytotic processes, which are largely determined by their size and surface properties (Iversen et al., 2011; Owens & Peppas, 2006). The technology used to create nanoparticles can be used to modify these features (Pinto Reis et al., 2006; Rao & Geckeler, 2011).

Nanocapsules or nanospheres can be produced, depending on the method of preparation and organic phase composition (Crucho, 2015). An aqueous or oily cavity containing the active chemicals is contained within a nanocapsule particle's core-shell morphology, which is encased in a polymer shell. Nanospheres have a matrix-like structure where the polymer and active ingredients are evenly distributed. By regulating the rates of polymer biodegradation and drug diffusion out of the polymer matrix, the traditional strategy for controlling drug release from PNPs is accomplished (Kamaly et al., 2016). Exogenous and endogenous cues that induce medication release have recently attracted a lot of attention since they are selective to the microenvironment of particular disorders (Crucho, 2015; Marin et al., 2013).

12.5.2 LIPOSOMES

Liposomes are tiny vesicles that have an internal aqueous area within one or more bilayer membranes made of phospholipids that can be either natural or manufactured. They are rarely immunogenic, generally low in toxicity, biocompatible, and biodegradable. Particle size can be controlled using a variety of methods, and the smallest liposomes are considered nanoparticulate drug carriers.

There are numerous approved and available liposome-based products (Chang & Yeh, 2012). To improve liposomes' therapeutic indices for oncology applications, numerous kinds of antineoplastic drugs have been added. They consist of vinca alkaloids (Krishna et al., 2001; Zhigaltsev et al., 2005), taxanes (Guo et al., 2005; Sharma et al., n.d., 1997), anthracyclines (Forssen et al., 1996; Mayer et al., n.d.), camptothecins, platinum analogs (Kim et al., 2001; Lu et al., 2005), camptothecins (Emerson, 2000; Pal et al., n.d.; Tardi et al., 2000), and antimetabolites (Cosco et al., 2009). Numerous liposomal anticancer medicines are in late-stage clinical development or are clinically authorized. The traditional and SSL-based formulations of doxorubicin (Myocet® and Doxil®), daunorubicin (DaunoXome®), vincristine (Marqibo®), and cytarabine (DepoCyte®) are among the goods that the Food and Drug Administration (FDA) has approved.

While in other instances, toxicity is decreased by avoiding vital normal tissues, liposome inclusion can sometimes boost the anticancer efficacy of the encapsulated medications by allowing for more selective delivery or targeting of the tumor tissue. In the end, cytotoxic medicines improved overall pharmacological qualities as a result of adjustment of their pharmacokinetic and pharmacodynamic (PD) features. Among the positive pharmacokinetic effects mediated by liposomes are the following: decreasing metabolism or inactivation of labile drugs in the plasma or tissues; extending drug circulating half-life by reducing drug removal (clearance) from the blood; reducing drug distribution to healthy tissues due to the particle size restriction for transport across healthy vascular endothelium (Matsumura & Maeda, 1986).

12.5.3 NIOSOMES

Niosomes are a one-of-a-kind bilayer lipid nanostructure created by the self-aggregation of a non-ionic surfactant. It was first created for cosmetic purposes by the L'Oreal corporation in 1975. They were employed as medicine delivery devices after five years of study in 1980. They can readily absorb medicinal chemicals, proteins, and genes, which may be loaded into the hydrophilic core, whereas lipid-soluble molecules, as previously indicated, are incorporated in the hydrophobic layer.

Funkhouser invented the term "theranostic" in 2002 as a new concept in nanotechnology. In nanostructures, these compounds have both medicinal and diagnostic characteristics. A growing variety of niosomal formulations with theranostic applications are being developed. Barlas et al. created a nanosystem that had niosomes that encapsulated gadolinium nanoparticles (GdNP) and protoporphyrin IX (Pp IX). These nanosystems improve the efficacy of radiation and photodynamic treatment in human alveolar type II (ATII) similar cells (A549) and human cervical cancer cell line (HeLa), whereas Pp IX was utilized to trace the niosome utilizing its fluorescence characteristic (Demir et al., 2018). Nowroozi et al. created a multifunctional niosome capable of encapsulating doxorubicin and quantum dots. This type of nanocluster.

12.6 FUTURE PROSPECTS

The use of nanotechnology in cancer is known as "nanooncology," and it covers both diagnostics and therapy (Jain, 2011). As a result, many lipid-based, polymer-based, inorganic, viral, and drug-conjugated nanoparticles are being investigated for possible application in cancer. Gold nanoshells, iron oxide nanocrystals, and quantum dots-based nanomedicines have already been created for application in cancer (Jabir et al., 2018). Drug delivery in the realm of Nano oncology might be passive or aggressive. Passive drug delivery relies on increased vascular permeability and retention to achieve drug accumulation on tumor cells, whereas active drug delivery relies on the accumulation of targeted nanoparticles at the site of interest via different molecular recognition forms such as lectin-carbohydrate, ligand-receptor, or antigen-antibody (Jabir et al., 2018; Lammers et al., 2008; Ventola, 2017; M. D. Wang et al., 2007).

Nanoparticles have the ability to modify medication pharmacokinetics and pharmacodynamics, hence increasing their therapeutic potential (Wicki et al., 2015). Despite the expanding number of nanomedicines in research investigations, only a tiny fraction of them make it to clinical use. This is impacted in part by tumor heterogeneity, where "one size fits all" processes are difficult to apply (Hua et al., 2018). Other factors include a lack of specificity, accumulation, and specificity, as well as the use of incorrect animal models, which results in failed translation into humans. Nanomedicines based on current FDA-approved pharmaceuticals must demonstrate benefits such as reduced toxicity and improved efficacy over the existing treatment to be authorized.

Nanomaterials are projected to outperform conventional cancer therapies such as surgical excision of tumors, chemotherapy, and radiation therapy in the future. Nanocarriers offer several benefits over free pharmaceuticals because they shield medications from early breakdown and premature interaction with biological surroundings while delivering drugs to target cells and/or tissues. The introduction of nanocarriers can enhance the pharmacokinetic and medication distribution profiles while also improving drug absorption and intracellular penetration in target cells/tissue. When evaluating a nanocarrier for use in medicine, it must be adequately described, biocompatible and biodegradable, water-soluble or form colloids under aqueous conditions, have a long shelf life, and have an extended circulation half-life. Nonetheless, it must target certain audiences.

However, it must target cells and/or tissues. The possible toxicity risks associated with the actual deployment of nanomaterials in patient clinical care are not insignificant and should be carefully evaluated. It would be preferable if nanoparticles could also be made to be biocompatible and biodegradable.

Furthermore, build-up in human off-target organs should be prevented, and clearance rates should be increased to ensure minimum injury during administration. In the creation of nanoparticles, nanomaterials provide a vast range of various combinations; nevertheless, we must bear in mind that they must be batch-to-batch similar, simple to assemble, and endure rigorous clinical tests to show their specificity and safety. Finally, there is the footprint.

12.7 CONCLUSION

In the current medical era, biomarkers and molecular medicine are replacing "one size fits all" medicine with personalized medicine (Kalia, 2013). As a result of this paradigm shift, personalized oncology must rapidly implement new validated biomarkers. Over the next decade, oncology will transition from a reactive to a proactive discipline – a discipline that is predictive, personalized, preventive, and participatory. Additionally, genomic and molecular diagnostics and interventions will be developed to implement pre-emptive medicine, which will improve prevention, early detection, and access to care. It is essential for healthcare oncology professionals to keep up to date on the latest tumor biomarkers, their optimal clinical use, as well as their side effects management.

REFERENCES

Abbasi Kajani, A., Haghjooy Javanmard, S., Asadnia, M., & Razmjou, A. (2021). Recent advances in nanomaterials development for nanomedicine and cancer. *ACS Applied Biomaterials*, 4(8), 5908–5925. 10.1021/ACSABM.1C00591

Adeel, M., Duzagac, F., Canzonieri, V., & Rizzolio, F. (2020). Self-therapeutic nanomaterials for cancer therapy: A review. *ACS Applied Nanomaterials*, 3(6), 4962–4971. 10.1021/ACSANM.0C00762

Anselmo, A. C., & Mitragotri, S. (2019). Nanoparticles in the clinic: An update. *Bioengineering & Translational Medicine*, 4(3). 10.1002/BTM2.10143

Bonvalot, S., Rutkowski, P. L., Thariat, J., Carrère, S., Ducassou, A., Sunyach, M. P., Agoston, P., Hong, A., Mervoyer, A., Rastrelli, M., Moreno, V., Li, R. K., Tiangco, B., Herraez, A. C., Gronchi, A., Mangel, L., Sy-Ortin, T., Hohenberger, P., de Baère, T., ... & Papai, Z. (2019). NBTXR3, a first-in-class radioenhancer hafnium oxide nanoparticle, plus radiotherapy versus radiotherapy alone in patients with locally advanced soft-tissue sarcoma (Act.In.Sarc): A multicentre, phase 2-3, randomised, controlled trial. *The Lancet. Oncology*, 20(8), 1148–1159. 10.1016/S1470-2045(19)30326-2

Chang, H. I., & Yeh, M. K. (2012). Clinical development of liposome-based drugs: Formulation, characterization, and therapeutic efficacy. *International Journal of Nanomedicine*, 7, 49–60. 10.2147/IJN.S26766

Cosco, D., Paolino, D., Muzzalupo, R., Celia, C., Citraro, R., Caponio, D., Picci, N., & Fresta, M. (2009). Novel PEG-coated niosomes based on bola-surfactant as drug carriers for 5-fluorouracil. *Biomedical Microdevices*, 11(5), 1115–1125. 10.1007/S10544-009-9328-2

Crucho, C. I. C. (2015). Stimuli-responsive polymeric nanoparticles for nanomedicine. *ChemMedChem*, 10(1), 24–38. 10.1002/CMDC.201402290

Demir, B., Barlas, F. B., Gumus, Z. P., Unak, P., & Timur, S. (2018). Theranostic niosomes as a promising tool for combined therapy and diagnosis: "All-in-one" approach. *ACS Applied Nano Materials*, 1, 2827–2835. 10.1021/acsanm.8b00468.

Emerson, D. (2000). Antitumor efficacy, pharmacokinetics, and biodistribution of NX 211: A low-clearance liposomal formulation of lurtotecan. *Clinical Cancer Research: An Official Journal of the American Association for Cancer Research.* https://www. academia.edu/86233125/Antitumor_efficacy_pharmacokinetics_and_biodistribution_ of_NX_211_a_low_clearance_liposomal_formulation_of_lurtotecan

Farokhzad, O. C., & Langer, R. (2009a). Impact of nanotechnology on drug delivery. *ACS Nano, 3*(1), 16–20. 10.1021/NN900002M/ASSET/IMAGES/MEDIUM/NN-2009-00002M_0003.GIF

Farokhzad, O. C., & Langer, R. (2009b). Impact of nanotechnology on drug delivery. *ACS Nano, 3*(1), 16–20. 10.1021/NN900002M

Forssen, E. A., Male-Brune, R., Adler-Moore, J. P., Lee, M. J. A., Schmidt, P. G., Krasieva, T. B., ... & Tromberg, B. J. (1996). Fluorescence imaging studies for the disposition of daunorubicin liposomes (DaunoXome) within tumor tissue. *Cancer Research, 56,* 2066–2075.

Guo, W., Johnson, J. L., Khan, S., Ahmad, A., & Ahmad, I. (2005). Paclitaxel quantification in mouse plasma and tissues containing liposome-entrapped paclitaxel by liquid chromatography-tandem mass spectrometry: Application to a pharmacokinetics study. *Analytical Biochemistry, 336*(2), 213–220. 10.1016/J.AB.2004.09.046

Hua, S., de Matos, M. B. C., Metselaar, J. M., & Storm, G. (2018). Current trends and challenges in the clinical translation of nanoparticulate nanomedicines: Pathways for translational development and commercialization. *Frontiers in Pharmacology, 9*(JUL). 10.3389/FPHAR.2018.00790/FULL

Huang, S., Shao, K., Kuang, Y., Liu, Y., Li, J., An, S., Guo, Y., Ma, H., He, X., & Jiang, C. (2013). Tumor targeting and microenvironment-responsive nanoparticles for gene delivery. *Biomaterials, 34*(21), 5294–5302. 10.1016/J.BIOMATERIALS.2013.03.043

Iversen, T. G., Skotland, T., & Sandvig, K. (2011). Endocytosis and intracellular transport of nanoparticles: Present knowledge and need for future studies. *Nano Today, 6*(2), 176–185. 10.1016/j.nantod.2011.02.003

Jabir, N. R., Anwar, K., Firoz, C. K., Oves, M., Kamal, M. A., & Tabrez, S. (2018). An overview on the current status of cancer nanomedicines. *Current Medical Research and Opinion, 34*(5), 911–921. 10.1080/03007995.2017.1421528

Jain, K. K. (2005). Role of nanobiotechnology in developing personalized medicine for cancer. *Technology in Cancer Research & Treatment, 4*(6), 645–650. 10.1177/1533 03460500400608

Jain, K. K. (2011). Nanobiotechnology and personalized medicine. *Progress in Molecular Biology and Translational Science, 104,* 325–354. 10.1016/B978-0-12-416020-0.00008-5

Kalia, M. (2013). Personalized oncology: Recent advances and future challenges. *Metabolism: Clinical and Experimental, 62* (Suppl. 1). 10.1016/J.METABOL.2012.08.016

Kamaly, N., Xiao, Z., Valencia, P. M., Radovic-Moreno, A. F., & Farokhzad, O. C. (2012). Targeted polymeric therapeutic nanoparticles: Design, development and clinical translation. *Chemical Society Reviews, 41*(7), 2971–3010. 10.1039/C2CS15344K

Kamaly, N., Yameen, B., Wu, J., & Farokhzad, O. C. (2016). Degradable controlled-release polymers and polymeric nanoparticles: Mechanisms of controlling drug release. *Chemical Reviews, 116*(4), 2602–2663. 10.1021/acs.chemrev.5b00346

Karimi-Maleh, H., Orooji, Y., Karimi, F., Alizadeh, M., Baghayeri, M., Rouhi, J., Tajik, S., Beitollahi, H., Agarwal, S., Gupta, V. K., Rajendran, S., Ayati, A., Fu, L., Sanati, A. L., Tanhaei, B., Sen, F., shabani-nooshabadi, M., Asrami, P. N., & Al-Othman, A. (2021). A critical review on the use of potentiometric based biosensors for biomarkers detection. *Biosensors & Bioelectronics, 184.* 10.1016/J.BIOS.2021.113252

Kim, E. S., Lu, C., Khuri, F. R., Tonda, M., Glisson, B. S., Liu, D., Jung, M., Hong, W. K., & Herbst, R. S. (2001). A phase II study of STEALTH cisplatin (SPI-77) in patients with advanced non-small cell lung cancer. *Lung Cancer (Amsterdam, Netherlands)*, *34*(3), 427–432. 10.1016/S0169-5002(01)00278-1

Krasia-Christoforou, T., & Georgiou, T. K. (2013). Polymeric theranostics: Using polymer-based systems for simultaneous imaging and therapy. *Journal of Materials Chemistry B*, *1*(24), 3002–3025. 10.1039/C3TB20191K

Krishna, R., Webb, M., Onge, G. S., & Mayer, L. (2001). Liposomal and nonliposomal drug pharmacokinetics after administration of liposome-encapsulated vincristine and their contribution to drug tissue distribution properties. *The Journal of Pharmacology and Experimental Therapeutics* September 2001, *298*(3): 1206–1212.

Kumar, A., Yadav, A. K., Kumar, D., & Mishra, V. (2023). Recent advancements in triazole-based click chemistry in cancer drug discovery and development. *SynOpen*, *07*, 186–208. 10.1055/s-0042-1751452.

Lammers, T., Hennink, W. E., & Storm, G. (2008). Tumour-targeted nanomedicines: Principles and practice. *British Journal of Cancer*, *99*(3), 392. 10.1038/SJ.BJC.6604483

Liang, M., Li, L. D., Li, L., & Li, S. (2022). Nanotechnology in diagnosis and therapy of gastrointestinal cancer. *World Journal of Clinical Cases*, *10*(16), 5146. 10.12998/WJCC.V10.I16.5146

Lin, G., Zhang, H., & Huang, L. (2015). Smart polymeric nanoparticles for cancer gene delivery. *Molecular Pharmaceutics*, *12*(2), 314–321. 10.1021/MP500656V

Lu, C., Perez-Soler, R., Piperdi, B., Walsh, G. L., Swisher, S. G., Smythe, W. R., Shin, H. J., Ro, J. Y., Feng, L., Truong, M., Yalamanchili, A., Lopez-Berestein, G., Hong, W. K., Khokhar, A. R., & Shin, D. M. (2005). Phase II study of a liposome-entrapped cisplatin analog (L-NDDP) administered intrapleurally and pathologic response rates in patients with malignant pleural mesothelioma. *Journal of Clinical Oncology*, *23*(15), 3495–3501. 10.1200/JCO.2005.00.802

Marin, E., Briceño, M. I., & Caballero-George, C. (2013). Critical evaluation of biodegradable polymers used in nanodrugs. *International Journal of Nanomedicine*, *8*, 3071–3091. 10.2147/IJN.S47186

Martinelli, C., Pucci, C., & Ciofani, G. (2019). Nanostructured carriers as innovative tools for cancer diagnosis and therapy. *APL Bioengineering*, *3*(1). 10.1063/1.5079943

Matsumura, Y., & Maeda, H. (1986). A new concept for macromolecular therapeutics in cancer chemotherapy: Mechanism of tumoritropic accumulation of proteins and the antitumor agent smancs. *Cancer Research*, *46*(12_Part_1), 6387–6392.

Mayer, L. D., Tai, L. C. L., Ko, S. C., Masin, D., Ginsberg, R. S., Cullis, P. R., & Bally, M. B. (n.d.). *Influence of vesicle size, lipid composition, and drug-to-lipid ratio on the biological activity of liposomal doxorubicin in mice1*. Retrieved December 20, 2022, from http://aacrjournals.org/cancerres/article-pdf/49/21/5922/2437232/cr0490215922.pdf

McGoron, A. J. (2020). Perspectives on the future of nanomedicine to impact patients: An analysis of US Federal Funding and Interventional Clinical Trials. *Bioconjugate Chemistry*, *31*(3), 436–447. 10.1021/ACS.BIOCONJCHEM.9B00818/ASSET/IMAGES/MEDIUM/BC9B00818_0011.GIF

Nagraik, R., Sharma, A., Kumar, D., Mukherjee, S., Sen, F., & Kumar, A. P. (2021). Amalgamation of biosensors and nanotechnology in disease diagnosis: Mini-review. *Sensors International*, *2*. 10.1016/J.SINTL.2021.100089

Owens, D. E., & Peppas, N. A. (2006). Opsonization, biodistribution, and pharmacokinetics of polymeric nanoparticles. *International Journal of Pharmaceutics*, *307*(1), 93–102. 10.1016/j.ijpharm.2005.10.010

Pal, A., Khan, S., Wang, Y., Kamath, N., Sarkar, A. K., Ahmad, A., Sheikh, S., Ali, S., Carbonaro, D., Zhang, A., & Ahmad, I. (n.d.). Preclinical safety, pharmacokinetics and antitumor efficacy profile of liposome-entrapped SN-38 formulation. *Ar.Iiarjournals.Org*. Retrieved December 20, 2022, from https://ar.iiarjournals.org/content/25/1A/331.short

Pinto Reis, C., Neufeld, R. J., Ribeiro, A. J., & Veiga, F. (2006). Nanoencapsulation I. Methods for preparation of drug-loaded polymeric nanoparticles. *Nanomedicine: Nanotechnology, Biology, and Medicine*, 2(1), 8–21. 10.1016/j.nano.2005.12.003

Rao, J. P., & Geckeler, K. E. (2011). Polymer nanoparticles: Preparation techniques and size-control parameters. *Progress in Polymer Science (Oxford)*, 36(7), 887–913. 10.1016/j.progpolymsci.2011.01.001

Ray, M., Lee, Y. W., Hardie, J., Mout, R., Yeşilbag Tonga, G., Farkas, M. E., & Rotello, V. M. (2018). CRISPRed macrophages for cell-based cancer immunotherapy. *Bioconjugate Chemistry*, 29(2), 445–450. 10.1021/ACS.BIOCONJCHEM.7B00768

Salahpour Anarjan, F. (2019). Active targeting drug delivery nanocarriers: Ligands. *Nano-Structures and Nano-Objects*, 19. 10.1016/j.nanoso.2019.100370

Shao, F., Zhang, M., Xu, L., Yin, D., Li, M., Jiang, Q., Zhang, Q., & Yang, Y. (2020). Multiboosting of cancer immunotherapy by a core-shell delivery system. *Molecular Pharmaceutics*, 17(1), 338–348. 10.1021/ACS.MOLPHARMACEUT.9B01113

Sharma, A., Mayhew, E., Bolcsak, L., Cavanaugh, C., Harmon, P., Janoff, A., & Bernacki, R. J. (1997). Activity of paclitaxel liposome formulations against human ovarian tumor xenografts. *International Journal of Cancer*, 71, 1097–0215. 10.1002/(SICI)1097-0215(19970328)71:1

Sharma, A., Mayhew, E., & Straubinger, R. M. 1993. Antitumor effect of taxol-containing liposomes in a taxol-resistant murine tumor model. *Cancer research 53*(24): 5877–5881.

Smith, B. R., & Gambhir, S. S. (2017). Nanomaterials for in vivo imaging. *Chemical Reviews*, 117(3), 901–986. 10.1021/ACS.CHEMREV.6B00073/ASSET/IMAGES/MEDIUM/CR-2016-000736_0047.GIF

Tardi, P., Choice, E., Masin, D., Redelmeier, T., Bally, M., & Madden, T. D. (2000). *Liposomal encapsulation of topotecan enhances anticancer efficacy in murine and human xenograft models*. https://tspace.library.utoronto.ca/handle/1807.1/72

Tosi, G., Costantino, L., Ruozi, B., Forni, F., & Vandelli, M. A. (2008). Polymeric nanoparticles for the drug delivery to the central nervous system. *Expert Opinion on Drug Delivery*, 5(2), 155–174. 10.1517/17425247.5.2.155

Tu, K., Deng, H., Kong, L., Wang, Y., Yang, T., Hu, Q., Hu, M., Yang, C., & Zhang, Z. (2020). Reshaping tumor immune microenvironment through acidity-responsive nanoparticles featured with CRISPR/Cas9-mediated programmed death-ligand 1 attenuation and chemotherapeutics-induced immunogenic cell death. *ACS Applied Materials & Interfaces*, 12(14), 16018–16030. 10.1021/ACSAMI.9B23084

Ventola, C. L. (2017). Progress in nanomedicine: Approved and investigational nanodrugs. *Pharmacy and Therapeutics*, 42(12), 742. /pmc/articles/PMC5720487/

Wang, M. D., Shin, D. M., Simons, J. W., & Nie, S. (2007). Nanotechnology for targeted cancer therapy. *Expert Review of Anticancer Therapy*, 7(6), 833–837. 10.1586/14737140.7.6.833

Wang, X., Tu, M., Tian, B., Yi, Y., Wei, Z. Z., & Wei, F. (2016). Synthesis of tumor-targeted folate conjugated fluorescent magnetic albumin nanoparticles for enhanced intra-cellular dual-modal imaging into human brain tumor cells. *Analytical Biochemistry*, 512, 8–17. 10.1016/J.AB.2016.08.010

Wicki, A., Witzigmann, D., Balasubramanian, V., & Huwyler, J. (2015). Nanomedicine in cancer therapy: Challenges, opportunities, and clinical applications. *Journal of Controlled Release: Official Journal of the Controlled Release Society*, 200, 138–157. 10.1016/J.JCONREL.2014.12.030

Xiong, X. Y., Gong, Y. C., Li, Z. L., Li, Y. P., & Guo, L. (2011). Active targeting behaviors of biotinylated pluronic/poly (lactic acid) nanoparticles in vitro through three-step biotin-avidin interaction. *Journal of Biomaterials Science, Polymer Edition*, 22(12), 1607–1619. 10.1163/092050610X519444

Yadav, N., Mudgal, D., Anand, R., Jindal, S., & Mishra, V. (2022). Recent development in nanoencapsulation and delivery of natural bioactives through chitosan scaffolds for various biological applications. *International Journal of Biological Macromolecules*, *220*, 537–572. 10.1016/j.ijbiomac.2022.08.098

Yadav, N., Mudgal, D., & Mishra, V. (2023). In-situ synthesis of ionic liquid-based-carbon quantum dots as fluorescence probe for hemoglobin detection. *Analytica Chimica Acta*, *1272*, 341–502. 10.1016/j.aca.2023.341502

Yadav, N., Mudgal, D., Mishra, S., Sehrawat, H., Singh, N. K., Sharma, K., Sharma, P. C., Singh, J., & Mishra, V. (2023). Development of ionic liquid-capped carbon dots derived from Tecoma stans (L.) Juss. ex Kunth: Combatting bacterial pathogens in diabetic foot ulcer pus swabs, targeting both standard and multi-drug resistant strains. *South African Journal of Botany*, *163*, 412–426. 10.1016/j.sajb.2023.10.063

Yadav, N., Gaikwad, R. P., Mishra, V., & Gawande, M. B. (2022). Synthesis and photocatalytic applications of functionalized carbon quantum dots. *Bulletin of the Chemical Society of Japan*, *95*, 1638–1679. 10.1246/bcsj.20220250

Zhang, Y., Li, M., Gao, X., Chen, Y., & Liu, T. (2019). Nanotechnology in cancer diagnosis: Progress, challenges and opportunities. *Journal of Hematology and Oncology*, *12*(1), 1–13. 10.1186/S13045-019-0833-3/FIGURES/2

Zhao, X., Yang, L., Li, X., Jia, X., Liu, L., Zeng, J., Guo, J., & Liu, P. (2015). Functionalized graphene oxide nanoparticles for cancer cell-specific delivery of antitumor drug. *Bioconjugate Chemistry*, *26*(1), 128–136. 10.1021/BC5005137

Zhigaltsev, I. V., Maurer, N., Akhong, Q. F., Leone, R., Leng, E., Wang, J., Semple, S. C., & Cullis, P. R. (2005). Liposome-encapsulated vincristine, vinblastine and vinorelbine: A comparative study of drug loading and retention. *Journal of Controlled Release*, *104*(1), 103–111. 10.1016/J.JCONREL.2005.01.010

Zhong, Y., Meng, F., Deng, C., & Zhong, Z. (2014). Ligand-directed active tumor-targeting polymeric nanoparticles for cancer chemotherapy. *Biomacromolecules*, *15*(6), 1955–1969. 10.1021/BM5003009/ASSET/IMAGES/MEDIUM/BM-2014-003009_0005.GIF

Zulfiqar, H., Hussain, S., Riaz, M., Saddiqa, A., Iqbal, M., Ali, J., Amjad, M., & Javaid, K. (2020). Nature of nanoparticles and their applications in targeted drug delivery. *Pakistan Journal of Science*, *72*(1): 30–36.

13 Rheumatoid Arthritis

Treatments Available at Present

Neeraj Rajdan, Bhavana Srivastava, and Kunal Sharma

13.1 INTRODUCTION

Rheumatoid arthritis (RA) is an inflammatory rheumatic disorder with a progressive course affecting articular and additional-articular systems resulting in pain, disability and mortality (Birch and Bhattacharya, 2010). Chronic infection in erosive joint harms, leading to impairment in the vast majority of patients (El Miedany et al., 2008; Combe, 2009). The onset of complaint is not analogous in all patients but varies in regard to type, number, and pattern of common involvement. The course of complaint may be also different according to the presence or absence of several variables including inheritable background, swollen joints, autoantibody in the serum and the severity of the inflammatory process (Gossec et al., 2010; Finckh, 2006).

The original presenting features of early RA don't mainly differ from other inflammatory arthritis. So prior to definite diagnosis patients with early RA are generally classified as undifferentiated arthritis which can be discerned from other inflammatory arthritis. Early RA was denoted to patients with complaint duration of lower than two years preferentially less than 12 months but presently most rheumatologists are willing to see patients with symptom duration of lower than six weeks. At present, "early" RA is regarded in patients with symptom duration < three months as an early complaint (Aletaha et al., 2002). The frequency rate reported in 2002 ranged from 0.5% to 1% of the population and had indigenous variation (Silman and Pearson, 2002) RA primarily affects the lining of the synovial joints and can beget progressive disability, premature death, and socioeconomic burdens. The clinical manifestations of symmetrical common involvement include arthralgia, swelling, redness, and indeed limiting the range of motion.

13.2 EARLY DIAGNOSIS AND ITS SIGNIFICANCE

Early diagnosis is considered the key improvement indicator for the most desirable outcome (i.e., reduced joint destruction, less radiologic progression, no functional disability, and disease-modifying antirheumatic drugs (DMARD)-free remission) as

DOI: 10.1201/9781003348672-13

well as cost-effectiveness as the first 12 weeks after early symptoms do is regarded as the optimal therapeutic window (van der Linden et al., 2010; Moura et al., 2015; Cho et al., 2019). Identification of RA at initial presentation and treatment at an earlier stage can affect the disease course, prevent the development of joint erosions or retard the progression of erosive disease (Finckh, A. et al., 2006; Goekoop-Ruiterman et al., 2007). Early diagnosis and treatment may affect disease outcomes even to a remissive state (Van der Helm-van Mil et al., 2008; Finckh, 2009). Recognizing early RA from non-RA at the onset of disease is not easier but there are limitations in the use of the American College of Rheumatology (ACR) revised criteria for early opinion. Due to insufficient clinical or laboratory investigations at the onset of arthritis, this criterion is not sensitive enough to identify early RA (Gossec et al., 2010; Arnett 1988). In a study of French cohorts, only 50.9% of RA favored with 1987 ACR revised criteria for diagnosis of RA within one year of onset (Gossec et al., 2010) still, in the absence of treatment inflammation will lead to articular damage and bone corrosion, particularly within the first two years of disease onset (Graudal, 2004). It initially affects small joints, progressing to larger joints, and ultimately the skin, eyes, heart, renal system, and lungs. Frequently, the bone and cartilage of joints are destroyed, and tendons and ligaments weaken (Lee et al., 2017). All this damage to the joints causes scars and bone corrosion, generally very painful for a patient. Common symptoms of RA include morning stiffness of the affected joints for> 30 min, fatigue, fever, and weight loss; joints that are tender, blown, and warm, and rheumatoid nodes under the skin. The onset of this complaint is generally from the age of 35 to 60 years, with absolution and exacerbation. It can also torment children indeed before the age of 16 years, referred to as juvenile RA (Juvenile Rheumatoid Arthritis), which is similar to RA except that the rheumatoid factor isn't set up (McInnes and Schett, 2011; Chaudhari, 2016; Picerno et al., 2015). In the West, the prevalence of RA is believed to be 1–2% (Picerno et al., 2015; Alamanos et al., 2006) and 1% worldwide (Chopra and Abdel-Nasser, 2008).

Regarding the current concept of "opportunity," early diagnosis of RA is essential for the initiation of treatment, or else disease will progress to more severe forms requiring more aggressive treatments (Van der Helm-van, Mil et al., 2008).

Application of recently developed individual criteria provided an opportunity to identify and treat those cases with early inflammatory arthritis who progress to future RA. Using these criteria can discriminate inflammatory arthritis who fulfill the 1987 ACR criteria in the future from those who do not develop RA. The 2010 criteria is an important diagnostic tool with advanced higher sensitivity and specificity compared to former ACR criteria. The new criteria classify a greater no of patients at an earlier phase with reasonable discriminative ability (Van der Linden et al., 2011).

13.3 PREDICTION OF EARLY RA

A patient with inflammatory arthritis may pass several stages from the onset of arthritis to a specific form of rheumatic conditions similar as RA. The first phase begins with the onset of arthritis, and alternate (second), is the period during which

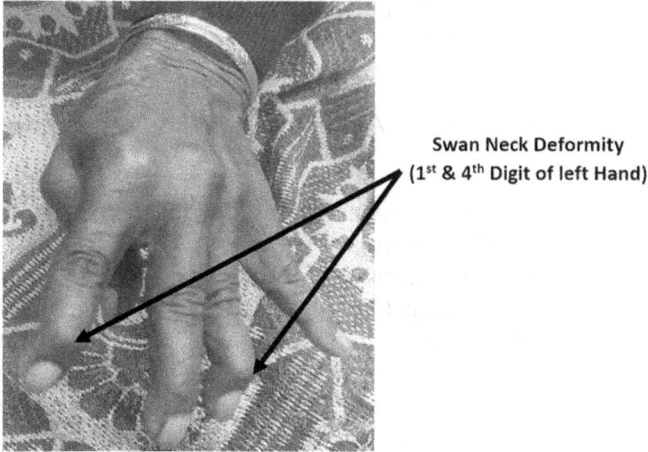

FIGURE 13.1 Classical picture of joint deformities associated with rheumatoid arthritis.

persistence and remission is determined. The third and the fourth phases are the evolution into a specific form of inflammatory arthritis and the outgrowth/ inflexibility of that arthritis. In some cases, these four phases follow in rapid sequence whereas in other cases the time course may prolong and continue for several months or years. Clinically, the diagnosis of RA can be differentiated from osteoarthritis (OA) as the affected areas in RA are the proximal interphalangeal (PIP) and metacarpophalangeal (MP) joints; OA generally affects the distal interphalangeal (DIP) joint (Figure 13.1). OA is the most common type of arthritis and is caused by wear and tear and rather than an autoimmune condition. It does not involve lungs, heart, or immune system. In addition, OA generally affects only one side of the body, as opposed to the symmetrical nature of RA. Another differentiating factor is that RA patients suffer from morning stiffness for at least ≥ 1 h. Patient with OA may have morning stiffness, but this generally resolves or decreases within 20–30 min (McGonagle et al., 2015).

13.4 PATHOGENESIS OF RHEUMATOID ARTHRITIS

There are two subtypes of RA according to the presence or absence of anti-citrullinated protein antibodies (ACPAs). Citrullination is catalyzed by the calcium-dependent enzyme peptidylarginine-deiminase (PAD), changing a positively charged arginine to a polar but neutral citrulline as the result of a post-translational modification. ACPAs can be detected in roughly 67% of RA cases and serve as an useful diagnostic reference for patients with early, undifferentiated arthritis and give an indication of likely disease progression through to RA (Nishimura et al., 2007; Bizzaro et al., 2013). The ACPA-positive subset of RA has a more aggressive clinical phenotype compared to ACPA-negative subset of RA. (Malmstrom et al., 2017). It has been reported that ACPA-negative RA has different genetics association patterns (Padyukov et al., 2011) and differential response of immune cells to citrullinated antigens (Schuerwegh et al., 2010) from those of ACPA-positive subset. This chapter briefly highlights the classic and current treatment options available to address the discomfort/ complications of RA.

13.4.1 STAGES OF RHEUMATOID ARTHRITIS

13.4.1.1 Triggering Stage

The appearance of ACPA is now extensively used to diagnose and predict RA due to its high specificity (> 97%) in clinical practice. ACPA occurs as a result of an abnormal antibody response to a range of citrullinated proteins, including fibrin, vimentin—"Barr Nuclear Antigen-1" (EBNA- 1), α- enolase, type II collagen, and histones, all of which are distributed throughout the whole body. ACPA production have been associated with genetics and environmental factors. The strongest genetics risk factor associated with ACPA-positive RA is found in, gene encoding HLADR, especially HLA- DR1 and HLA- DR4, also known as "Shared Epitopes" (SEs) (Raychaudhuri et al., 2012). It is thought that SE influences RA outgrowth via the product of ACPA and therefore represents a primary risk factor for ACPA products (Okada et al., 2014). The protein tyrosine phosphatase nonreceptor type 22 (PTPN22), which is a lymphoid-specific protein tyrosine phosphatase, has also drawn important attention because of polymorphisms associated with ACPA-positive RA with the contribution of PTPN22 to ACPA-positive RA among different racial ethnicities (Mori et al., 2005; Nabi et al., 2016; Goh et al., 2017). It may thus act as a potent stimulator of T-cell activation and in turn affect the ACPA product. Still, whether the product is directly linked to α1- antitrypsin insufficiency per se or results from altered autophagy induced by the mutant α1- antitrypsin requires further study. The increased response of the type I interferon gene associated with Th2-cell induction and B-cell proliferation correlates with ACPA product (Castaned- Delgado et al., 2017). Some researchers have recently compared the gene expression profiles between ACPA-positive RA and ACPA-negative RA patients (Padyukov et al., 2011; Ding et al., 2009). The critical solution to the puzzle is the association between the discovered genes and ACPA products. In addition, the risks of RA increase in individuals with a family history of RA.

The risk of developing RA was three times higher in first-degree cousins of RA patients indeed though familial factors impact RA in men and women equally. (Schiff et al., 2006; Frisell et al., 2013; Kuo et al., 2017). It is also reflected in a twin study presenting the recurrent risk at 9.5–13.1 in monozygotic co-twins and at 6.4–11.7 in dizygotic same-sexed co-twins as opposed to a background population threat at only 0.37% (Svendsen et al., 2013). Another study of 12,590 twins reveals that environment, lifestyle, and stochastic factors may also play more important places than genetics in ACPA products while inheritable factors are more responsible for the progression from ACPA-positive individuals to arthritis (Hensvold et al., 2015). The environment acts as a driving factor for ACPA products in RA an epigenetic regulation combines environment with genes. Gene-environment interaction influences the reactivity of autoantibodies to citrullinated antigens in RA (Van der Woude et al., 2010), ACPAs can be detected long before the onset of the common symptoms.

This phenomenon suggests that the joints may not be the triggering spot for autoimmunity. Lung exposure to noxious agents, silica dust, nano-sized silica, or carbon derived nanomaterials can trigger mucosal toll-like receptors (TLRs) that spark Ca2- intermediated PADs, but also antigen-presenting cells (APCs), similar as classical dendritic cells (DCs) and B cells (Stolt et al., 2010; Mohamed et al., 2012; Too et al., 2016). The co-atomer subunit α gene mutations could disrupt the endoplasmic reticulum (ER) Golgi transport and cause heritable autoimmune-mediated lung disease and arthritis. Thereby, providing a connection between the lung and the common conditions (Watkin et al., 2015), also smoking in the environment of the HLA-DR SE gene may trigger RA-specific vulnerable responses to citrullinated proteins (Klareskog et al., 2006). DNA methylation mediates smoking and genotype interaction in ANPA-positive RA (Meng et al., 2017). There is ample evidence for three contagious agents regarded as autoimmunity triggers in RA, such as; *Porphyromonas (P.) gingivalis, Aggregatibacter actino-mycetemcomitans (Aa)*, and *Epstein Barr Virus* (EBV). The periodontal space can also be a triggering site. In a clinic setting, 47% of the patients with RA showed evidence of former *Aa* infection compared with 11% in the control group. The pathogen *Aa* can secret leukotoxin A, and form pores in the neutrophil membranes that lead to neutrophil hyperactive citrullination, which results in the release of citrullinated autoantigens in the epoxies (Konig et al., 2016), *P. gingivalis* infection leads to citrullinated autoantigens and the ACPA product in two reported ways one way is about PAD, and arginine gingipains (Rgps), which can stick proteins at arginine remainders and citrullinate proteins producing further neoantigens (Wegner et al., 2010); and another is about neutrophil extracellular trap (NET) conformation convinced by the *P. gingivalis* during the process of NET-osis. ACPAs induce NET-osis and in turn, NET-osis provides citrullinated autoantigens (Khandpur et al., 2013). EBV can affect ACPA-producing B-cells, and disabled EBV control can be observed in RA (Alspaugh et al., 1981).

The intestinal tract is another mucosal organ implicated in the pathogenesis of RA because dysbiosis in RA patients can result from the abundance of certain rare bacterial lineages. It's well proven that gut microbiota may contribute to the pathogenesis of RA via multiple molecular mechanisms (Wu et al., 2016; Chen et al., 2016). Several studies have established the part of dietary factors in RA. The omega-3 fatty acids might not only lower the risk of ACPA products but also help the onset of arthritis after detecting ACPAs (Gan et al., 2017). A healthier diet can also make a contribution to reducing the threat of ACPA-positive RA at 55 years of age. (Hu et al., 2017)

In addition, hormonal levels have been implicated with the pathology of RA (Orellana et al., 2017; Alpizara, and Rodriguez et al., 2017), but the association with ACPA has not been firmly established. Differences in gene expression regulation through both micro-RNAs and long non-coding RNAs have been proposed to contribute to the pathogenesis of RA. The contribution of other epigenetic variations (e.g., sumoylation, histone methylation, histone acetylation, and deace-tylation) and their functional part in RA presently remain unclear.

Translation of the above observations to effective treatment and exploring their interaction with the genome is challenging but would be meaningful. It is of significance to clarify the detailed knowledge of each triggering factor in the triggering of RA so that tools can be developed to provide susceptibility score and early diagnosis, as well as to identify new molecular targets for an individualized drug.

13.4.1.2 Maturation Stage

This stage is initiated at the site of secondary lymphoid tissues or bone marrow. Epitope spreading refers to the development of vulnerable responses to endogenous epitopes performing from the release of self-antigens. The immune response to autoantigens may exist many years before disease onset and lay outside the joints. In this stage, epitope spreading and a gradually increased titer of ACPA can last several times before the onset of common symptoms (Van der Woude et al., 2010). Initial ACCP situations appear to be of great significance in predicting the interval time to disease onset. The production of ACPA reflects a break of immunological tolerance. As a result, numerous citrullination neoantigens would activate MHC class II-dependent T-cells that in turn would help B-cells produce further ACPA. ACPA can induce pain, bone loss, and inflammation in RA (Krishnamurthy et al., 2016; Wigerblad et al., 2016)

One study has linked two RA-specific autoantigens N-acetylglucosamine-6-sulfatase (GNS) and filamin A (FLNA) co-relate microbial with autoimmune responses in the joints (Pianta et al., 2017). Further, it has been proposed that citrullination plays a unique part during osteoclast isolation and ACPA- induced osteoclast activation which might explain important features of the gradual development of RA including why the joints are targeted. Other likely factors include biological features of the targeted autoantigen, original microvascular, neurologic, and biomechanical factors, and microtrauma-related mechanisms may further contribute (McInnes and Schett, 2011) (Figure 13.2).

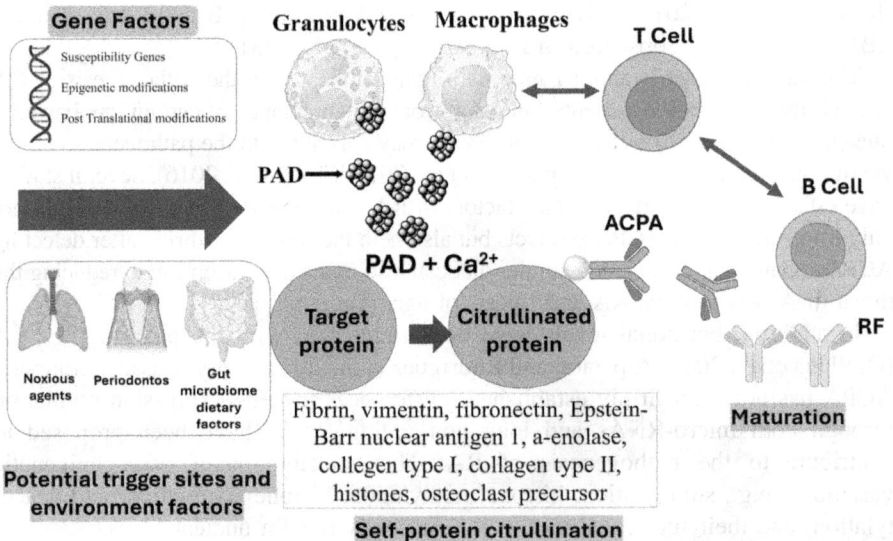

FIGURE 13.2 Pathogenesis and role of triggering factors in RA development (RA, rheumatoid arthritis; PAD, peptidyl-argininedeiminase; ACPA, anti-citrullinated protein antibodies; RF, rheumatoid factor).

RA can be triggered in the potential trigger sites (lung, oral, gut, *etc.*) by the interaction between the genes and environmental factors, which is characterized by the onset of self-protein citrullination resulting in the production of autoantibodies against citrullinated peptides. Lung exposure to noxious agents, infectious agents (*P. gingivalis*, *Aggregatibacter actinomycetemcomitans*, and *Epstein Barr virus*), gut microbiome, and dietary factors may induce the self-protein citrullination and maturation of ACPA. Citrullination is catalyzed by the calcium-dependent enzyme PAD, changing a positively charged arginine to a polar but neutral citrulline as the result of a post-translational modification. In RA, PAD can be secreted by the granulocyte and macrophage. ACPA occurs as a result of an abnormal antibody response to a range of citrullinated proteins, including fibrin, vimentin, fibronectin, *Epstein- Barr* Nuclear Antigen 1, α- enolase, type II collagen, and histones, all of which are distributed throughout the whole body. Many citrullination neoantigens would activate MHC class II-dependent T cells that in turn would help B cells produce more ACPA. The stage is also called loss of tolerance.

13.4.1.3 Targeting Stage

The involvement of RA in joints generally has a characteristic presentation with synovitis being in symmetrical small joints. Joint swelling is the external reflection of synovial membrane inflammation following immune activation. The normal synovial compartment is infiltrated by leukocytes and the synovial fluid is inundated with pro-inflammatory mediators that interact to produce an inflammatory cascade which is characterized by the interaction of fibroblast- such as synoviocytes (FLSs) with the cells of the innate immune system, including monocytes, macrophages, mast cells, DCs, and so on, as well as cells of adaptive immune system similar as T lymphocytes (cell-intermediated immunity) and B-cells (humoral immunity). The two immune systems and their interaction are intimately involved in the development of ACPA-positive RA, which results in the failed resolution of inflammation (habitual synovitis). Monocyte macrophages have been found to massively irritate synovial membranes (Burmester et al., 1983) and be central to the pathophysiology of inflammation. ACPA can enhance NF-kB exertion and TNF-α product in monocyte/macrophages via binding to surface-expressedcitrullinated Grp78 (Lu et al., 2010). α-Enolase on the surfaced of monocytes and macrophages induces the product of pro-inflammatory intercessors (Bae et al., 2012). The imbalances between proinflammatory M1-macrophage and anti-inflammatory M2-macrophage must also be considered in the context of inflammatory RA. (Quero et al., 2017) Indeed, a recent study reported that an imbalance in M1/ M2 monocytes contributes to osteoclastogenesis in RA cases, especially in ACPA-positive RA (Fukui et al., 2017). Further, the pro-inflammatory cytokine interleukin (IL)- 17 A in RA joint samples is localized primarily to mast cells based on one study (Hueber et al., 2010), and mast cells can be activated by ACPA and TLRs ligands (Suurmond et al., 2015).

The accumulation of DCs in the articular cavity has also been reported (Zvaifler et al., 1985). As an APC, especially myeloid DCs have been shown to induce T-cell isolation. A detailed understanding of how myeloid DCs serve in RA may give further effective RA treatment strategies. Other possible ingrain vulnerable pathways comprise neutrophil NETosis, natural killer cell activation, etc. On the other hand, many researcher place the adaptive vulnerable system at the center of RA complaint pathogenesis. Most interest in the contribution of T-cells has focused on their antigen-driven part and cytokine release of specific T-cell subsets. CD 4 effector T-cells are major drivers of abnormal impunity in RA by sustaining habitual synovitis and supporting autoantibody product and a lack of reactive oxygen species could boost pro-inflammatory T-cells, which throws light on the significance of energy metabolism inRA (Yang et al., 2016). As for B-cells, the research focuses on their antigen presentation, antibody formation and release, and cytokine release into the milieu. Thus, better understanding of the mechanisms of disordered innate immunity, including immune complex-intermediated complement activation, adaptive immune responses against self-antigens, and abnormal cytokine networks may open up new avenues to restore immunologic homeostasis (Figure 13.3).

Many cells and their cytokines play an important role in the development of RA. The synovial compartment is infiltrated by leukocytes and the synovial fluid is inundated with pro-inflammatory mediators which induces an inflammatory cascade followed by interactions of fibroblast-like synoviocytes including cells like mast cells, dendritic cells, macrophages, monocytes etc. which are cells of innate

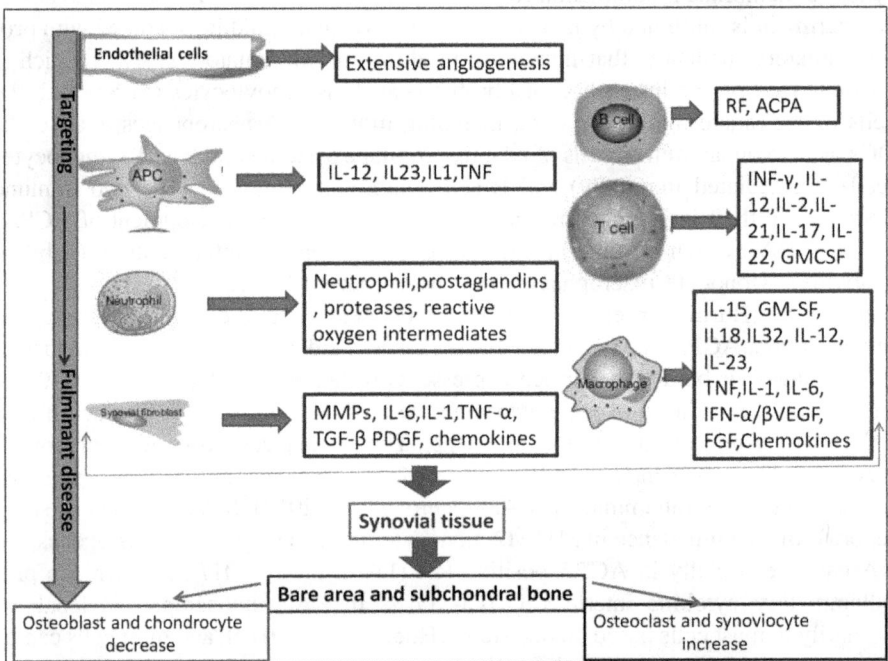

FIGURE 13.3 Role of different inflammatory mediators in the development of RA (IL, interleukin; TNF, tumor necrosis factor; MMP, matrix metalloproteinase; TGF, transforming growth factor; PDGF, platelet-derived growth factor; IFN, interferon; GM-CSF, granulocyte–macrophage colony-stimulating factor; VEGF, vascular endothelial growth factor; FGF, fibroblast growth factor).

immune system and along with adaptive immune systems like T-cells and B-cells. Endothelial cells play a role and contribute to the extensive angiogenesis. The fulminant stage comprises of hyperplastic synovium, bone erosion, cartilage damage and systemic consequences. Bone resorption virtually creates bone erosions which are usually found at spots where the synovial membrane inserts into the periosteum and is known as a bare area according to its anatomical features. The destruction of the subchondral bone can eventually result in the degeneration of the articular cartilage as the result of a decrease in osteoblasts and an increase in osteoclasts and synoviocytes into the periosteum.

13.4.1.4 Fulminant Stage

Hyperplastic synovium is characterized by a mixture of bone marrow-derivedmacrophages and specialized FLSs (Edwards, 1994). Synovial cells maintain the steady state of the joint by secreting hyaluronic acid and lubricin for common lubrication and function, as well as processing waste products. In RA, the dysfunction of FLS leads to hyperplastic synovium. The abnormal proliferation of FLS results from a loss of contact inhibition that plays a critical part in RA by producing inflammatory cytokines and proteinases, similar as matrix metalloproteinases (MMPs) and tissue inhibitors of metalloproteinases (TIMPs) that perpetuate joint destruction. They produce a medium that allows for the survival of T-cell and B-cell and neutrophil accumulation (Filer et al., 2006). Another cause regarding the hyperplastic synovium is probably due to the resistance to apoptosis associated with distinctive pathways. Similar pathways include abnormalities of tumor protein p53 function, which contributes to the synovial filling expansion and common destruction in RA (Aupperle et al., 1998); overexpression of heat shock protein 70 and enhanced activation of heat shock factor 1 in RA synovial tissues that foster the survival of FLS (Schett et al., 1998). The pathogenetic mouse model synoviolin/ Hrd1 triggers synovial cell outgrowth through its anti-apoptotic effects (Amano et al., 2003). It appears that synovial hyperplasia contains the proliferation of resident slow-cycling cells, similar to mesenchymal stromal/ stem cells and the infiltration of bone marrow-derived cells in lethally irradiated mice after bone marrow transplantation (Sergijenko et al., 2016). Although animal models of RA have been useful, they don't always reliably replicate the human disease phenotype, indeed less the ACPA-positive RA.

13.4.1.4.1 Cartilage Damage

Cartilage acts as a crucial element of synovial joints, consisting of chondrocytes and a thick and largely systematized extracellular matrix (ECM) synthesized by these chondrocytes and contains type II collagen and glycosaminoglycans (knaveries). The hyperplastic synovium causes major damage to the cartilage in RA through directed adhesion and invasion. Again, inflammatory signals, including those released from the ECM, can further stimulate FLS activity.

The mediators of cartilage damage include MMPs, a disintegrin-like metalloprotease with thrombospondin type 1 motifs 4 and 5 and cathepsins. MMPs are synthesized by FLS and can promote the disassembly of the type II collagen network causing biomechanical dysfunction. Membrane-type I MMP is imaged to be the predominant proteinase that degrades the collagenous cartilage matrix (Sabeh et al., 2010). Still, articular cartilage does not have enough regenerative eventually by itself. Accordingly, under the influence of synovial cytokines, particularly IL-1 and 17 A, and reactive nitrogen intermediates, the cartilage is progressively deprived of chondrocytes that undergo apoptosis (McInnes and Schett, 2011). This results in cartilage degradation demonstrable as joint space narrowing on radiography. These observation may help to explain why, RA is a site –specific manifestation of a systemic manifestation of autoimmune disease, in which early cartilage damage in context of altered immune system leads to specific cellular activation of FLS within the articular joints (Pap and Korb-Pap, 2015). Nevertheless, a better understanding of the mechanisms underlying cartilage damage is needed.

13.4.1.4.2   Bone Erosion

Bone loss is a pathological hallmark of RA and manifests as localized, periarticular and systemic bone loss. Bone loss is the result of the induction of osteoclasts and the repression of osteoblasts. "Peri-articular" bone loss most likely refers to cellular changes of the subchondral bone marrow, such as osteoclast differentiation and the formation of inflammatory infiltrates. It remains controversial whether inflammation or autoimmunity is a key driver for bone damage evidence for the traditional inflammatory theory is as follows tumor necrosis factor-alpha (TNF-α), IL-6, IL-1β, IL-17, and other inflammatory cytokines involved in RA could polypro-osteoclastogenic effects and suppress bone formation in the appropriate environment via adequate signals, similar as the receptor activator of nuclear factor kappa-B ligand (RANKL) and macrophage colony-stimulating factor (M- CSF) (Okamoto et al., 2017). These promote the influx and differentiation of the monocytes into osteoclasts in the context of inflammation (Pettit et al., 2006), while anti-inflammation curatives for RA arrest the progression of bone damage and vice versa.

The second possible pathway for bone loss in RA involves two mechanisms for autoimmunity that act as a trigger for structural bone damage. The first medium pertains to the formation of immune complex and Fc- receptor-intermediated osteoclast isolation. The second is the formation of anti-citrullinated vimentin antibodies against the most citrullinated protein, making osteoclasts the ideal antigenic targets for anti-citrullinated protein antibodies (ACPA). It is reported that ACPA list to osteoclast precursors induces osteoclastogenesis, bone resorption, and bone loss (Harre et al., 2012). Bone resorption virtually creates a hole, which is generally found at spot where the synovial membrane inserts into the periosteum, which is known as a bare area according to certain anatomical features. Subchondral bone plays a vital part in maintaining the homeostasis of weight-bearing joints, and the destruction of the subchondral bone can eventually affect the degeneration of the articular cartilage. In the early stages of RA, bone marrow edema is a common finding at the spot of subchondral bone in humans (Borrero et al., 2011), and aberrant transforming growth factor- β (TGF- β) in the subchondral bone is involved at the onset of RA common destruction in animal models (Xu et al., 2015).

13.4.2 SYSTEMIC CONSEQUENCES

Multiple studies have documented an elevated risk of cardiovascular events in RA patients (Arts et al., 2017). The mechanisms responsible for this risk may be related to cytokines that increase endothelial activation and potentially make atheromatous plaques unstable. Patients with active untreated RA have reduced total cholesterol, low-density and high-density cholesterol. (Myasoedova et al., 2010). RA also influences the brain by causing fatigue and reduced cognitive function; the lungs by causing inflammatory and fibrotic disease; the exocrine glands by causing secondary Sjogren's syndrome; the skeletal muscles by causing sarcopenia; and the bones by causing osteoporosis. Finally, RA patients may be at greater risk of cancer, especially hematologic and renal cancers (Chen et al., 2011). Abnormal values of the laboratory tests are the most typical features of RA. Erythrocyte sedimentation rate (ESR) and C-reactive protein (CRP) give information about the acute phase response. The position of CRP was shown to be correlated with the severity of the disease as well as radiographic changes (Grassi et al., 1998).

Autoantibodies such to RF, and anti-CCP are very helpful for the diagnosis of RA. Anti-CCP antibodies demonstrated a comparable sensitivity but a greater specificity than RF for the opinion of RA (Heidari et al., 2009). The combination of anti-CCP and RF increases diagnostic specificity for RA. The level of serum anti-CCP can be also helpful in predicting subsequent progression of UA to RA with high accuracy (Heidari et al., 2009). Anti-CCP exerts additional diagnostic ability in recognising seronegative RA (Quinn et al., 2006). Arthrocynthesis and synovial fluid analysis can be also helpful for diagnosing inflammatory arthritis as well as in differentiating inflammatory from non-inflammatory arthritis. Assessment of synovial fluid anti-CCP may be diagnostic individual in feting RA from non-RA arthritis. The diagnostic performance of synovial fluid anti-CCP was shown in a cross-sectional study. In this study, the identification of anti-CCP in the synovial fluid of cases with arthritis demonstrated high discriminative ability in recognizing RA from non-RA condition (Heidari et al., 2009). Acute phase reactants, similar to ESR and CRP are important tools for both evidence and inflexibility of inflammation in cases with arthritis. Increased levels of these inflammatory markers suggest higher disease activity. These tests may be also helpful in the evaluation of treatment efficacy. The situations of acute phase reactants drop in correlation with the effectiveness of treatment as reflected by a drop in DAS value (Heidari et al., 2007).

13.5 IMAGING

Radiographic signs of RA such as joint space narrowing, erosions and subluxation develop at a later stage of the RA process. Plain radiography is the standard method of investigating the extent of anatomic changes in RA patients there is few data regarding the value of conventional radiographic examination in recent-onset arthritis. Synovitis is the early finding of RA and is a strong predictor of bone erosion. Soft tissue swelling and mild juxta-articular osteoporosis may be the inital radiographic features of hand joints in early RA (Grassi et al., 1998). These findings are representative of synovitis but can not be shown on conventional radiographs in all patients and are not precise enough, and so are unreliable in the regular assessment of synovitis (Farrant et al., 2007). In particular, due to later occurence of radiographic changes, plain radiography is too insensitve for the discovery of bone erosion, which is a characteristic for the diagnosis of RA (Devauchelle-Pensec et al., 2002). In a study of very recent onset arthritis with symptom duration < 3 months, radiographic bone erosions were observed in 12.8% of initial radiographs compared with 27.6% after one year (Machold et al., 2002). In contrast, sonography and MRI are more sensitive and seem promising but can be used in limited centers. Sonography is a reliable technique to detect further erosion than radiography, especially in early RA (Wakefield et al., 2000). The senstivity of conventional radiography in the discovery of bone erosion in one study was 13%, whereas, the senstivity of MRI and sonography in the detection of bone erosion were 98% and 63% respectively (Rahmani et al., 2010). For these reasons, there is a trend toward early discovery of RA bone erosion by MRI especially in cases with early signs of arthritis. The presence of common erosion in undifferentiated arthritis (UdA) cases may be reflective of progression to RA. In a study by Tamai et al., 2009, patients with at least two MRI proven for symmetric synovitis or bone edema and/ or bone erosion progressed to RA at one year with a 79.7% positive predictive value and 75.9% specificity, 68% sensitivity. In early RA, sonography can detect lesser amounts of erosion and in a lesser number of patients than can radiography (Graudal, 2004). The introduction of MRI imaging provides more diagnostic facilities in early diagnosis of RA; and early differentiation of RA from non-RA disease. MRI findings may detect additional patients with true RA compared with ACR diagnostic criteria. In addition, MRI is more sensitive than clinical examination to detect synovitis of hands and wrists in RA (Goupille et al., 2001) (Table 13.1).

The goals of treatment for RA are to reduce joint inflammation and pain, maximize joint function, and prevent joint destruction and deformity. Treatment regimens consist of combinations of pharmaceuticals, weight-bearing exercise, educating patients about the disease, and rest.

13.6   DISEASE MODIFYING ANTIRHEUMATIC DRUGS (DMARDS)

These are a group of medicines, which commonly prescribed for patients of rheumatoid arthritis and have proven their efficacy to control joint destruction. These are broadly classified into three categories, such a, Conventional synthetic DMARDs (cs DMARDs) a relatively long onset of action, while faster actings are biological DMARDs (bDMARDs), and targeted synthetic DMARDs (tsDMARDs) (Grosser et al., 2022) (Table 13.2).

13.7   DRUGS FOR SYMPTOMATIC TREATMENT

13.7.1   First-Line Management: NSAIDs and Corticosteroids

The overall thing of first-line treatment is to relieve pain and reduce inflammation. Medications, considered to be fast- acting, are Nonsteroidal Anti-Inflammatory

TABLE 13.1

2010 American College of Rheumatology (ACR)/European League Against Rheumatism (ELAR) Classification Criteria for Rheumatoid Arthritis

Domains	Description	Number of Joints	Score
Joint involvement (Tender/ Swollen).	**Median Large Joint:** *e.g.* Shoulder, Elbow, Knee, and Ankle joints.	1 Large joint	0
	Other Joints: temporomaibular, acromioclavicular, sternoclavicular, *etc.*	2-10 Large joints	1
	Small Joints: *e.g., Metacarpophalangeal, Proximal interphalangeal,* 2nd–5th Metatarsophalangeal, Thumb interphalangeal, and Wrist joints	1-3 Small joints (± Large joints)	2
		4-10 Small joints (± Large joints)	3
		>10 joints (At least one small joint)	5
Duration of synovitis	<6 weeks		0
	≥6 weeks		1
Serology	No positive for either RF or anti-CCP		0
	At least one of these test positive at low titer		2
	At least one of these test positive at high titer		3
Acute Phase Reactant	Neither CRP nor ESR is abnormal		0
	Abnormal CRP or ESR		1

Score ≥ 6 Indicates Rhematoid Arthritis

Distal interphalangeal 1st carpometacarpal and 1st tarsometatarsal joints are excluded from assessment.

TABLE 13.2
Disease-Modifying Antirheumatic Drugs (DMARDs)

S.No.	Drug	Class or Action
1	Small Molecules	**Methotrexate** - Antifolate,
		Leflunomide - Pyrimidine synthase inhibitor,
		Hydroxychloroquine - Antimalarial,
		Minocycline - 5-Lipoxygenase inhibitor,
		Sulfasalazine - Salicylate,
		Azathioprine - Purine synthase inhibitor,
		Cyclosporine - Calcineurin inhibitor,
		Cyclophosphamide - Alkylating agent,
		Penicillamine -Chelating agent,
		Auranofin - Gold compound
2	Biologicals	**Adalimumab, Golimumab, Etanercept** - TNFα antagonist,
		Infliximab - IgGTNF receptor fusion protein (antiTNF),
		Certolizumab - Fab fragment toward TNFα,
		Abatacept - Tcell costimulation inhibitor (binds B7 protein on antigen-presenting cell),
		Rituximab - Ab toward CD20 (cytotoxic toward B cells),
		Anakinra - IL1 receptor antagonist,
		Tocilizumab - IL6 receptor antagonist,
		Tofacitinib - Janus kinase inhibitor

Drugs (NSAIDs) including acetyl-salicylate (Aspirin), Naproxen, Ibuprofen, and Etodolac. Aspirin is an effective anti-inflammatory for RA when used at high doses, due to the inhibition of prostaglandins. It is one of the oldest NSAIDs used for common pain. Side effects of aspirin at high doses include tinnitus, hair loss, and gastric intolerance. There are also other NSAIDs that are newer on the market than aspirin, and equally effective in alleviating pain. In addition, these drugs require few doses per day. NSAIDs work by inhibiting cyclo-oxygenase to inhibit the synthesis of prostaglandins, prostacyclin, and thromboxanes. Common side effects are nausea, abdominal pain, stomach ulcers, and gastrointestinal (GI) bleeding. These symptoms can be reduced if taken with food, antacids, proton pump inhibitors, or misoprostol. An indeed newer NSAID called celecoxib is a selective Cox-2 inhibitor that has lower risk of GI side effects (Ong et al., 2007).

Corticosteroids are a more potent anti-inflammatory drug than NSAIDs, but they come with fewer side effects. For this reason, they are only indicated for a short time at low doses, during exacerbations or flares of RA. Intra-articular injections of corticosteroids can be used for the local symptoms of inflammation (Combe et al., 2017). They work by preventing the release of phospholipids and decreasing the actions of eosinophils, thereby reducing inflammation. Their side effects include osteoporosis, weight gain, diabetes, and immunosuppression. Advising the patients to take calcium and vitamin D supplementation can protect them from the thinning of the bone. The side effects can be reduced by gradationally tapering doses as the condition improves. It is important to not suddenly discontinue injectables or oral corticosteroids as this can lead to suppression of the hypothalamic-pituitary-adrenal axis (HPA) or flares of RA (Liu et al., 2013).

13.7.2 OPIOID ANALGESICS

Whittle et al., (2012), addressed the question of the use of opioid analgesics for patients with pain due to RA and concluded that weak opioids are similar to codeine, dextropropoxyphene, and tramadol may play an effective role in the short-term relief of pain, but their adverse effects are overweigh the benefits. They recommend that other analgesics be considered as the first therapy to control intermittent painful episodes (Richards et al., 2012).

13.7.3 STEROIDS

Administration of steroids in combination with DMARDs or with biological therapies in early RA can induce an advanced rate of remission, control of radiological progression compared with DMARD alone. This authority provides better outgrowth and should be considered in all patients (Combe, 2009; Sizova, 2008). Systemic glucocorticoids are also effective in the short-term relief of pain and swelling, and thus, may be considered for these purposes but substantially as a temporary therapy (Combe, 2007). In addition, the combination of steroids with DMARDs therapy exerts a better effect on bone corrosion. Glucocorticoids (GCs) in RA give the advantage of a rapid onset of action, which prolongs the onset of csDMARDs efficacy, also, if GCs are substantially extensively used whenever clinicians need rapid relief for their patients with RA, their side effects must be kept into consideration still, the benefit/ risk ratio of GCs remains precarious and their modalities of use in RA remain controversial.

In this review, the latest European and US recommendations on GCs use in RA and use of GCs in current practice are discussed.

13.8 INTERNATIONAL RECOMMENDATIONS

13.8.1 EUROPEAN RECOMMENDATIONS

Recent updates of the European recommendations for the management of early arthritis and RA (Combe et al., 2017; Daien et al., 2017; Smolen et al., 2017) placed a lesser focus on the benefit of GCs remedy than the former performances. Short-term GCs therapy should now be considered as part of the initial treatment strategy, and later if the initial strategy has failed, as a bridging remedy if a change in a csDMARD is considered. GCs should be tapered as rapidly as is clinically feasible, long-term use of GCs should be avoided, GCs should be gradually reduced and stopped, generally within three months and only exceptionally by six months (Smolen et al., 2017). The term "low-cure" GCs was replaced by "short-term" GCs to take into account several current ways of using GCs, similar to parenteral bolus (Smolen et al., 2017).

13.8.2 US RECOMMENDATIONS

The 2015 American College of Rheumatology (ACR) guidelines for early and, established RA recommend adding GCs to DMARDs during disease flares, at the lowest dose and for the shortest period possible (Singh et al., 2016). In contrast with the European recommendations, adding GCs when a csDMARD is initiated depends on disease activity.

Taken together, these international recommendations agree on the use of GCs for disease flare and at the start of new csDMARD. Specific advice concerning dosage, duration, route of administration and strategies is limited and less consensual because reliable and detailed evidence is scarce.

For US recommendations, a dose <10 mg/ day is considered a low dose, and GCs should be tapered in less than three months, whereas for European recommendations, the threshold is 7.5 mg/ day, and GCs could be specified in combination with csDMARDs for over to six months outside, knowing that this duration is expert-driven (Gaujoux-Viala and Gossec, 2014). Despite these differences, international guidelines underline the importance of GCs but also advocate the use of GCs at the lowest accumulation dose possible because of the high awareness of potentially associated adverse effects.

In these sets of recommendations as well as in this review, GCs dosages are expressed in prednisone equivalent.

In contrast to the 2015 guideline (Singh et al., 2016), recommendations were not provided for subgroups defined by early versus late RA disease duration. This change was made because current disease activity, prior therapies used, and the presence of comorbidities were felt to be more relevant than disease duration for most treatment decisions. However, early diagnosis and treatment of RA are associated with improved outcomes and are thus an important overarching principle in its management (Burgers et al., 2019). Recommendations are intended for the general RA patient population and assume that patients do not have contra-indications to the options under consideration.

13.9 AMERICAN COLLEGE OF RHEUMATOLOGY GUIDELINE FOR THE TREATMENT OF RHEUMATOID ARTHRITIS 2021

Several guiding principles, definitions, and assumptions were established. Because poor prognostic factors (Albrecht and Zink, 2017) have had less impact than other factors on prior RA treatment recommendations. However, poor prognostic factors were considered as possible influential factors in physicians, and, on decision-making for the management of RA patients when developing recommendations.

TABLE 13.3

Disease-Modifying Antirheumatic Drugs (DMARDs) Initiation*

Recommendations	Certainty of evidence
• Initiation of treatment in DMARD-naive	
• Patients with moderate-to-high disease activity	
• Methotrexate monotherapy is **strongly** recommended over:	
Hydroxychloroquine or sulfasalazine, bDMARD or tsDMARD	Very low/low
monotherapy, Combination of methotrexate plus a non–TNF,	Very low/moderate
inhibitor bDMARD or tsDMARD	Low/very low
• Methotrexate monotherapy is **conditionally** recommended over:	
Leflunomide	Low
Dual or triple csDMARD therapy	Moderate
Combination of methotrexate plus a TNF inhibitornitiation of a	Low
csDMARD without short-term (<3 months) glucocorticoids is	Very low
conditionally recommended over initiation of a csDMARD with	
short-term glucocorticoids.	
Initiation of a csDMARD without longer-term (≥3 months) glucocorticoids	Moderate
is **strongly** recommended over initiation of a csDMARD with longer-term	
glucocorticoids	
• Initiation of treatment in DMARD-naive patients with low disease	
activity Hydroxychloroquine is **conditionally** recommended over other	
csDMARDs.	
Sulfasalazine is **conditionally** recommended over methotrexate.	Very low
Methotrexate is **conditionally** recommended over leflunomide.	Very low
Initiation of treatment in csDMARD-treated, but methotrexate-naive,	Very low
patients with moderate-to-High disease activity	
• Methotrexate monotherapy is **conditionally** recommended over the	Moderate/ Very low
combination of methotrexate plus a bDMARD or tsDMARD.**	

** The certainty of evidence is high for the combination of Methotrexate plus a TNF inhibitor and moderate for other bDMARDs

The Guiding Principles (Fraenkel et al. 2021) (Table 13.3)

- RA requires early evaluation, diagnosis, and management.
  - Treatment decisions should follow a shared decision-making process.
  - Treatment decisions should be reevaluated within a minimum of three months based on the efficacy and tolerability of the DMARD(s) chosen.
- Disease activity levels refer to those calculated using RA disease activity measures endorsed by the ACR-10.
- Recommendations are intended for the general RA patient population and assume that patients do not have contraindications to the options under consideration.

- Recommendations are limited to DMARDs approved by the US FDA for treatment of RA. *Such as,*
  - **csDMARDs:** Hydroxychloroquine, Sulfasalazine, Methotrexate, Leflunomide
  - **bDMARDs:** TNF inhibitors (etanercept, adalimumab, infliximab, golimumab, certolizumab pegol), T cell costimulatory inhibitor (abatacept), IL-6 receptor inhibitors (tocilizumab, sarilumab), anti-CD20 antibody (rituximab)† tsDMARDs: JAK inhibitors (tofacitinib, baricitinib, upadacitinib) (Anakinra was not included due to infrequent use for patients with RA).
  - **Triple therapy** refers to hydroxychloroquine, sulfasalazine, and either methotrexate or leflunomide.
- Serious infection refers to an infection requiring intravenous antibiotics or hospitalization.
  - Biosimilars are considered equivalent to FDA-approved Originator bDMARDs.
- Recommendations referring to bDMARDs exclude rituximab unless patients have had an inadequate response to TNF inhibitors (in order to be consistent with FDA approval) or have a history of lymphoproliferative disorder for which rituximab is an approved therapy.
- Treat-to-target refers to a systematic approach involving frequent monitoring of disease activity using validated instruments and modification of treatment to minimize disease activity with the goal of reaching a predefined target (low disease activity or remission).
- Target refers to low disease activity or remission.
- Recommendations specify that patients be at target (low disease activity or remission) for at least six months prior to tapering.
- Dose reduction refers to lowering the dose or increasing the dosing interval of a DMARD. Gradual discontinuation of a DMARD is defined as gradually lowering the dose of a DMARD and subsequently stopping it.

13.10 RECOMMENDATIONS FOR DMARD-NAÏVE PATIENTS WITH MODERATE-TO-HIGH DISEASE ACTIVITY

13.11 CURRENT PRACTICE

A recent study of an Australian cohort of patients with RA showed that the probability of GCs use throughout follow-up has decreased over time, from 55% in 2001 to 39% in 2012(p<0.001) (Black et al., 2017). In this cohort, current csDMARD use but not bDMARD use was associated with increased current GCs use. In a recent analysis considering the times from 1980 up to 2004, the reduction of an initial low dose, for long-term GCs remedy in RA, was set from 10.3 mg/ day up to 3.6 mg/ day (Pincus et al., 2013). In contrast, another experimental cohort study showed that the proportion of patients initiating GCs was higher in the group from 1995 to 2007 compared with the earlier group from 1980 to 1994 (68% vs

36%) but the cumulative dose didn't differ over the first time (Makol et al., 2014). GCs are still extensively used in RA. GCs appear to be used in approximately 50% of patients with RA, (Sokka et al., 2007) with varied duration and dosage among the studies. In the German CAPEA cohort of cases with early arthritis, 82% received Methotrexate (MTX) within the first months, 77% received GCs and 20% of these entered <75mg/d prednisone but $1/3^{rd}$ received> 20 mg/ day(Albrecht et al., 2015). After two years of follow-up, 12% of the patients received biologics, 52% were free of GCs and 41 were receiving < 5 mg/ day. In the French ESPOIR cohort of cases with early arthritis, 45% started GCs during the first six months and further than 50%received GCs at least once over 5 years after inclusion (Combe and Rincheval, 2015). Overall, the cure of GCs entered during follow-up was veritably low, the mean was 3.1 ± 2.9 mg/ day (Roubille et al., 2017). In the Canadian CATCH cohort of cases with RA, 42%were considered GCs users and the median oral daily dose was 5 mg(IQR2.5–10) (McKeown et al., 2012).

13.12   GLUCOCORTICOIDS EFFICACY

13.12.1   CLINICAL EFFICACY

For reasons of brevity only the most relevant and recent data on the clinical efficacy of GCs in RA published during the last six years (Table 13.4).

Disease Activity Score in 28 joints (DAS28) remission at 16 weeks was more frequently achieved with than without GCs, although not significantly (65 vs 47, p = 0.08). According to data at 1 and 2 years, the rates of remission were still advanced in the MTX GCs than MTX-only arm but showed non-significant differences in long-term effects of the disease as bony erosions and disease progression.

There are majority of studies suggest additional glucocorticoid therapy has shown beneficial effects at the time of aggravation or active episodes of Rheumatoid Arthritis in the long term. The available data primarily relate to GCs in addition to csDMARDs and not, or not specifically, to bDMARDs or tsDMARDs. also, the current literature concern mainly patients with early arthritis, and studies reporting on GCs efficacy in patients with established RA are clearly less frequent A study by (Buttgereit et al., 2013; Alten et al., 2015) in **CAPRA-2** trail, which was conducted in patients with an established Rheumatoid arthritis who had a disease duration of eight years were prescribed with a low dose (5 mg/kg) of prednisone along with one of the conventional DMARDs compared with placebo shown significant improvement in disease by 12 weeks of duration.

Similarly, another trial of **CareRA trial** by (Verschueren et al., 2015) found effects of Methotrexate with and without glucocorticoids therapy by randomization studies in two different arms, and on the basis of Disease Activity Score in 28 joints (DAS28) found rate of remission was higher in the MTX+GCs i.e. (30 mg/day prednisone decreased to 5 mg/ day in six weeks) than MTX-only arm although not significant. (Verschueren et al., 2017) (Table 13.5).

TABLE 13.4

Characteristics of Studies of the Clinical Efficacy of Glucocorticoids Published in the Last Six Years

Characteristics of studies of the clinical efficacy of glucocorticoids (Recent publication <6 years)

Study	Disease duration	Intervention	Period of evaluation	Outcomes	Results
Buttgereit et al (CAPRA-2)	Mean 8 years	MR prednisone (5 mg/day) (Gp 1) or PBO (Gp 2)+existing DMARDs	12 weeks	ACR 20	Gp 1: 48% Gp 2: 29%
Ajeganova et al (BARFOT at 10 years)	≤1 year	Initial groups of randomization: csDMARDs with (Gp 1) or w/o (Gp 2) GCs (7.5 mg/day)	10 years	Use of bDMARD	Gp 1: 15% Gp 2: 15%
Safy et al (CAMERA-II follow-up)	≤1 year	Initial groups of randomization: GCs (10 mg/day) (Gp 1) or PBO (Gp 2)+MTX	Median 6.6 years	Initiation of first bDMARD	Gp 1: 31% Gp 2: 50%*
Markusse et al (BeSt at 10 years)	≤2 years	Initial groups of randomization: MTX then substituted with csDMARDs (Gp 1) or MTX then addition of csDMARDs (Gp 2) or COBRA scheme=MTX+ SSZ+GCs (60 mg/day to 7.5 mg/day in 6 weeks) (Gp 3) or MTX+IFX (Gp 4)	10 years	DAS44 <1.6	Approx. 50% in each Gp
Verschueren et al (CareRA)	≤1 year	csDMARDs with (Gp 1) or w/o (Gp 2) GCs (30 mg/day to 5 mg/day in 6 weeks)	16 weeks	DAS28-CRP< 2.6	Gp 1: 65% Gp 2: 47%
Verschueren et al (CareRA at 1 year)	≤1 year	csDMARDs with (Gp 1) or w/o (Gp 2) GCs (30 mg/days to 5 mg/day in 6 weeks)	1 year	DAS28-CRP< 2.6	Gp 1: 67% Gp 2: 57%

TABLE 13.5

Modern Pharmacologic Therapies for Rheumatoid Arthritis

S. No.	Classification	Name	Mechanism of Action	Potential Mechanisms	Side Effect
A	Conventional synthetic DMARDs	Methotrexate	Analog of folic acid	Folate-dependent processes; Adenosine signaling; Methyl-donor production; Reactive oxygen species; Adhesion-molecule expression; Cytokine profiles Eicosanoids and MMPs.	Increased liver enzymes, pulmonary Damage (Brown et al., 2016)
		Leflunomide/ Teriflunomide	Pyrimidine synthesis inhibitor	DHODH-dependent pathway; Leukocyte adhesion; Rapidly dividing cells; NF-kB; Kinases; Interleukins; TGF-β.	Hypertension, diarrhea and nausea, Hepatotoxicity (Kasarello et al., 2017)
		Sulfasalazine	Anti-inflammatory and immunosuppression	Cyclooxygenase and PGE2; Leukotriene production and chemotaxis; Inflammatory cytokines (IL-1, IL-6, TNF-α); Adenosine signaling; NF-kB activation.	Gastrointestinal, central nervous system, and hematologic adverse effect. (Linares et al., 2011)
		Chloroquine /Hydroxychloroquine	Immunomodulatory effects	Toll-like receptors; Lysosomotropic action; Monocyte-derived proinflammatory cytokines; Antiinflammatory effects; Cellular immune reactions; T cell responses; Neutrophils; Cartilage metabolism and degradation.	Gastrointestinal tract, skin, central nervous system adverse effect and retinal toxicity. (Rainsford et al., 2015)

(Continued)

TABLE 13.5 (Continued)
Modern Pharmacologic Therapies for Rheumatoid Arthritis

S. No.	Classification	Name	Mechanism of Action	Potential Mechanisms	Side Effect
B (i)	**Biological DMARDs** **(b DMARDs)** Antibody-based therapies, TNF-α targeted Therapy	Infliximab Adalimumab Etanercept Golimumab Certolizumab pegol	TNF-α inhibitor	Phagocytosis and pro-inflammatory cytokines; Chemoattractant; Adhesion molecules and chemokines; Treg cell function; Function of osteoclasts, leukocytes, endothelial and synovial fibroblasts.	Infection (pneumonia and atypical tuberculosis) injection-site reaction Hypertension. Severe/anaphylactoid transfusion reaction. (Kim E Y and Moudgil K D, 2017)
(ii)	B-cell targeted Therapy	Rituximab Ofatumumab Belimumab Atacicept Tabalumab	B cell depleting Inhibitors of B cell function	Fc receptor gamma-mediated antibody-dependent cytotoxicity and phagocytosis; Complementmediated cell lysis; antigen presentation; B cell apoptosis; Depletion of CD4+ T cells.	Infection, hypertension, hypogammaglobulinemia, viral reactivation, vaccination responses. Late-onset neutropenia Severe/ anaphylactoid transfusion reaction. (Mota et al., 2017)
(iii)	T-cell targeted therapy	Abatacept Belatacept	CD28/CTLA4 system CD80/CD86	Autoantigen recognition; Immune cell infiltrate; T cells activation.	Infection, malignancy. (Mellado et al., 2015)
(iv)	Interleukin targeted therapy	Tocilizumab	IL-6 inhibition	Innate and the adaptive immune system perturbation; Acute-phase proteins	Infections (most notably skin and soft tissue), increases in serum cholesterol, transient decreases in neutrophil count and abnormal liver function. (Raimondo M G et al., 2017)

		Drug	Target	Function	Side effects / References
		Anakinra, Canakinumab, Rilonacept	IL-1 inhibition	Inflammatory responses; Matrixenzyme	Injection site reactions, infections, neutropenia, malignancy. (Cavalli and Dinarello, 2015)
		Secukinumab, Ixekizumab	IL-17 inhibition	Mitochondrial function; Autophagosome formation.	Infections, nasopharyngitis, candidiasis, neutropenia, safety data of mental health is limited. (Kim E K et al., 2017)
(v)	Growth and differentiation factors	Denosumab	RANKL inhibitor	Maturation and activation of osteoclast	Low Ca2+ and phosphate in the blood, muscle cramps, cellulitis, and numbness (Fassio A et al., 2017)
		Mavrilimumab	GM-CSF inhibitor	Activation, differentiation, and survival of macrophages, dendritic cells, and neutrophils; T helper 1/ 17 cell; modulation of pain pathways.	Safety file needs further research. (Burmester et al., 2017)
(vi)	Small molecules JAK pathway	Tofacitinib, Baricitinib, Filgotinib	JAK1 and JAK3 Inhibitor; JAK1 and JAK2 Inhibitor; JAKinhibitor	T-cell activation, pro-inflammatory cytokine production, synovial inflammation, and structural joint damage	Zoster infection (advice is to vaccinate beforehand) and other potential side-effects should be monitored carefully through further study (Yamaoka, 2016; Winthrop et al. 2017)
(vii)	Future drug and target	Toll like receptors; (Elshabrawy et al., 2017) Bruton's tyrosine kinase; (Whang and Chang, 2014) Phosphoinositide-3-kinasepathway; (Bartok et al., 2014) Transforming growth factor-beta; (Fechtner S et al.,2017) Neuropathways; (Cheung and McInnes, 2017) Dendritic cell (Benham et al., 2015)			

13.13   MODERN PHARMACOLOGIC THERAPIES FOR RHEUMATOID ARTHRITIS

The identification of a preclinical stage and a growing understanding of the natural history and mechanisms of RA development, alongside new potential therapeutic intervention, shape the prospect that RA might be prevented in the future (Deane, 2013). The current treatment principles for established RA involve symptomatic management and disease modification. A meta-analysis of 12 published studies confirmed that patients receiving delayed DMARDs therapy were at higher risk of developing radiographic joint space narrowing and bony erosions (Finckh et al., 2006).

In poorly controlled RA patients, bony erosion becomes evident on radiographs within two years of onset and these erosive changes are predictive of poor functional out come (Fuchs et al., 1989). In a patient with otherwise unexplained new-onset polyarthritis, an urgent referral to a rheumatologist is thus mandatory to confirm an RA diagnosis and early intiation of a DMARDs-based treatment plan aiming for disease remission with prevention of deformity. Oral corticosteroids are potent and effective anti-inflammatory drugs that may contribute to disease modification (Cohen and Emery, 2010).

However, this needs to be weighed up against its well-known adverse effects. Symptomatic management remains important throughout the disease progression and consists of everyday practical measures to deal with the primary symptoms of joint stiffness, similar to pain and fatigue. Exercise is important to support joint flexibility and function, while abstaining from smoking is a universal advice to all RA cases given its impact on antibody structure.

13.14   CONVENTIONAL SYNTHETIC DMARDS (CSDMARDS)

13.14.1   METHOTREXATE

MTX is a modified form of folate designed to have an increased affinity for dihydrofolate reductase (DHFR) compared with its parent molecule. MTX is the cornerstone in the treatment of RA either as a single agent or in combination with other DMARDs (Sanmarti et al., 2015). In a recent meta-analysis, MTX showed a substantial clinical and statistically significant benefit compared to a placebo in the short-term treatment of people with RA, although its use was associated with a 16% discontinuation rate due to adverse effects (Lopez-Olivo et al., 2012). Also, radiographic progression rates measured by an increase in erosions scores of more than three units were statistically significantly lower for patients in the MTX group (Rezaei et al., 2013). MTX has been proposed to share in the process of folate antagonism, adenosine signaling, the blocking of methyl-donor products involved in reactive oxygen species, downregulation of the adhesion molecule expression, modification of cytokine biographies, and the downregulation of eicosanoids and MMPs (Brown et al., 2016). Single nucleotide polymorphisms (SNP) analysis and genome-wide association studies (GWAS) have set up some SNPs related to MTX responsiveness.

For example, those located in the gamma-glutamyl hydrolase (GGH), 5-aminoimidazole-4-carboxamide (ATIC), and solute carrier molecule 19 member 1 (SLC19A1) genes (Owen et al., 2013). Nevertheless, the results from the studies are conflicting, and sufficiently large genomic studies are needed to further develop the understanding.

MTX for RA is administered as a low-dose (5–25 mg) weekly regimen with dosing conditional to the complaint state and side effects. Oral MTX has a more variable uptake than subcutaneous administration, which also leads to fewer significant side effects.

Subcutaneous MTX administration also demonstrated a greater bioavailability compared with oral MTX (Schiff, and Sadowski, 2017). It requires regular monitoring to optimize dosing and assess its immunosuppressive and hepatotoxic effects through frequent blood tests (monthly, initially). There are few well-established drug interactions including cotrimoxazole, which causes pancytopenia, combined with azathioprine or leflunomide, which causes liver and lung complications. NSAIDs can be safely used in conjunction with MTX for symptom control after over 30 years of routine use of the two agents. It is inconclusive that MTX enhances the risk of malignancy beyond the increased relative risk of neoplasia associated with RA per se (Lopez-Olivo et al., 2012). Despite this, the absolute risk is low. Adverse effects associated with the use of MTX also include the development of accelerated nodulosis, also known as MTX-induced accelerated nodulosis(MIAN), which occurs in (1–10) of patients on MTX (Maashari and Hamodat, 2016). However, most adverse effects can be reversed by supplementation with calcium or sodium folinate (Brown et al., 2016).

13.14.2 LEFLUNOMIDE

Leflunomide reduces inflammation in the joints of RA patients by inhibiting dihydroorotate enzymes essential for producing DNA and RNA, particularly in activated proliferation lymphocytes. At higher doses, the active metabolite teriflunomide also inhibits tyrosine kinases responsible for early T-cell and B-cell signaling (Herrmann, 2000).

Due to its different mechanism of action, Leflunomide is a valuable addition to the armamentarium of drug treatment for RA and is specified at a routine starting dose of 10 mg daily for the initial three days followed by 20 mg daily. Leflunomide has shown clinical, functional, and structural efficacy analogous to MTX (Smolen et al., 2014; Strand, et al., 1999); and has also been used effectively in combination with biological agents. Dose reduction to 10 mg daily should be considered if side effects occur, with the most common reported side effects being diarrhea, nausea, headache, rash, itching, loss of hair and body weight, hypertension, chest pain, palpitation, infection, and liver failure. It's therefore important to monitor gastrointestinal symptoms, allergic responses, alopecia, and liver function (Kalden et al., 2003; Schiff et al., 2000). There are many well-proven drug interactions, including cholestyramine that impairs the absorption of Leflunomide, rifampin side effects causing raised Leflunomide levels in the blood, and

Leflunomide infrequently increasing the anticoagulant effect of warfarin. Leflunomide showed deleterious effects on developing fetuses and suckling babies and thus should be avoided during gestation and lactation (Janssen and Genta, 2000; Schuna, 1998).

13.14.3 SULFASALAZINE (SSZ)

Owing to clinical trials, SSZ has been extensively available as a therapeutic agent for RA because of its anti-inflammatory and antimicrobial activities. SSZ has significant efficacy in reducing active joint counts and slowing radiographic progression, which is comparable to the effects of Leflunomide (Plosker, and Croom, 2005; Smolen et al., 1999). Its metabolites are sulfapyridine and 5-aminosalicylic acid (5-ASA). SSZ has the ability to increase the production of adenosine at the site of inflammation; inhibit osteoclast formation via modulatory effects on the receptor activator of nuclear factor κβ (RANK), osteoprotegerin, and RANKL inhibit TNF- α expression via the apoptosis of macrophages, (Rodenburg et al., 2000) and suppress B-cell function (Hirohata et al., 2002). Sulfapyridine may reduce IL-8 and monocyte chemotactic protein 1 (MCP- 1) secretion in inflammatory cytokines (Volin et al., 2002). The common adverse effects of SSZ include gastrointestinal and central nervous system toxicity, rash, liver function abnormalities, leukopenia and agranulocytosis, megaloblastic anemia, oligospermia, and infertility. The way to minimize the side effects is the slow initiation of drug therapy and the serial monitoring of specific laboratory tests. There are no major drug interactions reported but patients should be advised about the risk and benefit ratio with gestation (pregnancy) and breastfeeding (Ostensen, 1992).

13.14.4 HYDROXYCHLOROQUINE

In RA, hydroxychloroquine is designed to interfere with the interaction between T helper cells and antigen-presenting cells (APCs) that cause joint inflammation and decrease the production of pro-inflammatory cytokines, therefore reducing the overall inflammatory response (Sames et al., 2016). Whereas, the classical explanation is that, while hydroxychloroquine impaired phago/ lysosomal function, it also appears to work in a lysosome-independent manner by impacting intracellular TLRs, particularly TLR9, by inhibiting the product of TNF, and by interfering with the process of the conversion of the membrane-bound pro-TNF into soluable mature protein (Katz, and Russell, 2011). Hydroxychloroquine has a gradual onset action of two-to-six months, demonstrating enhancement of long-term functional outgrowth and retardation of radiographic damage (van der Heijde et al., 2000). The common adverse effects are generally gastrointestinal, dermatological, and ophthalmologic. High dose and long duration of use of hydroxychloroquine act as risk factors for retinal toxicity which may progress indeed after cessation of hydroxychloroquine. Thus, effective screening is important for early discovery of retinal toxicity (Kim et al., 2017).

13.15 BIOLOGICAL DMARDS (BDMARDS)

Although a somewhat vague description, bDMARDs are a group of drugs that target specific molecules or molecular pathways involved in RA inflammatory processes. A number of bDMARDs have been shown to have clinical and radiological efficacy in the management of RA. TNF-α-inhibiting agents were the original class of bDMARDs with newer agents targeting B lymphocyte antibodies CD- 20, IL6, and CD28 (Van Doornum et al., 2005) (Figure 13.4).

13.15.1 TNF-A INHIBITOR (TNFI)

TNF- α triggers inflammatory responses and is produced by activated monocytes, macrophages, and T lymphocytes. TNF- α acts through TNF receptors 1 and 2, which have some species specificity and different affinity with TNF- α. Through the interaction of TNFα and its receptors, key signaling pathways can be activated, similar to the NF- κB pathway, RANKL signaling, the extracellular signal-regulated kinase(ERK) signaling pathway, the tumor progression locus 2 (TPL2) pathway, and pro-apoptotic signaling. TNF- α has been proposed to mediate local bone destruction in inflammatory musculoskeletal disease due to the increased TNF- α levels in these conditions (Parameswaran and Patial, 2010). TNF has been involved

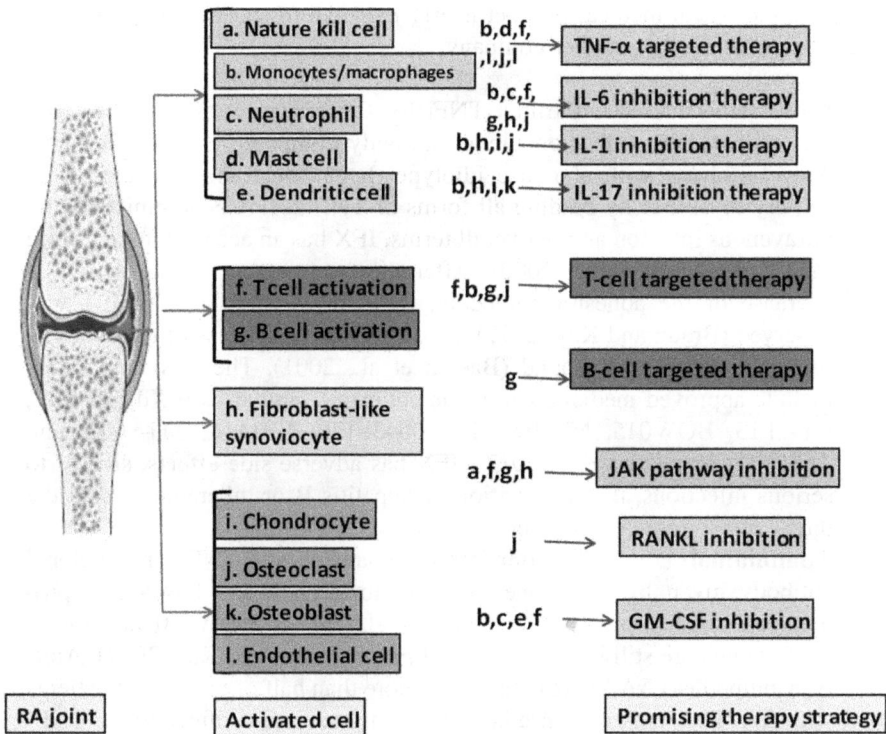

FIGURE 13.4 Cells and key receptors/pathways targeted by current therapy strategies.

in the process of endothelial cell activation, the induction of metalloproteinases and adhesion molecules, angiogenesis, and the regulation of fibroblast/keratinocyte/ enterocyte chondrocyte/osteoclast activation, as well as other inflammatory cytokines.

Current evidence implies that TNF- α antagonists may improve arterial stiffness in RA (Dulai et al., 2012). A substantial proportion of work-disabled patients with RA who start anti-TNF treatment regain work capability (Olofsson et al., 2017). Compared with patients with RA receiving DMARD therapy, TNFi can decrease the risk of myocardial infarction (Low et al., 2017). In the last 15 years, knowledge on the efficacy and toxicity of the TNFi has been published and was mainly gathered through regional or national registries created after these drugs reached the market. Based on currently available literature, TNFi has thus become the first choice of bDMARDs treatment in RA patients not responding to, or intolerant of a conventional sDMARD treatment (Smolen et al., 2014). Despite differences in biochemical and pharmacological properties of the five presently approved TNFi, there does not seem to be a clinically meaningful difference between them in terms of efficacy and safety. In a large cohort of RA patients, anti-TNF-α therapy does not increase the risk of serious bacterial infections compared with MTX treatment (Schneeweiss et al., 2007). This leaves the choice of TNFi mainly dependent on practicalities, similar to dosing frequency or mode, or on wider economical considerations. In recent years, numerous biosimilar medications have been developed, and some have formerly been approved. A biosimilar (bio-originator) refers to a biological medical product nearly identical to an original product that's frequently produced by another company.

- **Infliximab** (IFX) was the first TNFi for RA treatment and consists of a recombinant chimeric monoclonal antibody composed of a human anti-body backbone with a mouse idiotype. It can neutralize the biological activity of TNF-α by binding all forms of TNF-α. IFX is administered by intravenous infusion and in overall terms, IFX has an acceptable long-term safety profile (Schaible, 2000). After the treatment with IFX in RA, a decrease of the adhesion molecule, IL-1, IL-6, IL-8, and MCP-1 was observed (Braun and Kay, 2017) also, a reduced thickness of the synovial lining layer could be found (Baeten et al., 2001). The IFX biosimilars include approved medicines in some countries, similar as IFXdyyb, SB2, CT- P13, BOW015, NI- 071, PF- 06438179/ GP1111, STI- 002, and ABP710 (Braun and Kay, 2017). IFX has adverse side effects, similar to serious infections, the reactivation of hepatitis B or tuberculosis, and the threat of carcinoma and other cancers.
- **Adalimumab** (Ada) is a completely humanized anti-TNF-α monoclonal antibody given by subcutaneous route fortnightly and has a less pro-nounced toxicity profile (Weinblatt et al., 2003). BOW100 and ONS-3035, which are still in the preclinical phase (Braun and Kay, 2017). Anti-Ada antibodies (AAA) are detected in more than half of the treated patients with RA. The AAA response is highly restricted and confined to the TNF-α binding region of Ada, thereby neutralizing its therapeutic efficacy and contributing to a loss of clinical efficacy (Van Schouwenburg et al., 2013).

Ada is proven to be a potent antirheumatic agent to achieve remission and inhibit radiological progression. Furthermore, combination therapy with MTX is superior to monotherapy. The Ada biosimilars include drugs approved by some countries, such as ABP 501 (Cohen et al., 2017) Adfrar, and ZRC-3197 (Braun and Kay, 2017). Ada has adverse side effects, such as skin reactions, latent infections, and cardiac failure.

- **Etanercept** is a recombinant protein composed of an immunoglobulin backbone and two naturally occurring soluble human 75-kDa TNF receptors. It is given by subcutaneous route twice weekly with toxicity profiles similar to IFX and Ada (Moreland et al., 1999). Etanercept has shown sustained efficacy and function in rapidly decreasing radiographic progression in elderly and younger patients with RA (Genovese et al., 2005). The number of patients achieving clinical remission with etanercept varies between 50% and 75% in the literature. Etanercept biosimilars include the approved drugs SB4 and GP2015.113 (Braun and Kay, 2017).
- **Golimumab** is a human IgG1 kappa monoclonal antibody that binds to both the soluble and transmembrane bioactive forms of human TNF-α. It is administered once monthly by subcutaneous injection. While the short-term safety profile is reasonable with no differences in total adverse side effects, including serious infections, cancers, tuberculosis, or deaths. However, long-term surveillance studies are needed for further safety assessment (Singh et al., 2010).

One hundred milligrams of Golimumab showed numerically higher incidences of serious infections, demyelinating events, and lymphoma than 50 mg of Golimubab does (Kay et al., 2015). The Golimumab biosimilars include the BOW100 and ONS-3035, which are still in the preclinical phase (Braun and Kay, 2017).

- **Certolizumab pegol** is an anti-TNF-α antibody Fab antibody that is chemically linked to polyethylene glycol and neutralizes membrane-associated and soluble TNF- α. It is administered every two weeks by subcutaneous injection and is well tolerated. Certolizumab pegol biosimilars include the PF-688, a drug still in preclinical phase testing (Braun and Kay, 2017). Significant side effects in 2% of people who take certolizumab pegol.
- Incidentally TNFi (namely onercept and lenercept) failed clinical trials. However, TNF inhibitors have radically altered the approach to treating RA and have become an integral part of the management of RA. Medical professionals before prescribing the patients should have introductory knowledge of its adverse side effects.
- Nonetheless, the inactivation of TNF signaling by rationally designed dominant-negative TNF variants needs further investigation (Steed et al., 2003).
- **Rituximab** is a genetically engineered chimeric monoclonal antibody that targets CD20-positive B lymphocytes from early pre-B cells to latterly in the differentiation process, but it is absent in terminally differentiated plasma cells. The binding to CD20 enables rituximab to deplete

subpopulations of B lymphocytes by way of cell-mediation complement-dependent cytotoxicity, and the promotion of apoptosis and growth arrest. B lymphocytes may contribute to the initiation and maintenance of the inflammatory cascade by their action on antigen presentation and through the production of pro-inflammatory cytokines, including IL- 1,-4,-6,-8,-10, and-12, TNF-α vascular endothelial growth factor, MCP, macrophage migration inhibitory factor, and the autoantibodies rheumatoid factor (RF) and ACPA.

- It has been proposed that Rituximab has an effect on CD4+ cells, converting substantial T-cell reduction in RA (Melet et al., 2013). Rituximab plus MTX demonstrated significant and sustained effects on reducing disease progression in RA patients who had a preliminarily inadequate response to TNFi (Cohen et al., 2010). The Rituximab biosimilars include drugs BCD-020, Maball, and MabTas, which have been approved by some countries (Braun and Kay, 2017). The side effects reported include hypogammaglobulinemia, infection, late-onset neutropenia, and mucocutaneous reactions. Rituximab treatment has been linked with rare cases of progressive multifocal leuko-encephalopathy (PML).

- **Belimumab** is a monoclonal anti-B lymphocyte stimulator (BLyS) antibody. It binds to soluble human BLyS with high affinity and inhibits its biological activity. BLyS is elevated in the serum and synovial fluid of patients with RA and is associated with increased RF situations. The BLyS mechanism of action is important in the survival of B-cells, and its inhibition can lead to the apoptosis of autoimmune B-cell clones (Cancro, 2009). Belimumab was not effective in phase II clinical trials for RA. Other promising CD-20 targeting antibodies (obinutuzumab, ibritumomab, ocaratuzumab) need further clinical trials. The strategy of depth of reduction of B cell populations may not be the better way compared with the inhibition of B-cell modulatory cytokines.

- **Abatacept** is a T-cell co-stimulation modulator and a completely soluble human protein that consists of the extracellular domain of human CTLA-4, which is linked to the modified Fc part of human IgG1. T-cells insinuate into the synovial joint and increase the level of pro-inflammatory cytokines similar to interferon-γ and IL-17, causing synovial cartilage and bone destruction. Upon antigen recognition, T-cells bear a co-stimulatory signal for full activation. Like the natural CTLA4 patch, abatacept interferes with CD80/ CD86 with advanced avidity than CD28. Unlike other biologics medicines, it does not inhibit inflammatory proteins but blocks the communication between these cells by attaching to their surface. It is available in an infusible or injectable form and is administered to patients who have an inadequate response to one or more DMARDs. The data available on abatacept suggests the threat of serious infections when used together with the TNF- α blocker (Moreland et al., 2006). Its side effects include headaches, common cold, sore throat, nausea, and infection. By discrepancy, targeting T cells using ciclosporin, anti-CD4 antibodies, anti-CD5 antibodies, or alemtuzumab hasn't yielded clinically robust responses in patients. The function of T cells and its subsets needs to be further redefined (McInnes and Schett, 2017). Other T-cell specifics, similar to ALX- 0061, Sirukumab, Clazakizumab, Olokizumab, are still in the clinical trial phase.

13.15.2 IL-6 INHIBITORS

- **Tocilizumab(TCZ)** is a humanized monoclonal antibody that targets the IL-6 receptor, which is found on cell surfaces and in circulation. IL-6 is produced by various cell types, including T-cells, B-cells, monocytes, fibroblasts, and endothelial and synovial cells. It has two receptors mIL- 6 R (CD 126) and sIL- 6 R. In the pathology of RA, IL-6 can stimulate pannus conformation through increased vascular endothelial growth factor expression and increase bone resorption as a result of osteoclastogenesis, as well as oxidative stress in leukocytes (Ruiz-Limon et al., 2017; Navarro-Millan et al., 2012). TCZ is available in subcutaneous and intravenous formulations. Its immunogenicity risk is low (Burmester et al., 2017). Decreases in neutrophil counts in patients taking TCZ do not appear to be associated with serious infections (Moots et al., 2017).
- **Sirukumab,** a human monoclonal antibody binding to the IL-6 with high affinity, also shows satisfied outgrowth with an anticipated safety profile in a clinical phase 3 study (Aletaha et al., 2017). It provides another valuable chance to explore the effect of cytokine inhibition in RA rather than cytokine receptor inhibition. The most common adverse effects observed in clinical trials were upper respiratory tract infections, nasopharyngitis, headaches, and high blood pressure. The candidates of IL-6 inhibitors presently witnessing clinical trials include sarilumab, ALX- 0061, MEDI5117, clazakizumab, and olokizumab. Clinical trial data are promising and suggest that anti-IL-6 agents could be a promising remedy (Weinblatt et al., 2015; Kim et al., 2015).

13.15.3 IL-1 INHIBITORS

IL-1 is a cytokine that has the capability of immune and proinflammatory action. There are two specific immunoglobulin-like membrane-bound IL-1 receptors, IL-1RI and IL-1RII. At the cell surface, IL-RII, in discrepancy to IL-1RI, does not transmit signals and acts rather as a bait receptor that binds and inhibits IL-1. In serum, both IL-1 receptors can bind IL-1, thereby regulating the bioavailability of the cytokine (Boissier, 2011).

Anakinra is a non-glycosylated recombinant form of the IL-1 receptor antagonist used as a once-daily injectable. It is different from the native human protein by having a fresh N-terminal methionine. It decreases the exertion of IL-1α and IL-1β by binding to the IL-1 receptor. Its disadvantage includes the demand for daily injections, and an itchy rash may be observed at the injection site. It can be used as a mono-therapy agent or in combination with DMARDs. Still, anakinra should not be used in combination with anti-TNF agents. Its side effects include gastrointestinal tract, allergies and infection of the upper respiratory tract; therefore, regular monitoring is important. Interestingly, RA patients receiving anakinra improved cardiac contractility indeed within three hours of a single administration (Ikonomidis et al., 2009). Thus, Anakinra should be considered for patients with severe or refractory pericardial complaints and (or) heart failure (Schatz et al., 2016). The benefits of IL-1 inhibition in this population are worth further exploration.

Other IL cytokines and their receptors have been studied as the potential target IL-17 (Secukinumab) was finished in a phase III study displaying improvement in patients with active RA who had an inadequate response to TNF impediments (Blanco et al., 2017). Still, IL-12/23 blockade, ustekinumab, did not show a satisfying outcome despite being combined with MTX in a randomized phase II study (Smolen et al., 2017). The medicines targeting IL-7, 15, 18, 21, 32, and 33 are also in a clinical trial.

13.15.4 OSTEOCLAST ISOLATION FACTOR

Denosumab (DMab) is a human monoclonal IgG2 antibody that inhibits bone resorption by binding and inhibiting the receptor activator of the NF-kB ligand (RANKL), an essential cytokine for osteoclastogenesis and bone resorption. Compactly, RANKL is an essential survival factor RANKL- expressing Th17 cells intervene in bone resorption. In addition, RANKL secreted by memory B cells promotes bone corrosion in RA. Incipiently, RANKL was known to induce immune tolerance by promoting the differentiation of Treg cells. It's conceivable that RANKL antagonists may influence immune regulation. The interplay of activated immune cells, synovial cell hyperplasia, and cytokine fosters an osteoclastogenic environment fueled by TNF- α and RANKL. Indeed, the presence of original and systemic bone loss in RA patients raised the possibility that the inhibition of RANKL may be an effective strategy to limit pathologic bone resorption (Chiu, and Ritchlin, 2017). It has been proved that combining denosumab with DMARDs may be considered for RA patients with progressive bone resorption (Yue et al., 2017). Evidence from two phase II trials and one randomized observational trial indicate that DMab inhibits focal and systemic bone loss in RA. Phase III trials are needed to discern the magnitude of the inhibitory effect on bone resorption and help to establish an optimal dose. The side effects include low calcium and phosphate levels in the blood, muscle cramps, cellulitis, and numbness. Eventually, DMab may prove to be a promising medicine in the treatment of RA (Chiu, and Ritchlin, 2017). Besides the phase IIb study of a new granulocyte–macrophage colony-stimulating factor (GM-CSF) receptor nascence monoclonal antibody, mavrilimumab, showed a meaningful response by representing a new mechanism (Burmester et al., 2017).

13.16 SMALL MOLECULE DMARDS

Small-molecule DMARDs revolutionized RA treatment. Numerous cytokines use the Janus kinase(JAK) and signal transducer and activator of recap(STAT) pathway to exert their effect in the pathology of RA, rendering them amenable to therapeutic blockade with Jakinibs which have proven effective for the treatment of RA (Venkatesha et al., 2014).

- **Jakinibs** are being developed, and targeting STATs as well as other intracellular signaling pathways may be a future avenue for the treatment of RA, although substantial challenges remain.
- **Tofacitinib** is the first of a new class of oral drugs to have synthetic small molecules that interfere with specific signal transduction pathways and is the third class of DMARD (tsDMARDs) in RA treatment. It created the way for JAK inhibition in RA.
- Tofacitinib preferentially inhibits JAK-3 and-1 over JAK-2. With an oral bioavailability of 74% and mean elimination half-life of three hours, tofacitinib is metabolized via cytochrome P450 3A4 (CYP3A4) with 30% renal excretion; 5 mg as a twice daily dose of Tofacitinib has recently been approved by the FDA for moderate to severe RA refractory to DMARDs based on recent efficacy studies, with the onset benefits associated with the treatment being earlier (Strand et al., 2016). Common adverse side effects were related to infection, hematologic and hepatic diseases, and association of tofacitinib, with carcinogenicity and infections debatable.
- **Baricitinib** is an orally administered molecular that inhibits JAK-1 and-2. It has moderate activity on tyrosine kinase 2 (TYK2) and negligible activity on JAK- 3 in both enzymatic and cellular assays. Baricitinib also proved effective in radiological progression.
- **Peficitinib** showed a 14 times advanced selectivity for JAK-1/-3 over JAK-2. Filgotinib is a highly selective inhibitor of JAK- 1 over JAK- 2, JAK- 3, and TYK2 in biochemical and cell assays. ABT- 494 is also a JAK- 1 selective Jakinib.
- **Decernotinib** widely inhibits JAK3 over the other JAK family members in both enzyme and cellular assays. The new Jakinibs is more restricted JAK isoform selectivity is now between phases 2 and 3 of clinical development. It is advised that jakinibs will require clinical and laboratory vigilance (Semerano et al., 2016).

13.17 SURGERY

Common surgery in patients with RA reached a peak in the 1990s. Still, a 2010 study showed decreased rates of joint surgery in RA patients 40–59 years of age. In contrast, patients older than 60 years had increased rates of surgery (Louie, and Ward, 2010). Surgery is a last resort for the treatment of RA. Indications include intractable common pain or functional decline due to joint destruction after all nonsurgical approaches have failed. At this point, the disease is considered "end-stage". The goal of surgical management is to relieve the pain of the patients and restore the function of the joints. A patient requiring surgical treatment should be evaluated based on their customized requirements because there are numerous different types of surgery.

A tenosynovectomy involves the excision of an inflamed tendon sheath or repairing a recent tendon rupture, most commonly in the hand (Chung, and Pushman, 2011). Radiosynovectomy is an alternative to surgical synovectomy; it involves intra-articular injection of small radioactive patches, is cost-effective, and can treat multiple joints simultaneously. (Knut, 2015) Repair of ruptured tendons can also be done through arthroscopy, generally in the rotator cuff of the shoulder. Excision of inflamed synovium via arthroscopy or open synovectomy is no longer generally used due to the availability of more effective options. Another surgical option is osteotomy. In this procedure, weight-bearing bones are realigned to correct valgus or varus scars, generally in the knee (Puddu et al., 2010). Joint fusion can be done to stabilize joints that aren't easily replaceable as the ankle, wrist, thumb, and cervical spine.

A procedure for soft-tissue release can be done to correct severe contractures around joints causing a decreased range of motion this is an older procedure that is not generally employed (Brooks and Hariharan, 2013). Small joint implant arthroplasty can be done to reduce pain and ameliorate hand function most commonly in the metacarpophalangeal joints. Metatarsal-head excision arthroplasty is done to palliate severe forefoot pain.

Lastly a total joint replacement involves removing the damaged joint and replacing it with a metallic, plastic, or ceramic prosthesis. This is most commonly done in the shoulder, elbow, wrist, knee, and ankle (Pajarinen, 2014). The major contraindication for surgical joint replacement is the presence of active systemic articular infection.

13.18   OTHER THERAPIES

It has been set up that, in contrast to suggestions in the history, there are no specific foods that patients with RA should avoid. The idea that diet can "aggravate" symptoms is no longer accepted as true (Halstead, and Stoten, 2010) Home remedies have been proven to be helpful for patients suffering from RA, although they aren't as effective as DMARDs. Fish oil and omega-3 fatty acid supplements are beneficial for the short-term treatment of RA. Cumin has been shown to have anti-inflammatory effects in patients. Calcium and vitamin D supplementation can be helpful in preventing osteoporosis. Incipiently, folic acid can help to help the side effects of MTX. Patients with RA also profit from physical and occupational benefits. It's recommended that they perform exercise regularly to maintain common mobility and strengthen the muscles around the joints. Movement exercises that are less traumatic for joints but good for muscle strength include swimming, yoga, and *tai chi*.

Applying heat- and cold- packs ahead and after exercise minimizes painful symptoms. Studies are being done on different types of connective tissue collagen, to more understand and reduce RA disease activity. Lastly, with the scientific advancements and enhanced understanding of molecular mechanisms, newer and better treatment options should come available in the near future (Cooney et al., 2011; Zitnay et al., 2017; Burska et al., 2014; Nakamura et al., 2016; Smolen et al., 2016).

13.19   FUTURE PERSPECTIVES

With a better understanding of the pathophysiology of RA, new therapeutic approaches are arising to provide precise medication to RA patients. Still, the function and adverse side effects of these medicines will need to be precisely estimated and used correctly by individuals. Gene therapy means treating RA by inserting a gene into a patient's cells rather than using medicines (Naldini, 2015). Targeting gene therapy in RA is a treatment strategy that is still in the very early stages of development but could lead to new possibilities because of treating the disease at its root.

The availability of Notch1 targeting siRNA delivery nanoparticles (Kim et al., 2015) and TNF-α gene silencing using polymerized siRNA/ Thiolated Glycol Chitosan Nanoparticles(Lee et al., 2014) has been tested fairly successfully in an animal model.

To prevent disease onset or relapses, smoking cessation or avoiding body exposure to environmental factors is presumably the easiest and most cost-effective system. Autoimmunity develops a year before the onset of inflammatory disease which can be considered as a golden period for preventing complaint progression. Re-establishing vulnerable forbearance and immunological homeostasis are ambitious pretensions in the way to overcome the disease. T-cells and B-cells can be targeted by specific medicines in the future to achieve seroconversion or delay the onset of common destruction. Reduction of the function of APCs and revision of the pro-inflammatory properties of antibodies are being further developed (Lundstrom et al., 2017). There's also a great interest in the new approaches that have the possibility of getting therapeutic targets, similar to TLRs; Bruton's tyrosine kinase; phosphoinositide-3-kinase pathway; TGF-β; neuro pathways, and DCs. Bruton's tyrosine kinase is involved in various signaling pathways downstream of the pre-B-cell receptor and formula FcR, which is a promising therapeutic target for RA (Whang and Chang, 2014). The safety and tolerability of the intravenous infusions of expanded adipose-derived stem cells in refractory RA have been reported (Álvaro-Gracia et al., 2017). Besides this, new pathologic insight will support new avenues for therapeutic development.

13.20   CONCLUSION

RA is a debilitating, chronic, inflammatory disease capable of causing joint damage as well as long-term disability. Early diagnosis and intervention are essential for the prevention of serious damage and loss of essential bodily functions. The treating clinicians should consider adhering to treat-to-target recommendations by first outlining the aim and also implementing the protocols to achieve and assess them (Smolen et al., 2016). Furthermore, early referral to a clinician can help to ensure better treatment issues. With advances in the field of molecular drugs, we have a better understanding of disease mechanisms which can be helpful in the designing of further effective treatments. Old treatment modalities have been optimized and new bones have been produced. Gene array analysis is proving beneficial in finding out which patients will be more responsive to specific therapy. This customization will allow for more rapid treatment as well as decrease the disease progression during the experimental phase to seek an applicable treatment for a particular patient. Gene array analysis is also being used to determine which patients are at greater risk for more aggressive forms of RA. It is foreseen that treatment methods will face tremendous improvements in the management of RA.

REFERENCES

Al Maashari, R., & Hamodat, M. M. (2016). Methotrexate-induced panniculitis in a patient with rheumatoid arthritis. *Acta dermatovenerologica Alpina, Pannonica, et Adriatica, 25*(4), 79–81. 10.15570/actaapa.2016.23

Alamanos, Y., Voulgari, P. V., & Drosos, A. A. (2006). Incidence and prevalence of rheumatoid arthritis, based on the 1987 American College of Rheumatology criteria: A systematic review. *Seminars in Arthritis and Rheumatism, 36*(3), 182–188. 10.1016/j.semarthrit.2006.08.006

Albrecht, K., Callhoff, J., Schneider, M., & Zink, A. (2015). High variability in glucocorticoid starting doses in patients with rheumatoid arthritis: Observational data from an early arthritis cohort. *Rheumatology International, 35*(8), 1377–1384. 10.1007/s00296-015-3229-x

Albrecht, K., & Zink, A. (2017). Poor prognostic factors guiding treatment decisions in rheumatoid arthritis patients: A review of data from randomized clinical trials and cohort studies. *Arthritis Research Therapy, 19*(68), 2–8. 10.1186/s13075-017-1266-4

Aletaha, D., Bingham, C. O., 3rd, Tanaka, Y., Agarwal, P., Kurrasch, R., Tak, P. P., & Popik, S. (2017). Efficacy and safety of sirukumab in patients with active rheumatoid arthritis refractory to anti-TNF therapy (SIRROUND-T): A randomised, double-blind, placebo-controlled, parallel-group, multinational, phase 3 study. *Lancet (London, England), 389*(10075), 1206–1217. 10.1016/S0140-6736(17)30401-4

Aletaha, D., Eberl, G., Nell, V. P., Machold, K. P., & Smolen, J. S. (2002). Practical progress in realisation of early diagnosis and treatment of patients with suspected rheumatoid arthritis: Results from two matched questionnaires within three years. *Annals of the Rheumatic Diseases, 61*(7), 630–634. 10.1136/ard.61.7.630

Alpizar-Rodriguez, D., Mueller, R. B., Möller, B., Dudler, J., Ciurea, A., Zufferey, P., Kyburz, D., Walker, U. A., von Mühlenen, I., Roux-Lombard, P., Mahler, M., Lamacchia, C., Courvoisier, D. S., Gabay, C., & Finckh, A. (2017). Female hormonal factors and the development of anti-citrullinated protein antibodies in women at risk of rheumatoid arthritis. *Rheumatology (Oxford, England), 56*(9), 1579–1585. 10.1093/rheumatology/kex239

Alspaugh, M. A., Henle, G., Lennette, E. T., & Henle, W. (1981). Elevated levels of antibodies to Epstein-Barr virus antigens in sera and synovial fluids of patients with rheumatoid arthritis. *The Journal of Clinical Investigation, 67*(4), 1134–1140. 10.1172/jci110127

Alten, R., Grahn, A., Holt, R. J., Rice, P., & Buttgereit, F. (2015). Delayed-release prednisone improves fatigue and health-related quality of life: Findings from the CAPRA-2 double-blind randomised study in rheumatoid arthritis. *RMD Open, 1*(1), e000134. 10.1136/rmdopen-2015-000134

Álvaro-Gracia, J. M., Jover, J. A., García-Vicuña, R., Carreño, L., Alonso, A., Marsal, S., Blanco, F., Martínez-Taboada, V. M., Taylor, P., Martín-Martín, C., DelaRosa, O., Tagarro, I., & Díaz-González, F. (2017). Intravenous administration of expanded allogeneic adipose-derived mesenchymal stem cells in refractory rheumatoid arthritis (Cx611): Results of a multicentre, dose escalation, randomised, single-blind, placebo-controlled phase Ib/IIa clinical trial. *Annals of the Rheumatic Diseases, 76*(1), 196–202. 10.1136/annrheumdis-2015-208918

Amano, T., Yamasaki, S., Yagishita, N., Tsuchimochi, K., Shin, H., Kawahara, K., Aratani, S., Fujita, H., Zhang, L., Ikeda, R., Fujii, R., Miura, N., Komiya, S., Nishioka, K., Maruyama, I., Fukamizu, A., & Nakajima, T. (2003). Synoviolin/Hrd1, an E3 ubiquitin ligase, as a novel pathogenic factor for arthropathy. *Genes & Development, 17*(19), 2436–2449. 10.1101/gad.1096603

Arnett, F. C., Edworthy, S. M., Bloch, D. A., McShane, D. J., Fries, J. F., Cooper, N. S., Healey, L. A., Kaplan, S. R., Liang, M. H., & Luthra, H. S. (1988). The American Rheumatism Association 1987 revised criteria for the classification of rheumatoid arthritis. *Arthritis and Rheumatism, 31*(3), 315–324. 10.1002/art.1780310302

Arts, E. E., Fransen, J., Den Broeder, A. A., van Riel, P. L. C. M., & Popa, C. D. (2017). Low disease activity (DAS28≤3.2) reduces the risk of first cardiovascular event in rheumatoid arthritis: A time-dependent Cox regression analysis in a large cohort study. *Annals of the Rheumatic Diseases, 76*(10), 1693–1699. 10.1136/annrheumdis-2016-210997

Aupperle, K. R., Boyle, D. L., Hendrix, M., Seftor, E. A., Zvaifler, N. J., Barbosa, M., & Firestein, G. S. (1998). Regulation of synoviocyte proliferation, apoptosis, and invasion by the p53 tumor suppressor gene. *The American Journal of Pathology, 152*(4), 1091–1098.

Bae, S., Kim, H., Lee, N., Won, C., Kim, H. R., Hwang, Y. I., Song, Y. W., Kang, J. S., & Lee, W. J. (2012). α-Enolase expressed on the surfaces of monocytes and macrophages induces robust synovial inflammation in rheumatoid arthritis. *Journal of Immunology, 189*(1), 365–372. 10.4049/jimmunol.1102073

Baeten, D., Kruithof, E., Van den Bosch, F., Demetter, P., Van Damme, N., Cuvelier, C., De Vos, M., Mielants, H., Veys, E. M., & De Keyser, F. (2001). Immunomodulatory effects of anti-tumor necrosis factor alpha therapy on synovium in spondyloarthropathy: Histologic findings in eight patients from an open-label pilot study. *Arthritis and Rheumatism, 44*(1), 186–195. 10.1002/1529-0131(200101)44:1<186::AID-ANR25 >3.0.CO;2-B

Bartok, B., Hammaker, D., & Firestein, G. S. (2014). Phosphoinositide 3-kinase δ regulates migration and invasion of synoviocytes in rheumatoid arthritis. *Journal of Immunology, 192*(5), 2063–2070. 10.4049/jimmunol.1300950

Benham, H., Nel, H. J., Law, S. C., Mehdi, A. M., Street, S., Ramnoruth, N., Pahau, H., Lee, B. T., Ng, J., Brunck, M. E., Hyde, C., Trouw, L. A., Dudek, N. L., Purcell, A. W., O'Sullivan, B. J., Connolly, J. E., Paul, S. K., Lê Cao, K. A., & Thomas, R. (2015). Citrullinated peptide dendritic cell immunotherapy in HLA risk genotype-positive rheumatoid arthritis patients. *Science Translational Medicine, 7*(290), 290ra87. 10.112 6/scitranslmed.aaa9301

Birch, J. T., & Bhattacharya, S. (2010). Emerging trends in diagnosis and treatment of rheumatoid arthritis. *Primary Care, 37*(4), 779–vii. 10.1016/j.pop.2010.07.001

Bizzaro, N., Bartoloni, E., Morozzi, G., Manganelli, S., Riccieri, V., Sabatini, P., Filippini, M., Tampoia, M., Afeltra, A., Sebastiani, G., Alpini, C., Bini, V., Bistoni, O., Alunno, A., Gerli, R., & Forum Interdisciplinare per la Ricerca nelle Malattie Autoimmuni (FIRMA Group) (2013). Anti-cyclic citrullinated peptide antibody titer predicts time to rheumatoid arthritis onset in patients with undifferentiated arthritis: Results from a 2-year prospective study. *Arthritis Research & Therapy, 15*(1), R16. 10.1186/ar4148

Black, R. J., Lester, S., Buchbinder, R., Barrett, C., Lassere, M., March, L., Whittle, S., & Hill, C. L. (2017). Factors associated with oral glucocorticoid use in patients with rheumatoid arthritis: A drug use study from a prospective national biologics registry. *Arthritis Research & Therapy, 19*(1), 253. 10.1186/s13075-017-1461-3

Blanco, F. J., Möricke, R., Dokoupilova, E., Codding, C., Neal, J., Andersson, M., Rohrer, S., & Richards, H. (2017). Secukinumab in active rheumatoid arthritis: A phase III randomized, double-blind, active comparator- and placebo-controlled study. *Arthritis & Rheumatology (Hoboken, N.J.), 69*(6), 1144–1153. 10.1002/art.40070

Boissier, M. C. (2011). Cell and cytokine imbalances in rheumatoid synovitis. *Joint Bone Spine*, *78*(3), 230–234. 10.1016/j.jbspin.2010.08.017

Borrero, C. G., Mountz, J. M., & Mountz, J. D. (2011). Emerging MRI methods in rheumatoid arthritis. *Nature Reviews. Rheumatology*, *7*(2), 85–95. 10.1038/nrrheum.2 010.173

Braun, J., & Kay, J. (2017). The safety of emerging biosimilar drugs for the treatment of rheumatoid arthritis. *Expert Opinion on Drug Safety*, *16*(3), 289–302. 10.1080/1474 0338.2017.1273899

Brooks, F., & Hariharan, K. (2013). The rheumatoid forefoot. *Current Reviews in Musculoskeletal Medicine*, *6*(4), 320–327. 10.1007/s12178-013-9178-7

Brown, P. M., Pratt, A. G., & Isaacs, J. D. (2016). Mechanism of action of methotrexate in rheumatoid arthritis, and the search for biomarkers. *Nature Reviews. Rheumatology*, *12*(12), 731–742. 10.1038/nrrheum.2016.175

Burgers, L. E., Raza, K., & van der Helm-van Mil, A. H. (2019). Window of opportunity in rheumatoid arthritis – Definitions and supporting evidence: From old to new perspectives. *RMD Open*, *5*(1), e000870. 10.1136/rmdopen-2018-000870

Burmester, G. R., Choy, E., Kivitz, A., Ogata, A., Bao, M., Nomura, A., Lacey, S., Pei, J., Reiss, W., Pethoe-Schramm, A., Mallalieu, N. L., Wallace, T., Michalska, M., Birnboeck, H., Stubenrauch, K., & Genovese, M. C. (2017). Low immunogenicity of tocilizumab in patients with rheumatoid arthritis. *Annals of the Rheumatic Diseases*, *76*(6), 1078–1085. 10.1136/annrheumdis-2016-210297

Burmester, G. R., Dimitriu-Bona, A., Waters, S. J., & Winchester, R. J. (1983). Identification of three major synovial lining cell populations by monoclonal antibodies directed to Ia antigens and antigens associated with monocytes/macrophages and fibroblasts. *Scandinavian Journal of Immunology*, *17*(1), 69–82. 10.1111/j.1365-3083.1983.tb00767.x

Burska, A. N., Roget, K., Blits, M., Soto Gomez, L., van de Loo, F., Hazelwood, L. D., Verweij, C. L., Rowe, A., Goulielmos, G. N., van Baarsen, L. G., & Ponchel, F. (2014). Gene expression analysis in RA: Towards personalized medicine. *The Pharmacogenomics Journal*, *14*(2), 93–106. 10.1038/tpj.2013.48

Buttgereit, F., Mehta, D., Kirwan, J., Szechinski, J., Boers, M., Alten, R. E., Supronik, J., Szombati, I., Romer, U., Witte, S., & Saag, K. G. (2013). Low-dose prednisone chronotherapy for rheumatoid arthritis: A randomised clinical trial (CAPRA-2). *Annals of the Rheumatic Diseases*, *72*(2), 204–210. 10.1136/annrheumdis-2011-201067

Cancro M. P. (2009). Signalling crosstalk in B cells: Managing worth and need. *Nature Reviews. Immunology*, *9*(9), 657–661. 10.1038/nri2621

Castañeda-Delgado, J. E., Bastián-Hernandez, Y., Macias-Segura, N., Santiago-Algarra, D., Castillo-Ortiz, J. D., Alemán-Navarro, A. L., Martínez-Tejada, P., Enciso-Moreno, L., Garcia-De Lira, Y., Olguín-Calderón, D., Trouw, L. A., Ramos-Remus, C., & Enciso-Moreno, J. A. (2017). Type I interferon gene response is increased in early and established rheumatoid arthritis and correlates with autoantibody production. *Frontiers in Immunology*, *8*, 285. 10.3389/fimmu.2017.00285

Cavalli, G., & Dinarello, C. A. (2015). Treating rheumatological diseases and co-morbidities with interleukin-1 blocking therapies. *Rheumatology (Oxford, England)*, *54*(12), 2134–2144. 10.1093/rheumatology/kev269

Chaudhari, K., Rizvi, S., & Syed, B. A. (2016). Rheumatoid arthritis: Current and future trends. *Nature Reviews. Drug Discovery*, *15*(5), 305–306. 10.1038/nrd.2016.21

Chen, J., Wright, K., Davis, J. M., Jeraldo, P., Marietta, E. V., Murray, J., Nelson, H., Matteson, E. L., & Taneja, V. (2016). An expansion of rare lineage intestinal microbes characterizes rheumatoid arthritis. *Genome Medicine*, *8*(1), 43. 10.1186/s13073-016-0299-7

Chen, Y. J., Chang, Y. T., Wang, C. B., & Wu, C. Y. (2011). The risk of cancer in patients with rheumatoid arthritis: A nationwide cohort study in Taiwan. *Arthritis and Rheumatism*, *63*(2), 352–358. 10.1002/art.30134

Cheung, T. T., & McInnes, I. B. (2017). Future therapeutic targets in rheumatoid arthritis? *Seminars in Immunopathology*, *39*(4), 487–500. 10.1007/s00281-017-0623-3

Chiu, Y. G., & Ritchlin, C. T. (2017). Denosumab: Targeting the RANKL pathway to treat rheumatoid arthritis. *Expert Opinion on Biological Therapy*, *17*(1), 119–128. 10.1080/14712598.2017.1263614

Cho, S. K., Kim, D., Won, S., Lee, J., Choi, C. B., Choe, J. Y., Hong, S. J., Jun, J. B., Kim, T. H., Koh, E., Lee, H. S., Lee, J., Yoo, D. H., Yoon, B. Y., Bae, S. C., & Sung, Y. K. (2019). Factors associated with time to diagnosis from symptom onset in patients with early rheumatoid arthritis. *The Korean Journal of Internal Medicine*, *34*(4), 910–916. 10.3904/kjim.2017.113

Chopra, A., & Abdel-Nasser, A. (2008). Epidemiology of rheumatic musculoskeletal disorders in the developing world. *Best Practice & Research. Clinical Rheumatology*, *22*(4), 583–604. 10.1016/j.berh.2008.07.001

Chung, K. C., & Pushman, A. G. (2011). Current concepts in the management of the rheumatoid hand. *The Journal of Hand Surgery*, *36*(4), 736–747. 10.1016/j.jhsa.2011.01.019

Cohen, S., & Emery, P. (2010). The American College of Rheumatology/European League Against Rheumatism criteria for the classification of rheumatoid arthritis: A game changer. *Arthritis Rheumatology*, *62*(9), 2592–2594. 10.1002/art.27583

Cohen, S. B., Keystone, E., Genovese, M. C., Emery, P., Peterfy, C., Tak, P. P., Cravets, M., Shaw, T., & Hagerty, D. (2010). Continued inhibition of structural damage over 2 years in patients with rheumatoid arthritis treated with rituximab in combination with methotrexate. *Annals of the Rheumatic Diseases*, *69*(6), 1158–1161. 10.1136/ard.2009.119222

Cohen, S., Genovese, M. C., Choy, E., Perez-Ruiz, F., Matsumoto, A., Pavelka, K., Pablos, J. L., Rizzo, W., Hrycaj, P., Zhang, N., Shergy, W., & Kaur, P. (2017). Efficacy and safety of the biosimilar ABP 501 compared with adalimumab in patients with moderate to severe rheumatoid arthritis: A randomised, double-blind, phase III equivalence study. *Annals of the Rheumatic Diseases*, *76*(10), 1679–1687. 10.1136/annrheumdis-2016-210459

Combe, B. (2007). Early rheumatoid arthritis: Strategies for prevention and management. *Best Practice & Research. Clinical Rheumatology*, *21*(1), 27–42. 10.1016/j.berh.2006.08.011

Combe, B. (2009). Progression in early rheumatoid arthritis. *Best Practice & Research. Clinical Rheumatology*, *23*(1), 59–69. 10.1016/j.berh.2008.11.006

Combe, B., & Rincheval, N. (2015). Early lessons from the recent-onset rheumatoid arthritis cohort ESPOIR. *Joint Bone Spine*, *82*(1), 13–17. 10.1016/j.jbspin.2014.07.003

Combe, B., Landewe, R., Daien, C. I., Hua, C., Aletaha, D., Álvaro-Gracia, J. M., Bakkers, M., Brodin, N., Burmester, G. R., Codreanu, C., Conway, R., Dougados, M., Emery, P., Ferraccioli, G., Fonseca, J., Raza, K., Silva-Fernández, L., Smolen, J. S., Skingle, D., Szekanecz, Z., ... & van Vollenhoven, R. (2017). 2016 update of the EULAR recommendations for the management of early arthritis. *Annals of the Rheumatic Diseases*, *76*(6), 948–959. 10.1136/annrheumdis-2016-210602

Cooney, J. K., Law, R. J., Matschke, V., Lemmey, A. B., Moore, J. P., Ahmad, Y., Jones, J. G., Maddison, P., & Thom, J. M. (2011). Benefits of exercise in rheumatoid arthritis. *Journal of Aging Research*, *2011*, 681640. 10.4061/2011/681640

Daien, C. I., Hua, C., Combe, B., & Landewe, R. (2017). Non-pharmacological and pharmacological interventions in patients with early arthritis: A systematic literature review informing the 2016 update of EULAR recommendations for the management of early arthritis. *RMD Open*, *3*(1), e000404. 10.1136/rmdopen-2016-000404

Deane, K. D. (2013). Can rheumatoid arthritis be prevented? *Best Practice & Research. Clinical Rheumatology*, *27*(4), 467–485. 10.1016/j.berh.2013.09.002

Devauchelle-Pensec, V., Saraux, A., Alapetite, S., Colin, D., & Le Goff, P. (2002). Diagnostic value of radiographs of the hands and feet in early rheumatoid arthritis. *Joint Bone Spine*, *69*(5), 434–441. 10.1016/s1297-319x(02)00427-x

Ding, B., Padyukov, L., Lundström, E., Seielstad, M., Plenge, R. M., Oksenberg, J. R., Gregersen, P. K., Alfredsson, L., & Klareskog, L. (2009). Different patterns of associations with anti-citrullinated protein antibody-positive and anti-citrullinated protein antibody-negative rheumatoid arthritis in the extended major histocompatibility complex region. *Arthritis and Rheumatism*, *60*(1), 30–38. 10.1002/art.24135

Dulai, R., Perry, M., Twycross-Lewis, R., Morrissey, D., Atzeni, F., & Greenwald, S. (2012). The effect of tumor necrosis factor-α antagonists on arterial stiffness in rheumatoid arthritis: A literature review. *Seminars in Arthritis and Rheumatism*, *42*(1), 1–8. 10. 1016/j.semarthrit.2012.02.002

Edwards J. C. (1994). The nature and origins of synovium: Experimental approaches to the study of synoviocyte differentiation. *Journal of Anatomy*, *184*(Pt 3), 493–501.

El Miedany, Y., Youssef, S., Mehanna, A. N., & El Gaafary, M. (2008). Development of a scoring system for assessment of outcome of early undifferentiated inflammatory synovitis. *Joint Bone Spine*, *75*(2), 155–162. 10.1016/j.jbspin.2007.04.021

Elshabrawy, H. A., Essani, A. E., Szekanecz, Z., Fox, D. A., & Shahrara, S. (2017). TLRs, future potential therapeutic targets for RA. *Autoimmunity Reviews*, *16*(2), 103–113. 10.1016/j.autrev.2016.12.003

Fraenkel, L., Bathon, J. M., England, B. R., St Clair, E. W., Arayssi, T., Carandang, K., Deane, K. D., Genovese, M., Huston, K. K., Kerr, G., Kremer, J., Nakamura, M. C., Russell, L. A., Singh, J. A., Smith, B. J., Sparks, J. A., Venkatachalam, S., Weinblatt, M. E., Al-Gibbawi, M., Baker, J. F., ... & Akl, E. A. (2021). 2021 American College of rheumatology guideline for the treatment of rheumatoid arthritis. *Arthritis Care & Research*, *73*(7), 924–939. 10.1002/acr.24596

Farrant, J. M., O'Connor, P. J., & Grainger, A. J. (2007). Advanced imaging in rheumatoid arthritis. Part 1: Synovitis. *Skeletal Radiology*, *36*(4), 269–279. 10.1007/s00256-006-0219-9

Fassio, A., Rossini, M., Viapiana, O., Idolazzi, L., Vantaggiato, E., Benini, C., & Gatti, D. (2017). New strategies for the prevention and treatment of systemic and local bone loss; from pathophysiology to clinical application. *Current Pharmaceutical Design*, *23*(41), 6241–6250. 10.2174/1381612823666170713104431

Fechtner, S., Fox, D. A., & Ahmed, S. (2017). Transforming growth factor β activated kinase 1: A potential therapeutic target for rheumatic diseases. *Rheumatology (Oxford, England)*, *56*(7), 1060–1068. 10.1093/rheumatology/kew301

Filer, A., Parsonage, G., Smith, E., Osborne, C., Thomas, A. M., Curnow, S. J., Rainger, G. E., Raza, K., Nash, G. B., Lord, J., Salmon, M., & Buckley, C. D. (2006). Differential survival of leukocyte subsets mediated by synovial, bone marrow, and skin fibroblasts: Site-specific versus activation-dependent survival of T cells and neutrophils. *Arthritis and Rheumatism*, *54*(7), 2096–2108. 10.1002/art.21930

Finckh A. (2009). Early inflammatory arthritis versus rheumatoid arthritis. *Current Opinion in Rheumatology*, *21*(2), 118–123. 10.1097/BOR.0b013e3283235ac4

Finckh, A., Liang, M. H., van Herckenrode, C. M., & de Pablo, P. (2006). Long-term impact of early treatment on radiographic progression in rheumatoid arthritis: A meta-analysis. *Arthritis and Rheumatism*, *55*(6), 864–872. 10.1002/art.22353

Frisell, T., Holmqvist, M., Källberg, H., Klareskog, L., Alfredsson, L., & Askling, J. (2013). Familial risks and heritability of rheumatoid arthritis: Role of rheumatoid factor/anti-citrullinated protein antibody status, number and type of affected relatives, sex, and age. *Arthritis and Rheumatism*, *65*(11), 2773–2782. 10.1002/art.38097

Fuchs, H. A., Kaye, J. J., Callahan, L. F., Nance, E. P., & Pincus, T. (1989). Evidence of significant radiographic damage in rheumatoid arthritis within the first 2 years of disease. *The Journal of Rheumatology*, *16*(5), 585–591.

Fukui, S., Iwamoto, N., Takatani, A., Igawa, T., Shimizu, T., Umeda, M., Nishino, A., Horai, Y., Hirai, Y., Koga, T., Kawashiri, S. Y., Tamai, M., Ichinose, K., Nakamura, H.,

Origuchi, T., Masuyama, R., Kosai, K., Yanagihara, K., & Kawakami, A. (2018). M1 and M2 monocytes in rheumatoid arthritis: A contribution of imbalance of M1/M2 monocytes to osteoclastogenesis. *Frontiers in Immunology*, *8*, 1958. 10.3389/fimmu. 2017.01958

Gan, R. W., Bemis, E. A., Demoruelle, M. K., Striebich, C. C., Brake, S., Feser, M. L., Moss, L., Clare-Salzler, M., Holers, V. M., Deane, K. D., & Norris, J. M. (2017). The association between omega-3 fatty acid biomarkers and inflammatory arthritis in an anti-citrullinated protein antibody positive population. *Rheumatology (Oxford, England)*, *56*(12), 2229–2236. 10.1093/rheumatology/kex360

Gaujoux-Viala, C., & Gossec, L. (2014). When and for how long should glucocorticoids be used in rheumatoid arthritis? International guidelines and recommendations. *Annals of the New York Academy of Sciences*, *1318*, 32–40. 10.1111/nyas.12452

Genovese, M. C., Bathon, J. M., Fleischmann, R. M., Moreland, L. W., Martin, R. W., Whitmore, J. B., Tsuji, W. H., & Leff, J. A. (2005). Long term safety, efficacy, and radiographic outcome with etanercept treatment in patients with early rheumatoid arthritis. *The Journal of Rheumatology*, *32*(7), 1232–1242.

Goekoop-Ruiterman, Y. P., de Vries-Bouwstra, J. K., Allaart, C. F., van Zeben, D., Kerstens, P. J., Hazes, J. M., Zwinderman, A. H., Peeters, A. J., de Jonge-Bok, J. M., Mallée, C., de Beus, W. M., de Sonnaville, P. B., Ewals, J. A., Breedveld, F. C., & Dijkmans, B. A. (2007). Comparison of treatment strategies in early rheumatoid arthritis: A randomized trial. *Annals of Internal Medicine*, *146*(6), 406–415. 10.7326/0003-4819-146-6-200703200-00005

Goh, L. L., Yong, M. Y., See, W. Q., Chee, E. Y. W., Lim, P. Q., Koh, E. T., Leong, K. P., & TTSH RA Study Group (2017). NLRP1, PTPN22 and PADI4 gene polymorphisms and rheumatoid arthritis in ACPA-positive Singaporean Chinese. *Rheumatology International*, *37*(8), 1295–1302. 10.1007/s00296-017-3762-x

Gossec, L., Combescure, C., Rincheval, N., Saraux, A., Combe, B., & Dougados, M. (2010). Relative clinical influence of clinical, laboratory, and radiological investigations in early arthritis on the diagnosis of rheumatoid arthritis. Data from the French Early Arthritis Cohort ESPOIR. *The Journal of Rheumatology*, *37*(12), 2486–2492. 10.3899/jrheum.100267

Goupille, P., Roulot, B., Akoka, S., Avimadje, A. M., Garaud, P., Naccache, L., Le Pape, A., & Valat, J. P. (2001). Magnetic resonance imaging: A valuable method for the detection of synovial inflammation in rheumatoid arthritis. *The Journal of Rheumatology*, *28*(1), 35–40.

Grassi, W., De Angelis, R., Lamanna, G., & Cervini, C. (1998). The clinical features of rheumatoid arthritis. *European Journal of Radiology*, *27*(Suppl 1), S18–S24. 10.1016/s0720-048x(98)00038-2

Graudal N. (2004). The natural history and prognosis of rheumatoid arthritis: Association of radiographic outcome with process variables, joint motion and immune proteins. *Scandinavian Journal of Rheumatology. Supplement*, *118*, 1–38. 10.1080/03009740310004847

Grosser, T. et al. (2022). Pharmacotherapy of inflammation, fever, pain, and gout. In Brunton, Laurence L., Hilal-Dandan Randa, Knollmann, Björn C. (eds). *The Pharmacological Basis of Therapeutics*, 14th edn, McGraw Hill Publishers, New York. p. 1478.

Halstead, J. A., & Stoten, S. (2010). *Orthopedic Nursing: Caring for Patients with Musculoskeletal Disorders*. Bridgewater: Western Schools.

Harre, U., Georgess, D., Bang, H., Bozec, A., Axmann, R., Ossipova, E., Jakobsson, P. J., Baum, W., Nimmerjahn, F., Szarka, E., Sarmay, G., Krumbholz, G., Neumann, E., Toes, R., Scherer, H. U., Catrina, A. I., Klareskog, L., Jurdic, P., & Schett, G. (2012). Induction of osteoclastogenesis and bone loss by human autoantibodies against citrullinated vimentin. *The Journal of Clinical Investigation*, *122*(5), 1791–1802. 10.1172/JCI60975

Heidari B. (2007). The value of changes in CRP and ESR for predicting treatment response in rheumatoid arthritis. *Rheumatology International, 10*(1), 23–28. 10.1111/j.1479-8077. 2007.00250.x

Heidari, B., Abedi, H., Firouzjahi, A., & Heidari, P. (2009). Diagnostic value of synovial fluid anti-cyclic citrullinated peptide antibody for rheumatoid arthritis. *Rheumatology International, 30*(11), 1465–1470. 10.1007/s00296-009-1171-5

Hensvold, A. H., Magnusson, P. K., Joshua, V., Hansson, M., Israelsson, L., Ferreira, R., Jakobsson, P. J., Holmdahl, R., Hammarström, L., Malmström, V., Askling, J., Klareskog, L., & Catrina, A. I. (2015). Environmental and genetic factors in the development of anticitrullinated protein antibodies (ACPAs) and ACPA-positive rheumatoid arthritis: An epidemiological investigation in twins. *Annals of the Rheumatic Diseases, 74*(2), 375–380. 10.1136/annrheumdis-2013-203947

Herrmann, M. L., Schleyerbach, R., & Kirschbaum, B. J. (2000). Leflunomide: An immunomodulatory drug for the treatment of rheumatoid arthritis and other autoimmune diseases. *Immunopharmacology, 47*(2-3), 273–289. 10.1016/s0162-3109(00)00191-0

Hirohata, S., Ohshima, N., Yanagida, T., & Aramaki, K. (2002). Regulation of human B cell function by sulfasalazine and its metabolites. *International Immunopharmacology, 2*(5), 631–640. 10.1016/s1567-5769(01)00186-2

Hu, Y., Sparks, J. A., Malspeis, S., Costenbader, K. H., Hu, F. B., Karlson, E. W., & Lu, B. (2017). Long-term dietary quality and risk of developing rheumatoid arthritis in women. *Annals of the Rheumatic Diseases, 76*(8), 1357–1364. 10.1136/annrheumdis-2016-210431

Hueber, A. J., Asquith, D. L., Miller, A. M., Reilly, J., Kerr, S., Leipe, J., Melendez, A. J., & McInnes, I. B. (2010). Mast cells express IL-17A in rheumatoid arthritis synovium. *Journal of Immunology, 184*(7), 3336–3340. 10.4049/jimmunol.0903566

Ikonomidis, I., Tzortzis, S., Lekakis, J., Paraskevaidis, I., Andreadou, I., Nikolaou, M., Kaplanoglou, T., Katsimbri, P., Skarantavos, G., Soucacos, P., & Kremastinos, D. T. (2009). Lowering interleukin-1 activity with anakinra improves myocardial deformation in rheumatoid arthritis. *Heart (British Cardiac Society), 95*(18), 1502–1507. 10.1136/hrt.2009.168971

Janssen, N. M., & Genta, M. S. (2000). The effects of immunosuppressive and anti-inflammatory medications on fertility, pregnancy, and lactation. *Archives of Internal Medicine, 160*(5), 610–619. 10.1001/archinte.160.5.610

Kalden, J. R., Schattenkirchner, M., Sörensen, H., Emery, P., Deighton, C., Rozman, B., & Breedveld, F. (2003). The efficacy and safety of leflunomide in patients with active rheumatoid arthritis: A five-year follow-up study. *Arthritis and Rheumatism, 48*(6), 1513–1520. 10.1002/art.11015

Kasareło, K., Cudnoch-Jędrzejewska, A., Członkowski, A., & Mirowska-Guzel, D. (2017). Mechanism of action of three newly registered drugs for multiple sclerosis treatment. *Pharmacological Reports: PR, 69*(4), 702–708. 10.1016/j.pharep.2017.02.017

Katz, S. J., & Russell, A. S. (2011). Re-evaluation of antimalarials in treating rheumatic diseases: Re-appreciation and insights into new mechanisms of action. *Current Opinion in Rheumatology, 23*(3), 278–281. 10.1097/BOR.0b013e32834456bf

Kay, J., Fleischmann, R., Keystone, E., Hsia, E. C., Hsu, B., Mack, M., Goldstein, N., Braun, J., & Kavanaugh, A. (2015). Golimumab 3-year safety update: An analysis of pooled data from the long-term extensions of randomised, double-blind, placebo-controlled trials conducted in patients with rheumatoid arthritis, psoriatic arthritis or ankylosing spondylitis. *Annals of the Rheumatic Diseases, 74*(3), 538–546. 10.1136/annrheumdis-2013-204195

Khandpur, R., Carmona-Rivera, C., Vivekanandan-Giri, A., Gizinski, A., Yalavarthi, S., Knight, J. S., Friday, S., Li, S., Patel, R. M., Subramanian, V., Thompson, P., Chen, P., Fox, D. A., Pennathur, S., & Kaplan, M. J. (2013). NETs are a source of citrullinated autoantigens and stimulate inflammatory responses in rheumatoid arthritis. *Science Translational Medicine, 5*(178), 178ra40. 10.1126/scitranslmed.3005580

Kim, E. K., Kwon, J. E., Lee, S. Y., Lee, E. J., Kim, D. S., Moon, S. J., Lee, J., Kwok, S. K., Park, S. H., & Cho, M. L. (2017). IL-17-mediated mitochondrial dysfunction impairs apoptosis in rheumatoid arthritis synovial fibroblasts through activation of autophagy. *Cell Death & Disease*, *8*(1), e2565. 10.1038/cddis.2016.490

Kim, E. Y., & Moudgil, K. D. (2017). Immunomodulation of autoimmune arthritis by pro-inflammatory cytokines. *Cytokine*, *98*, 87–96. 10.1016/j.cyto.2017.04.012

Kim, M. J., Park, J. S., Lee, S. J., Jang, J., Park, J. S., Back, S. H., Bahn, G., Park, J. H., Kang, Y. M., Kim, S. H., Kwon, I. C., Jo, D. G., & Kim, K. (2015). Notch1 targeting siRNA delivery nanoparticles for rheumatoid arthritis therapy. *Journal of Controlled Release: Official Journal of the Controlled Release Society*, *216*, 140–148. 10.1016/j.jconrel.2015.08.025

Klareskog, L., Stolt, P., Lundberg, K., Källberg, H., Bengtsson, C., Grunewald, J., Rönnelid, J., Harris, H. E., Ulfgren, A. K., Rantapää-Dahlqvist, S., Eklund, A., Padyukov, L., & Alfredsson, L. (2006). A new model for an etiology of rheumatoid arthritis: Smoking may trigger HLA-DR (shared epitope)-restricted immune reactions to autoantigens modified by citrullination. *Arthritis and Rheumatism*, *54*(1), 38–46. 10.1002/art.21575

Knut, L. (2015). Radiosynovectomy in the therapeutic management of arthritis. *World Journal of Nuclear Medicine*, *14*(1), 10–15. 10.4103/1450-1147.150509

Konig, M. F., Abusleme, L., Reinholdt, J., Palmer, R. J., Teles, R. P., Sampson, K., Rosen, A., Nigrovic, P. A., Sokolove, J., Giles, J. T., Moutsopoulos, N. M., & Andrade, F. (2016). Aggregatibacter actinomycetemcomitans-induced hypercitrullination links periodontal infection to autoimmunity in rheumatoid arthritis. *Science Translational Medicine*, *8*(369), 369ra176. 10.1126/scitranslmed.aaj1921

Krishnamurthy, A., Joshua, V., Haj Hensvold, A., Jin, T., Sun, M., Vivar, N., Ytterberg, A. J., Engström, M., Fernandes-Cerqueira, C., Amara, K., Magnusson, M., Wigerblad, G., Kato, J., Jiménez-Andrade, J. M., Tyson, K., Rapecki, S., Lundberg, K., Catrina, S. B., Jakobsson, P. J., Svensson, C., ... & Catrina, A. I. (2016). Identification of a novel chemokine-dependent molecular mechanism underlying rheumatoid arthritis-associated autoantibody-mediated bone loss. *Annals of the Rheumatic Diseases*, *75*(4), 721–729. 10.1136/annrheumdis-2015-208093

Kuo, C. F., Grainge, M. J., Valdes, A. M., See, L. C., Yu, K. H., Shaw, S. W. S., Luo, S. F., Zhang, W., & Doherty, M. (2017). Familial aggregation of rheumatoid arthritis and co-aggregation of autoimmune diseases in affected families: A nationwide population-based study. *Rheumatology (Oxford, England)*, *56*(6), 928–933. 10.1093/rheumatology/kew500

Lee, J. E., Kim, I. J., Cho, M. S., & Lee, J. (2017). A case of rheumatoid vasculitis Involving hepatic artery in early rheumatoid arthritis. *Journal of Korean Medical Science*, *32*(7), 1207–1210. 10.3346/jkms.2017.32.7.1207

Lee, S. J., Lee, A., Hwang, S. R., Park, J. S., Jang, J., Huh, M. S., Jo, D. G., Yoon, S. Y., Byun, Y., Kim, S. H., Kwon, I. C., Youn, I., & Kim, K. (2014). TNF-α gene silencing using polymerized siRNA/thiolated glycol chitosan nanoparticles for rheumatoid arthritis. *Molecular Therapy: The Journal of the American Society of Gene Therapy*, *22*(2), 397–408. 10.1038/mt.2013.245

Linares, V., Alonso, V., & Domingo, J. L. (2011). Oxidative stress as a mechanism underlying sulfasalazine-induced toxicity. *Expert Opinion on Drug Safety*, *10*(2), 253–263. 10.1517/14740338.2011.529898

Liu, D., Ahmet, A., Ward, L., Krishnamoorthy, P., Mandelcorn, E. D., Leigh, R., Brown, J. P., Cohen, A., & Kim, H. (2013). A practical guide to the monitoring and management of the complications of systemic corticosteroid therapy. *Allergy, Asthma, and Clinical Immunology: Official Journal of the Canadian Society of Allergy and Clinical Immunology*, *9*(1), 30. 10.1186/1710-1492-9-30

Lopez-Olivo, M. A., Tayar, J. H., Martinez-Lopez, J. A., Pollono, E. N., Cueto, J. P., Gonzales-Crespo, M. R., Fulton, S., & Suarez-Almazor, M. E. (2012). Risk of malignancies in patients with rheumatoid arthritis treated with biologic therapy: A meta-analysis. *JAMA*, *308*(9), 898–908. 10.1001/2012.jama.10857

Louie, G. H., & Ward, M. M. (2010). Changes in the rates of joint surgery among patients with rheumatoid arthritis in California, 1983–2007. *Annals of the Rheumatic Diseases*, *69*(5), 868–871. 10.1136/ard.2009.112474

Low, A. S., Symmons, D. P., Lunt, M., Mercer, L. K., Gale, C. P., Watson, K. D., Dixon, W. G., Hyrich, K. L., & British Society for Rheumatology Biologics Register for Rheumatoid Arthritis (BSRBR-RA) and the BSRBR Control Centre Consortium (2017). Relationship between exposure to tumour necrosis factor inhibitor therapy and incidence and severity of myocardial infarction in patients with rheumatoid arthritis. *Annals of the Rheumatic Diseases*, *76*(4), 654–660. 10.1136/annrheumdis-2016-209784

Lu, M. C., Lai, N. S., Yu, H. C., Huang, H. B., Hsieh, S. C., & Yu, C. L. (2010). Anti-citrullinated protein antibodies bind surface-expressed citrullinated Grp78 on mono-cyte/macrophages and stimulate tumor necrosis factor alpha production. *Arthritis and Rheumatism*, *62*(5), 1213–1223. 10.1002/art.27386

Lundström, S. L., Hensvold, A. H., Rutishauser, D., Klareskog, L., Ytterberg, A. J., Zubarev, R. A., & Catrina, A. I. (2017). IgG Fc galactosylation predicts response to methotrexate in early rheumatoid arthritis. *Arthritis Research & Therapy*, *19*(1), 182. 10.1186/s13075-017-1389-7

Machold, K. P., Stamm, T. A., Eberl, G. J., Nell, V. K., Dunky, A., Uffmann, M., & Smolen, J. S. (2002). Very recent onset arthritis—clinical, laboratory, and radiological findings during the first year of disease. *The Journal of Rheumatology*, *29*(11), 2278–2287.

Makol, A., Davis, J. M., 3rd, Crowson, C. S., Therneau, T. M., Gabriel, S. E., & Matteson, E. L. (2014). Time trends in glucocorticoid use in rheumatoid arthritis: Results from a population-based inception cohort, 1980–1994 versus 1995–2007. *Arthritis Care & Research*, *66*(10), 1482–1488. 10.1002/acr.22365

Malmström, V., Catrina, A. I., & Klareskog, L. (2017). The immunopathogenesis of seropositive rheumatoid arthritis: From triggering to targeting. *Nature Reviews. Immunology*, *17*(1), 60–75. 10.1038/nri.2016.124

Markusse, I. M., Akdemir, G., Dirven, L., Goekoop-Ruiterman, Y. P., van Groenendael, J. H., Han, K. H., Molenaar, T. H., Le Cessie, S., Lems, W. F., van der Lubbe, P. A., Kerstens, P. J., Peeters, A. J., Ronday, H. K., de Sonnaville, P. B., Speyer, I., Stijnen, T., Ten Wolde, S., Huizinga, T. W., & Allaart, C. F. (2016). Long-term outcomes of patients with recent-onset rheumatoid arthritis after 10 years of tight controlled treatment: A randomized trial. *Annals of Internal Medicine*, *164*(8), 523–531. 10.7326/M15-0919

McGonagle, D., Hermann, K. G., & Tan, A. L. (2015). Differentiation between osteoarthritis and psoriatic arthritis: Implications for pathogenesis and treatment in the biologic therapy era. *Rheumatology (Oxford, England)*, *54*(1), 29–38. 10.1093/rheumatology/keu328

McInnes, I. B., & Schett, G. (2011). The pathogenesis of rheumatoid arthritis. *The New England Journal of Medicine*, *365*(23), 2205–2219. 10.1056/NEJMra1004965

McInnes, I. B., & Schett, G. (2017). Pathogenetic insights from the treatment of rheumatoid arthritis. *Lancet (London, England)*, *389*(10086), 2328–2337. 10.1016/S0140-6736 (17)31472-1

McKeown, E., Bykerk, V. P., De Leon, F., Bonner, A., Thorne, C., Hitchon, C. A., Boire, G., Haraoui, B., Ferland, D. S., Keystone, E. C., Pope, J. E., & CATCH Investigators (2012). Quality assurance study of the use of preventative therapies in glucocorticoid-induced osteoporosis in early inflammatory arthritis: Results from the CATCH cohort. *Rheumatology (Oxford, England)*, *51*(9), 1662–1669. 10.1093/rheumatology/kes079

Mélet, J., Mulleman, D., Goupille, P., Ribourtout, B., Watier, H., & Thibault, G. (2013). Rituximab-induced T cell depletion in patients with rheumatoid arthritis: Association with clinical response. *Arthritis and Rheumatism*, *65*(11), 2783–2790. 10.1002/art. 38107

Mellado, M., Martínez-Muñoz, L., Cascio, G., Lucas, P., Pablos, J. L., & Rodríguez-Frade, J. M. (2015). T cell migration in rheumatoid arthritis. *Frontiers in Immunology*, 6, 384. 10.3389/fimmu.2015.00384

Meng, W., Zhu, Z., Jiang, X., Too, C. L., Uebe, S., Jagodic, M., Kockum, I., Murad, S., Ferrucci, L., Alfredsson, L., Zou, H., Klareskog, L., Feinberg, A. P., Ekström, T. J., Padyukov, L., & Liu, Y. (2017). DNA methylation mediates genotype and smoking interaction in the development of anti-citrullinated peptide antibody-positive rheumatoid arthritis. *Arthritis Research & Therapy*, 19(1), 71. 10.1186/s13075-017-1276-2

Mohamed, B. M., Verma, N. K., Davies, A. M., McGowan, A., Crosbie-Staunton, K., Prina-Mello, A., Kelleher, D., Botting, C. H., Causey, C. P., Thompson, P. R., Pruijn, G. J., Kisin, E. R., Tkach, A. V., Shvedova, A. A., & Volkov, Y. (2012). Citrullination of proteins: A common post-translational modification pathway induced by different nanoparticles in vitro and in vivo. *Nanomedicine (London, England)*, 7(8), 1181–1195. 10.2217/nnm.11.177

Moots, R. J., Sebba, A., Rigby, W., Ostor, A., Porter-Brown, B., Donaldson, F., Dimonaco, S., Rubbert-Roth, A., van Vollenhoven, R., & Genovese, M. C. (2017). Effect of tocilizumab on neutrophils in adult patients with rheumatoid arthritis: Pooled analysis of data from phase 3 and 4 clinical trials. *Rheumatology (Oxford, England)*, 56(4), 541–549. 10.1093/rheumatology/kew370

Moreland, L. W., Schiff, M. H., Baumgartner, S. W., Tindall, E. A., Fleischmann, R. M., Bulpitt, K. J., Weaver, A. L., Keystone, E. C., Furst, D. E., Mease, P. J., Ruderman, E. M., Horwitz, D. A., Arkfeld, D. G., Garrison, L., Burge, D. J., Blosch, C. M., Lange, M. L., McDonnell, N. D., & Weinblatt, M. E. (1999). Etanercept therapy in rheumatoid arthritis: A randomized, controlled trial. *Annals of Internal Medicine*, 130(6), 478–486. 10.7326/0003-4819-130-6-199903160-00004

Moreland, L., Bate, G., & Kirkpatrick, P. (2006). Abatacept. *Nature Reviews. Drug Discovery*, 5(3), 185–186. 10.1038/nrd1989

Mori, M., Yamada, R., Kobayashi, K., Kawaida, R., & Yamamoto, K. (2005). Ethnic differences in allele frequency of autoimmune-disease-associated SNPs. *Journal of Human Genetics*, 50(5), 264–266. 10.1007/s10038-005-0246-8

Mota, P., Reddy, V., & Isenberg, D. (2017). Improving B-cell depletion in systemic lupus erythematosus and rheumatoid arthritis. *Expert Review of Clinical Immunology*, 13(7), 667–676. 10.1080/1744666X.2017.1259068

Moura, C. S., Abrahamowicz, M., Beauchamp, M. E., Lacaille, D., Wang, Y., Boire, G., Fortin, P. R., Bessette, L., Bombardier, C., Widdifield, J., Hanly, J. G., Feldman, D., Maksymowych, W., Peschken, C., Barnabe, C., Edworthy, S., Bernatsky, S., & CAN-AIM (2015). Early medication use in new-onset rheumatoid arthritis may delay joint replacement: Results of a large population-based study. *Arthritis Research & Therapy*, 17(1), 197. 10.1186/s13075-015-0713-3

Myasoedova, E., Crowson, C. S., Kremers, H. M., Fitz-Gibbon, P. D., Therneau, T. M., & Gabriel, S. E. (2010). Total cholesterol and LDL levels decrease before rheumatoid arthritis. *Annals of the Rheumatic Diseases*, 69(7), 1310–1314. 10.1136/ard. 2009.122374

Nabi, G., Akhter, N., Wahid, M., Bhatia, K., Mandal, R. K., Dar, S. A., Jawed, A., & Haque, S. (2016). Meta-analysis reveals PTPN22 1858C/T polymorphism confers susceptibility to rheumatoid arthritis in Caucasian but not in Asian population. *Autoimmunity*, 49(3), 197–210. 10.3109/08916934.2015.1134514

Nakamura, S., Suzuki, K., Iijima, H., Hata, Y., Lim, C. R., Ishizawa, Y., Kameda, H., Amano, K., Matsubara, K., Matoba, R., & Takeuchi, T. (2016). Identification of baseline gene expression signatures predicting therapeutic responses to three biologic agents in rheumatoid arthritis: A retrospective observational study. *Arthritis Research & Therapy*, 18, 159. 10.1186/s13075-016-1052-8

Naldini L. (2015). Gene therapy returns to centre stage. *Nature, 526*(7573), 351–360. 10.1038/nature15818

Navarro-Millán, I., Singh, J. A., & Curtis, J. R. (2012). Systematic review of tocilizumab for rheumatoid arthritis: A new biologic agent targeting the interleukin-6 receptor. *Clinical Therapeutics, 34*(4), 788–802.e3. 10.1016/j.clinthera.2012.02.014

Nishimura, K., Sugiyama, D., Kogata, Y., Tsuji, G., Nakazawa, T., Kawano, S., Saigo, K., Morinobu, A., Koshiba, M., Kuntz, K. M., Kamae, I., & Kumagai, S. (2007). Meta-analysis: Diagnostic accuracy of anti-cyclic citrullinated peptide antibody and rheumatoid factor for rheumatoid arthritis. *Annals of Internal Medicine, 146*(11), 797–808. 10.7326/0003-4819-146-11-200706050-00008

Okada, Y., Kim, K., Han, B., Pillai, N. E., Ong, R. T., Saw, W. Y., Luo, M., Jiang, L., Yin, J., Bang, S. Y., Lee, H. S., Brown, M. A., Bae, S. C., Xu, H., Teo, Y. Y., de Bakker, P. I., & Raychaudhuri, S. (2014). Risk for ACPA-positive rheumatoid arthritis is driven by shared HLA amino acid polymorphisms in Asian and European populations. *Human Molecular Genetics, 23*(25), 6916–6926. 10.1093/hmg/ddu387

Okamoto, K., Nakashima, T., Shinohara, M., Negishi-Koga, T., Komatsu, N., Terashima, A., Sawa, S., Nitta, T., & Takayanagi, H. (2017). Osteoimmunology: The conceptual framework unifying the immune and skeletal systems. *Physiological Reviews, 97*(4), 1295–1349. 10.1152/physrev.00036.2016

Olofsson, T., Petersson, I. F., Eriksson, J. K., Englund, M., Nilsson, J. A., Geborek, P., Jacobsson, L. T. H., Askling, J., Neovius, M., & ARTIS Study Group (2017). Predictors of work disability after start of anti-TNF therapy in a national cohort of Swedish patients with rheumatoid arthritis: Does early anti-TNF therapy bring patients back to work? *Annals of the Rheumatic Diseases, 76*(7), 1245–1252. 10.1136/annrheumdis-2016-210239

Ong, C. K., Lirk, P., Tan, C. H., & Seymour, R. A. (2007). An evidence-based update on nonsteroidal anti-inflammatory drugs. *Clinical Medicine & Research, 5*(1), 19–34. 10.3121/cmr.2007.698

Orellana, C., Saevarsdottir, S., Klareskog, L., Karlson, E. W., Alfredsson, L., & Bengtsson, C. (2017). Oral contraceptives, breastfeeding and the risk of developing rheumatoid arthritis: Results from the Swedish EIRA study. *Annals of the Rheumatic Diseases, 76*(11), 1845–1852. 10.1136/annrheumdis-2017-211620

Ostensen, M. (1992). Treatment with immunosuppressive and disease modifying drugs during pregnancy and lactation. *American Journal of Reproductive Immunology, 28*(3–4), 148–152. 10.1111/j.1600-0897.1992.tb00778.x

Owen, S. A., Hider, S. L., Martin, P., Bruce, I. N., Barton, A., & Thomson, W. (2013). Genetic polymorphisms in key methotrexate pathway genes are associated with response to treatment in rheumatoid arthritis patients. *The Pharmacogenomics Journal, 13*(3), 227–234. 10.1038/tpj.2012.7

Padyukov, L., Seielstad, M., Ong, R. T., Ding, B., Rönnelid, J., Seddighzadeh, M., Alfredsson, L., Klareskog, L., & Epidemiological Investigation of Rheumatoid Arthritis (EIRA) study group (2011). A genome-wide association study suggests contrasting associations in ACPA-positive versus ACPA-negative rheumatoid arthritis. *Annals of the Rheumatic Diseases, 70*(2), 259–265. 10.1136/ard.2009.126821

Pajarinen, J., Lin, T. H., Sato, T., Yao, Z., & Goodman, S. B. (2014). Interaction of materials and biology in total joint replacement – successes, challenges and future directions. *Journal of Materials Chemistry. B, 2*(41), 7094–7108. 10.1039/C4TB01005A

Pap, T., & Korb-Pap, A. (2015). Cartilage damage in osteoarthritis and rheumatoid arthritis – two unequal siblings. *Nature Reviews. Rheumatology, 11*(10), 606–615. 10.1038/nrrheum.2015.95

Parameswaran, N., & Patial, S. (2010). Tumor necrosis factor-α signaling in macrophages. *Critical Reviews in Eukaryotic Gene Expression*, *20*(2), 87–103. 10.1615/critreveukargeneexpr.v20.i2.10

Pettit, A. R., Walsh, N. C., Manning, C., Goldring, S. R., & Gravallese, E. M. (2006). RANKL protein is expressed at the pannus-bone interface at sites of articular bone erosion in rheumatoid arthritis. *Rheumatology (Oxford, England)*, *45*(9), 1068–1076. 10.1093/rheumatology/kel045

Pianta, A., Arvikar, S. L., Strle, K., Drouin, E. E., Wang, Q., Costello, C. E., & Steere, A. C. (2017). Two rheumatoid arthritis-specific autoantigens correlate microbial immunity with autoimmune responses in joints. *The Journal of Clinical Investigation*, *127*(8), 2946–2956. 10.1172/JCI93450

Picerno, V., Ferro, F., Adinolfi, A., Valentini, E., Tani, C., & Alunno, A. (2015). One year in review: The pathogenesis of rheumatoid arthritis. *Clinical and Experimental Rheumatology*, *33*(4), 551–558.

Pincus, T., Sokka, T., Castrejón, I., & Cutolo, M. (2013). Decline of mean initial prednisone dosage from 10.3 to 3.6 mg/day to treat rheumatoid arthritis between 1980 and 2004 in one clinical setting, with long-term effectiveness of dosages less than 5 mg/day. *Arthritis Care & Research*, *65*(5), 729–736. 10.1002/acr.21899

Plosker, G. L., & Croom, K. F. (2005). Sulfasalazine: A review of its use in the management of rheumatoid arthritis. *Drugs*, *65*(13), 1825–1849. 10.2165/00003495-200565130-00008

Puddu, G., Cipolla, M., Cerullo, G., Franco, V., & Giannì, E. (2010). Which osteotomy for a valgus knee? *International Orthopaedics*, *34*(2), 239–247. 10.1007/s00264-009-0820-3

Quero, L., Hanser, E., Manigold, T., Tiaden, A. N., & Kyburz, D. (2017). TLR2 stimulation impairs anti-inflammatory activity of M2-like macrophages, generating a chimeric M1/M2 phenotype. *Arthritis Research & Therapy*, *19*(1), 245. 10.1186/s13075-017-1447-1

Quinn, M. A., Gough, A. K., Green, M. J., Devlin, J., Hensor, E. M., Greenstein, A., Fraser, A., & Emery, P. (2006). Anti-CCP antibodies measured at disease onset help identify seronegative rheumatoid arthritis and predict radiological and functional outcome. *Rheumatology (Oxford, England)*, *45*(4), 478–480. 10.1093/rheumatology/kei203

Rahmani, M., Chegini, H., Najafizadeh, S. R., Azimi, M., Habibollahi, P., & Shakiba, M. (2010). Detection of bone erosion in early rheumatoid arthritis: Ultrasonography and conventional radiography versus non-contrast magnetic resonance imaging. *Clinical Rheumatology*, *29*(8), 883–891. 10.1007/s10067-010-1423-5

Raimondo, M. G., Biggioggero, M., Crotti, C., Becciolini, A., & Favalli, E. G. (2017). Profile of sarilumab and its potential in the treatment of rheumatoid arthritis. *Drug Design, Development and Therapy*, *11*, 1593–1603. 10.2147/DDDT.S100302

Rainsford, K. D., Parke, A. L., Clifford-Rashotte, M., & Kean, W. F. (2015). Therapy and pharmacological properties of hydroxychloroquine and chloroquine in treatment of systemic lupus erythematosus, rheumatoid arthritis and related diseases. *Inflammopharmacology*, *23*(5), 231–269. 10.1007/s10787-015-0239-y

Raychaudhuri, S., Sandor, C., Stahl, E. A., Freudenberg, J., Lee, H. S., Jia, X., Alfredsson, L., Padyukov, L., Klareskog, L., Worthington, J., Siminovitch, K. A., Bae, S. C., Plenge, R. M., Gregersen, P. K., & de Bakker, P. I. (2012). Five amino acids in three HLA proteins explain most of the association between MHC and seropositive rheumatoid arthritis. *Nature Genetics*, *44*(3), 291–296. 10.1038/ng.1076

Rezaei, H., Saevarsdottir, S., Geborek, P., Petersson, I. F., van Vollenhoven, R. F., & Forslind, K. (2013). Evaluation of hand bone loss by digital X-ray radiogrammetry as a complement to clinical and radiographic assessment in early rheumatoid arthritis: results from the SWEFOT trial. *BMC Musculoskeletal Disorders*, *14*, 79. 10.1186/1471-2474-14-79

Richards, B. L., Whittle, S. L., van der Heijde, D. M., & Buchbinder, R. (2012). The efficacy and safety of antidepressants in inflammatory arthritis: A cochrane systematic review. *The Journal of Rheumatology. Supplement, 90*, 21–27. 10.3899/jrheum.120338

Rodenburg, R. J., Ganga, A., van Lent, P. L., van de Putte, L. B., & van Venrooij, W. J. (2000). The antiinflammatory drug sulfasalazine inhibits tumor necrosis factor alpha expression in macrophages by inducing apoptosis. *Arthritis and Rheumatism, 43*(9), 1941–1950. 10.1002/1529-0131(200009)43:9<1941::AID-ANR4>3.0.CO;2-O

Roubille, C., Rincheval, N., Dougados, M., Flipo, R. M., Daurès, J. P., & Combe, B. (2017). Seven-year tolerability profile of glucocorticoids use in early rheumatoid arthritis: Data from the ESPOIR cohort. *Annals of the Rheumatic Diseases, 76*(11), 1797–1802. 10.1136/annrheumdis-2016-210135

Ruiz-Limón, P., Ortega, R., Arias de la Rosa, I., Abalos-Aguilera, M. D. C., Perez-Sanchez, C., Jimenez-Gomez, Y., Peralbo-Santaella, E., Font, P., Ruiz-Vilches, D., Ferrin, G., Collantes-Estevez, E., Escudero-Contreras, A., López-Pedrera, C., & Barbarroja, N. (2017). Tocilizumab improves the proatherothrombotic profile of rheumatoid arthritis patients modulating endothelial dysfunction, NETosis, and inflammation. *Translational Research: The Journal of Laboratory and Clinical Medicine, 183*, 87–103. 10.1016/j.trsl.2016.12.003

Sabeh, F., Fox, D., & Weiss, S. J. (2010). Membrane-type I matrix metalloproteinase-dependent regulation of rheumatoid arthritis synoviocyte function. *Journal of Immunology, 184*(11), 6396–6406. 10.4049/jimmunol.0904068

Sames, E., Paterson, H., & Li, C. (2016). Hydroxychloroquine-induced agranulocytosis in a patient with long-term rheumatoid arthritis. *European Journal of Rheumatology, 3*(2), 91–92. 10.5152/eurjrheum.2015.0028

Sanmartí, R., García-Rodríguez, S., Álvaro-Gracia, J. M., Andreu, J. L., Balsa, A., Cáliz, R., Fernández-Nebro, A., Ferraz-Amaro, I., Gómez-Reino, J. J., González-Álvaro, I., Martín-Mola, E., Martínez-Taboada, V. M., Ortiz, A. M., Tornero, J., Marsal, S., & Moreno-Muelas, J. V. (2015). 2014 update of the Consensus Statement of the Spanish Society of Rheumatology on the use of biological therapies in rheumatoid arthritis. *Reumatologia Clinica, 11*(5), 279–294. 10.1016/j.reuma.2015.05.001

Schaible, T. F. (2000). Long term safety of infliximab. *Canadian Journal of Gastroenterology = Journal canadien de gastroenterologie, 14*(Suppl C), 29C–32C. 10.1155/2000/698523

Schatz, A., Trankle, C., Yassen, A., Chipko, C., Rajab, M., Abouzaki, N., & Abbate, A. (2016). Resolution of pericardial constriction with Anakinra in a patient with effusive-constrictive pericarditis secondary to rheumatoid arthritis. *International Journal of Cardiology, 223*, 215–216. 10.1016/j.ijcard.2016.08.131

Schett, G., Redlich, K., Xu, Q., Bizan, P., Gröger, M., Tohidast-Akrad, M., Kiener, H., Smolen, J., & Steiner, G. (1998). Enhanced expression of heat shock protein 70 (hsp70) and heat shock factor 1 (HSF1) activation in rheumatoid arthritis synovial tissue. Differential regulation of hsp70 expression and hsf1 activation in synovial fibroblasts by proinflammatory cytokines, shear stress, and anti-inflammatory drugs. *The Journal of Clinical Investigation, 102*(2), 302–311. 10.1172/JCI2465

Schiff, M. H., & Sadowski, P. (2017). Oral to subcutaneous methotrexate dose-conversion strategy in the treatment of rheumatoid arthritis. *Rheumatology International, 37*(2), 213–218. 10.1007/s00296-016-3621-1

Schiff, M. H., Strand, V., Oed, C., & Loew-Friedrich, I. (2000). Leflunomide: Efficacy and safety in clinical trials for the treatment of rheumatoid arthritis. *Drugs of Today, 36*(6), 383–394. 10.1358/dot.2000.36.6.584259

Schiff, M. H., Yu, E. B., Weinblatt, M. E., Moreland, L. W., Genovese, M. C., White, B., Singh, A., Chon, Y., & Woolley, J. M. (2006). Long-term experience with etanercept in the treatment of rheumatoid arthritis in elderly and younger patients: Patient-reported outcomes from multiple controlled and open-label extension studies. *Drugs & Aging*, 23(2), 167–178. 10.2165/00002512-200623020-00006

Schneeweiss, S., Setoguchi, S., Weinblatt, M. E., Katz, J. N., Avorn, J., Sax, P. E., Levin, R., & Solomon, D. H. (2007). Anti-tumor necrosis factor alpha therapy and the risk of serious bacterial infections in elderly patients with rheumatoid arthritis. *Arthritis and Rheumatism*, 56(6), 1754–1764. 10.1002/art.22600

Schuerwegh, A. J., Ioan-Facsinay, A., Dorjée, A. L., Roos, J., Bajema, I. M., van der Voort, E. I., Huizinga, T. W., & Toes, R. E. (2010). Evidence for a functional role of IgE anticitrullinated protein antibodies in rheumatoid arthritis. *Proceedings of the National Academy of Sciences of the United States of America*, 107(6), 2586–2591. 10.1073/pnas.0913054107

Schuna, A. A. (1998). Update on treatment of rheumatoid arthritis. *Journal of the American Pharmaceutical Association*, 38(6), 728–737. 10.1016/s1086-5802(16)30394-1

Semerano, L., Decker, P., Clavel, G., & Boissier, M. C. (2016). Developments with investigational Janus kinase inhibitors for rheumatoid arthritis. *Expert Opinion on Investigational Drugs*, 25(12), 1355–1359. 10.1080/13543784.2016.1249565

Sergijenko, A., Roelofs, A. J., Riemen, A. H. K. (2016) Bone marrow contribution to synovial hyperplasia following joint surface injury. *Arthritis Research Therapy*, 18(166), 2–11. 10.1186/s13075-016-1060-8

Silman, A. J., & Pearson, J. E. (2002). Epidemiology and genetics of rheumatoid arthritis. *Arthritis Research*, 4(Suppl 3), S265–S272. 10.1186/ar578

Singh, J. A., Noorbaloochi, S., & Singh, G. (2010). Golimumab for rheumatoid arthritis. *The Cochrane Database of Systematic Reviews*, (1), CD008341. 10.1002/14651858.CD008341

Singh, J. A., Saag, K. G., Bridges, S. L., Jr, Akl, E. A., Bannuru, R. R., Sullivan, M. C., Vaysbrot, E., McNaughton, C., Osani, M., Shmerling, R. H., Curtis, J. R., Furst, D. E., Parks, D., Kavanaugh, A., O'Dell, J., King, C., Leong, A., Matteson, E. L., Schousboe, J. T., Drevlow, B., … & McAlindon, T. (2016). 2015 American College of Rheumatology Guideline for the Treatment of Rheumatoid Arthritis. *Arthritis & Rheumatology*, 68(1), 1–26. 10.1002/art.39480

Singh, J. A., Saag, K. G., Bridges, S. L., Jr, Akl, E. A., Bannuru, R. R., Sullivan, M. C., Vaysbrot, E., McNaughton, C., Osani, M., Shmerling, R. H., Curtis, J. R., Furst, D. E., Parks, D., Kavanaugh, A., O'Dell, J., King, C., Leong, A., Matteson, E. L., Schousboe, J. T., Drevlow, B., … American College of Rheumatology (2016). 2015 American College of Rheumatology Guideline for the Treatment of Rheumatoid Arthritis. *Arthritis Care & Research*, 68(1), 1–25. 10.1002/acr.22783

Sizova L. (2008). Approaches to the treatment of early rheumatoid arthritis with disease-modifying antirheumatic drugs. *British Journal of Clinical Pharmacology*, 66(2), 173–178. 10.1111/j.1365-2125.2008.03222.x

Smolen, J. S., Agarwal, S. K., Ilivanova, E., Xu, X. L., Miao, Y., Zhuang, Y., Nnane, I., Radziszewski, W., Greenspan, A., Beutler, A., & Baker, D. (2017). A randomised phase II study evaluating the efficacy and safety of subcutaneously administered ustekinumab and guselkumab in patients with active rheumatoid arthritis despite treatment with methotrexate. *Annals of the Rheumatic Diseases*, 76(5), 831–839. 10.1136/annrheumdis-2016-209831

Smolen, J. S., Breedveld, F. C., Burmester, G. R., Bykerk, V., Dougados, M., Emery, P., Kvien, T. K., Navarro-Compán, M. V., Oliver, S., Schoels, M., Scholte-Voshaar, M., Stamm, T., Stoffer, M., Takeuchi, T., Aletaha, D., Andreu, J. L., Aringer, M., Bergman, M., Betteridge, N., Bijlsma, H., …van der Heijde, D. (2016). Treating rheumatoid arthritis to target: 2014 update of the recommendations of an international task force. *Annals of the Rheumatic Diseases*, 75(1), 3–15. 10.1136/annrheumdis-2015-207524

Smolen, J. S., Kalden, J. R., Scott, D. L., Rozman, B., Kvien, T. K., Larsen, A., Loew-Friedrich, I., Oed, C., & Rosenburg, R. (1999). Efficacy and safety of leflunomide compared with placebo and sulphasalazine in active rheumatoid arthritis: A double-blind, randomised, multicentre trial. European Leflunomide Study Group. *Lancet*, *353*(9149), 259–266. 10.1016/s0140-6736(98)09403-3

Smolen, J. S., Landewé, R., Breedveld, F. C., Buch, M., Burmester, G., Dougados, M., Emery, P., Gaujoux-Viala, C., Gossec, L., Nam, J., Ramiro, S., Winthrop, K., de Wit, M., Aletaha, D., Betteridge, N., Bijlsma, J. W., Boers, M., Buttgereit, F., Combe, B., Cutolo, M., ... & van der Heijde, D. (2014). EULAR recommendations for the management of rheumatoid arthritis with synthetic and biological disease-modifying antirheumatic drugs: 2013 update. *Annals of the Rheumatic Diseases*, *73*(3), 492–509. 10.1136/annrheumdis-2013-204573

Sokka, T., Kautiainen, H., Toloza, S., Mäkinen, H., Verstappen, S. M., Lund Hetland, M., Naranjo, A., Baecklund, E., Herborn, G., Rau, R., Cazzato, M., Gossec, L., Skakic, V., Gogus, F., Sierakowski, S., Bresnihan, B., Taylor, P., McClinton, C., Pincus, T., & QUEST-RA Group (2007). QUEST-RA: Quantitative clinical assessment of patients with rheumatoid arthritis seen in standard rheumatology care in 15 countries. *Annals of the Rheumatic Diseases*, *66*(11), 1491–1496. 10.1136/ard.2006.069252

Steed, P. M., Tansey, M. G., Zalevsky, J., Zhukovsky, E. A., Desjarlais, J. R., Szymkowski, D. E., Abbott, C., Carmichael, D., Chan, C., Cherry, L., Cheung, P., Chirino, A. J., Chung, H. H., Doberstein, S. K., Eivazi, A., Filikov, A. V., Gao, S. X., Hubert, R. S., Hwang, M., Hyun, L., ... & Dahiyat, B. I. (2003). Inactivation of TNF signaling by rationally designed dominant-negative TNF variants. *Science*, *301*(5641), 1895–1898. 10.1126/science.1081297

Stolt, P., Yahya, A., Bengtsson, C., Källberg, H., Rönnelid, J., Lundberg, I., Klareskog, L., Alfredsson, L., & EIRA Study Group (2010). Silica exposure among male current smokers is associated with a high risk of developing ACPA-positive rheumatoid arthritis. *Annals of the Rheumatic Diseases*, *69*(6), 1072–1076. 10.1136/ard.2009.114694

Strand, V., Cohen, S., Schiff, M., Weaver, A., Fleischmann, R., Cannon, G., Fox, R., Moreland, L., Olsen, N., Furst, D., Caldwell, J., Kaine, J., Sharp, J., Hurley, F., & Loew-Friedrich, I. (1999). Treatment of active rheumatoid arthritis with leflunomide compared with placebo and methotrexate. Leflunomide Rheumatoid Arthritis Investigators Group. *Archives of Internal Medicine*, *159*(21), 2542–2550. 10.1001/archinte.159.21.2542

Strand, V., Lee, E. B., Fleischmann, R., Alten, R. E., Koncz, T., Zwillich, S. H., Gruben, D., Wilkinson, B., Krishnaswami, S., & Wallenstein, G. (2016). Tofacitinib versus methotrexate in rheumatoid arthritis: Patient-reported outcomes from the randomised phase III ORAL Start trial. *RMD Open*, *2*(2), e000308. 10.1136/rmdopen-2016-000308

Suurmond, J., Rivellese, F., Dorjée, A. L., Bakker, A. M., Rombouts, Y. J., Rispens, T., Wolbink, G., Zaldumbide, A., Hoeben, R. C., Huizinga, T. W., & Toes, R. E. (2015). Toll-like receptor triggering augments activation of human mast cells by anti-citrullinated protein antibodies. *Annals of the Rheumatic Diseases*, *74*(10), 1915–1923. 10.1136/annrheumdis-2014-205562

Svendsen, A. J., Kyvik, K. O., Houen, G., Junker, P., Christensen, K., Christiansen, L., Nielsen, C., Skytthe, A., & Hjelmborg, J. V. (2013). On the origin of rheumatoid arthritis: The impact of environment and genes – a population based twin study. *PLoS One*, *8*(2), e57304. 10.1371/journal.pone.0057304

Tamai, M., Kawakami, A., Uetani, M., Takao, S., Arima, K., Iwamoto, N., Fujikawa, K., Aramaki, T., Kawashiri, S. Y., Ichinose, K., Kamachi, M., Nakamura, H., Origuchi, T., Ida, H., Aoyagi, K., & Eguchi, K. (2009). A prediction rule for disease outcome in patients with undifferentiated arthritis using magnetic resonance imaging of the wrists and finger joints and serologic autoantibodies. *Arthritis and Rheumatism*, *61*(6), 772–778. 10.1002/art.24711

Too, C. L., Muhamad, N. A., Ilar, A., Padyukov, L., Alfredsson, L., Klareskog, L., Murad, S., Bengtsson, C., & MyEIRA Study Group (2016). Occupational exposure to textile dust increases the risk of rheumatoid arthritis: Results from a Malaysian population-based case-control study. *Annals of the Rheumatic Diseases*, *75*(6), 997–1002. 10.1136/annrheumdis-2015-208278

van der Heijde, D. M., van Riel, P. L., Nuver-Zwart, I. H., & van de Putte, L. B. (2000). Alternative methods for analysis of radiographic damage in a randomized, double blind, parallel group clinical trial comparing hydroxychloroquine and sulfasalazine. *The Journal of Rheumatology*, *27*(2), 535–539.

Van der Helm-van Mil, A. H., Detert, J., le Cessie, S., Filer, A., Bastian, H., Burmester, G. R., Huizinga, T. W., & Raza, K. (2008). Validation of a prediction rule for disease outcome in patients with recent-onset undifferentiated arthritis: Moving toward individualized treatment decision-making. *Arthritis and Rheumatism*, *58*(8), 2241–2247. 10.1002/art.23681

Van der Linden, M. P., Knevel, R., Huizinga, T. W., & van der Helm-van Mil, A. H. (2011). Classification of rheumatoid arthritis: Comparison of the 1987 American College of Rheumatology criteria and the 2010 American College of Rheumatology/European League against Rheumatism criteria. *Arthritis and Rheumatism*, *63*(1), 37–42. 10.1002/art.30100

Van der Linden, M. P., le Cessie, S., Raza, K., van der Woude, D., Knevel, R., Huizinga, T. W., & van der Helm-van Mil, A. H. (2010). Long-term impact of delay in assessment of patients with early arthritis. *Arthritis and Rheumatism*, *62*(12), 3537–3546. 10.1002/art.27692

van der Woude, D., Alemayehu, W. G., Verduijn, W., de Vries, R. R., Houwing-Duistermaat, J. J., Huizinga, T. W., & Toes, R. E. (2010). Gene-environment interaction influences the reactivity of autoantibodies to citrullinated antigens in rheumatoid arthritis. *Nature genetics*, *42*(10), 814–816. 10.1038/ng1010-814

Van Doornum, S., McColl, G., & Wicks, I. P. (2005). Tumour necrosis factor antagonists improve disease activity but not arterial stiffness in rheumatoid arthritis. *Rheumatology*, *44*(11), 1428–1432. 10.1093/rheumatology/kei033

van Schouwenburg, P. A., van de Stadt, L. A., de Jong, R. N., van Buren, E. E., Kruithof, S., de Groot, E., Hart, M., van Ham, S. M., Rispens, T., Aarden, L., Wolbink, G. J., & Wouters, D. (2013). Adalimumab elicits a restricted anti-idiotypic antibody response in autoimmune patients resulting in functional neutralisation. *Annals of the Rheumatic Diseases*, *72*(1), 104–109. 10.1136/annrheumdis-2012-201445

Venkatesha, S. H., Dudics, S., Acharya, B., & Moudgil, K. D. (2014). Cytokine-modulating strategies and newer cytokine targets for arthritis therapy. *International Journal of Molecular Sciences*, *16*(1), 887–906. 10.3390/ijms16010887

Verschueren, P., De Cock, D., Corluy, L., Joos, R., Langenaken, C., Taelman, V., Raeman, F., Ravelingien, I., Vandevyvere, K., Lenaerts, J., Geens, E., Geusens, P., Vanhoof, J., Durnez, A., Remans, J., Vander Cruyssen, B., Van Essche, E., Sileghem, A., De Brabanter, G., Joly, J., …CareRA study group (2015). Patients lacking classical poor prognostic markers might also benefit from a step-down glucocorticoid bridging scheme in early rheumatoid arthritis: Week 16 results from the randomized multicenter CareRA trial. *Arthritis Research & Therapy*, *17*(1), 97. 10.1186/s13075-015-0611-8

Verschueren, P., De Cock, D., Corluy, L., Joos, R., Langenaken, C., Taelman, V., Raeman, F., Ravelingien, I., Vandevyvere, K., Lenaerts, J., Geens, E., Geusens, P., Vanhoof, J., Durnez, A., Remans, J., Vander Cruyssen, B., Van Essche, E., Sileghem, A., De Brabanter, G., Joly, J., … & Westhovens, R. (2017). Effectiveness of methotrexate with step-down glucocorticoid remission induction (COBRA Slim) versus other intensive treatment strategies for early rheumatoid arthritis in a treat-to-target approach: 1-year results of CareRA, a randomised pragmatic open-label superiority trial. *Annals of the Rheumatic Diseases, 76*(3), 511–520. 10.1136/annrheumdis-2016-209212

Volin, M. V., Campbell, P. L., Connors, M. A., Woodruff, D. C., & Koch, A. E. (2002). The effect of sulfasalazine on rheumatoid arthritic synovial tissue chemokine production. *Experimental and Molecular Pathology, 73*(2), 84–92. 10.1006/exmp.2002.2460

Wakefield, R. J., Gibbon, W. W., Conaghan, P. G., O'Connor, P., McGonagle, D., Pease, C., Green, M. J., Veale, D. J., Isaacs, J. D., & Emery, P. (2000). The value of sonography in the detection of bone erosions in patients with rheumatoid arthritis: A comparison with conventional radiography. *Arthritis and Rheumatism, 43*(12), 2762–2770. 10. 1002/1529-0131(200012)43:12<2762::AID-ANR16>3.0.CO;2-#

Watkin, L. B., Jessen, B., Wiszniewski, W., Vece, T. J., Jan, M., Sha, Y., Thamsen, M., Santos-Cortez, R. L., Lee, K., Gambin, T., Forbes, L. R., Law, C. S., Stray-Pedersen, A., Cheng, M. H., Mace, E. M., Anderson, M. S., Liu, D., Tang, L. F., Nicholas, S. K., Nahmod, K., ... & Shum, A. K. (2015). COPA mutations impair ER-Golgi transport and cause hereditary autoimmune-mediated lung disease and arthritis. *Nature Genetics, 47*(6), 654–660. 10.1038/ng.3279

Wegner, N., Wait, R., Sroka, A., Eick, S., Nguyen, K. A., Lundberg, K., Kinloch, A., Culshaw, S., Potempa, J., & Venables, P. J. (2010). Peptidylarginine deiminase from Porphyromonas gingivalis citrullinates human fibrinogen and α-enolase: Implications for autoimmunity in rheumatoid arthritis. *Arthritis and Rheumatism, 62*(9), 2662–2672. 10.1002/art.27552

Weinblatt, M. E., Keystone, E. C., Furst, D. E., Moreland, L. W., Weisman, M. H., Birbara, C. A., Teoh, L. A., Fischkoff, S. A., & Chartash, E. K. (2003). Adalimumab, a fully human anti-tumor necrosis factor alpha monoclonal antibody, for the treatment of rheumatoid arthritis in patients taking concomitant methotrexate: The ARMADA trial. *Arthritis and Rheumatism, 48*(1), 35–45. 10.1002/art.10697

Weinblatt, M. E., Mease, P., Mysler, E., Takeuchi, T., Drescher, E., Berman, A., Xing, J., Zilberstein, M., Banerjee, S., & Emery, P. (2015). The efficacy and safety of subcutaneous clazakizumab in patients with moderate-to-severe rheumatoid arthritis and an inadequate response to methotrexate: Results from a multinational, phase IIb, randomized, double-blind, placebo/active-controlled, dose-ranging study. *Arthritis & Rheumatology, 67*(10), 2591–2600. 10.1002/art.39249

Whang, J. A., & Chang, B. Y. (2014). Bruton's tyrosine kinase inhibitors for the treatment of rheumatoid arthritis. *Drug Discovery Today, 19*(8), 1200–1204. 10.1016/j.drudis.2014. 03.028

Whittle, S. L., Colebatch, A. N., Buchbinder, R., Edwards, C. J., Adams, K., Englbrecht, M., Hazlewood, G., Marks, J. L., Radner, H., Ramiro, S., Richards, B. L., Tarner, I. H., Aletaha, D., Bombardier, C., Landewé, R. B., Müller-Ladner, U., Bijlsma, J. W., Branco, J. C., Bykerk, V. P., da Rocha Castelar Pinheiro, G., ... & van der Heijde, D. (2012). Multinational evidence-based recommendations for pain management by pharmacotherapy in inflammatory arthritis: Integrating systematic literature research and expert opinion of a broad panel of rheumatologists in the 3e Initiative. *Rheumatology, 51*(8), 1416–1425. 10.1093/rheumatology/kes032

Wigerblad, G., Bas, D. B., Fernades-Cerqueira, C., Krishnamurthy, A., Nandakumar, K. S., Rogoz, K., Kato, J., Sandor, K., Su, J., Jimenez-Andrade, J. M., Finn, A., Bersellini Farinotti, A., Amara, K., Lundberg, K., Holmdahl, R., Jakobsson, P. J., Malmström, V., Catrina, A. I., Klareskog, L., & Svensson, C. I. (2016). Autoantibodies to citrullinated proteins induce joint pain independent of inflammation via a chemokine-dependent mechanism. *Annals of the Rheumatic Diseases, 75*(4), 730–738. 10.1136/ annrheumdis-2015-208094

Winthrop, K. L., Wouters, A. G., Choy, E. H., Soma, K., Hodge, J. A., Nduaka, C. I., Biswas, P., Needle, E., Passador, S., Mojcik, C. F., & Rigby, W. F. (2017). The safety and immunogenicity of live zoster vaccination in patients with rheumatoid arthritis before starting Tofacitinib: A randomized phase II trial. *Arthritis & Rheumatology*, *69*(10), 1969–1977. 10.1002/art.40187

Wu, X., He, B., Liu, J., Feng, H., Ma, Y., Li, D., Guo, B., Liang, C., Dang, L., Wang, L., Tian, J., Zhu, H., Xiao, L., Lu, C., Lu, A., & Zhang, G. (2016). Molecular insight into gut microbiota and rheumatoid arthritis. *International Journal of Molecular Sciences*, *17*(3), 431. 10.3390/ijms17030431

Xu, X., Zheng, L., Bian, Q., Xie, L., Liu, W., Zhen, G., Crane, J. L., Zhou, X., & Cao, X. (2015). Aberrant activation of TGF-β in subchondral bone at the onset of rheumatoid arthritis joint destruction. *Journal of Bone and Mineral Research: The Official Journal of the American Society for Bone and Mineral Research*, *30*(11), 2033–2043. 10.1002/jbmr.2550

Yamaoka, K. (2016). Janus kinase inhibitors for rheumatoid arthritis. *Current Opinion in Chemical Biology*, *32*, 29–33. 10.1016/j.cbpa.2016.03.006

Yang, Z., Shen, Y., Oishi, H., Matteson, E. L., Tian, L., Goronzy, J. J., & Weyand, C. M. (2016). Restoring oxidant signaling suppresses proarthritogenic T cell effector functions in rheumatoid arthritis. *Science Translational Medicine*, *8*(331), 331ra38. 10.1126/scitranslmed.aad7151

Yue, J., Griffith, J. F., Xiao, F., Shi, L., Wang, D., Shen, J., Wong, P., Li, E. K., Li, M., Li, T. K., Zhu, T. Y., Hung, V. W., Qin, L., & Tam, L. S. (2017). Repair of bone erosion in rheumatoid arthritis by denosumab: A high-resolution peripheral quantitative computed tomography study. *Arthritis Care & Research*, *69*(8), 1156–1163. 10.1002/acr.23133

Zitnay, J., Li, Y., Qin, Z. et al. (2017). Molecular level detection and localization of mechanical damage in collagen enabled by collagen hybridizing peptides. *Nature Communication*, *8*, 14913. 10.1038/ncomms14913

Zvaifler, N. J., Steinman, R. M., Kaplan, G., Lau, L. L., & Rivelis, M. (1985). Identification of immunostimulatory dendritic cells in the synovial effusions of patients with rheumatoid arthritis. *The Journal of Clinical Investigation*, *76*(2), 789–800. 10.1172/JCI112036

14 Newer Approaches in Managing Rheumatoid Arthritis

Yashendra Sethi and Kunal Sharma

14.1 INTRODUCTION

Rheumatoid arthritis (RA) is a systemic chronic inflammatory disease of auto-immune etiology, characterized by poly-articular disease mainly affecting the hands and feet. The pathological changes in RA include immune cell infiltration, synovial hyperplasia, pannus formation, and destruction of articular cartilage and bone. Despite the developments over past decades, the exact etiology remains abstruse. The genetic environmental factors and stochastic factors are taken to be the main culprits, but the disease seems an interplay of a multitude of factors. The patients usually experience morning stiffness and may land into necrosis, granulation, or fibrosis of articular surfaces leading to deformity (Huang et al., 2021).

14.2 CRITERIA FOR DIAGNOSIS

The 390 American College of Rheumatology (ACR) and European League against Rheumatism (EULAR) described a classification for RA (Aletaha et al., 2010), which is as follows:

- 2–10 large joints: 1
- 1–3 small joints (±large joints): 2
- 4–10 small joints (±large joints): 3
- >10 joints (≥1 small joint + any others): 5
- Negative Rheumatoid Factor (RF) and negative Anti-Citrullinated Peptide Antibody (ACPA): 0
- Low-positive RF and/or ACPA ≤3× upper limit of normal for local laboratory assay: 2
- High-positive RF and/or ACPA >3× upper limit of normal: 3
- Abnormal erythrocyte sedimentation rate (ESR) and/or abnormal C-reactive protein (CRP): 1
- Normal CRP and normal ESR: 0
- Patient-reported pain, swelling, and tenderness ≥6 weeks: 1

Patients with a score ≥ 6 are classified as RA.

DOI: 10.1201/9781003348672-14

14.3 BIOMARKERS

New biomarkers are being discovered as a result of advances in our understanding of the pathophysiology of RA processes and the increased interest in exploring the biomarkers associated with various disease phases. The current state of the utilization of biomarkers in the diagnosis, prognosis, and management of RA. The ACR 367 criteria labeled only one biomarker, RF. Consequentially, four biomarkers (RF, ACPA, ESR, CRP) have found their ground.

RFs are autoantibodies directed against the Fc portion of immunoglobulin (Ig) G. In clinical practice, IgM RF is most commonly measured although IgA and IgG RF also exist. RF is found in up to 80% of RA patients but can occur in a myriad of other inflammatory conditions that trigger chronic antigenic stimulation, limiting its specificity.

Autoantibodies to citrullinated protein epitopes have been a focus of biomarker research in RA for many years. Amongst ACPAs, the assay for anti-cyclic citrullinated peptide (anti-CCP2) is widely clinically available and has excellent diagnostic and prognostic value. High titer RF and anti-CCP2 antibodies are both associated with an increased risk of erosive joint damage; anti-CCP2 antibodies may confer a higher risk than RF. High titer anti-CCP2 is associated with better clinical response to certain biologics (rituximab, abatacept) and thus may aid clinicians in personalizing therapy for the greatest chance of response. ESR is an indirect measure of the levels of acute-phase reactants (mainly fibrinogen). ESR levels are influenced by several factors, such as the size, shape, and number of red blood cells, as well as other plasma constituents like immunoglobulins. Elevated ESR levels may be caused by systemic or local inflammatory processes, infection, malignancy, tissue injury, end-stage renal disease, nephrotic syndrome, and obesity. CRP is an acute-phase reactant in the pentraxin protein family, which comprises pattern-recognition molecules involved in the innate immune response. CRP occurs in both acute and chronic inflammatory states, infectious and noninfectious. In the RA synovium, there is an overabundance of pro-inflammatory cytokines that stimulate the production of CRP by the liver, thus making it an attractive candidate as a disease activity biomarker. However, CRP measurement in RA is not foolproof (Shapiro, 2021).

Recently a lot of new biomarkers like antibodies against mutated citrullinated vimentin (anti-MCV), antibodies against carbamylated proteins (anti-CarP), and 14-3-3 eta protein have also become available, which have been added to the armory. Other biomarkers include serum amyloid A-4 protein (SAA4), retinol-binding protein-4 (RBP4), angiotensinogen (AGT) and vitamin D-binding protein (VDBP), Glycoprotein YKL-40, etc. (Mun et al., 2021). Other biomarkers such as anti-CCP, anti-MCV, 14-3-3 eta, cartilage oligomeric matrix protein (COMP), survivin and calprotectin have been correlated to treatment response (Morozzi et al., 2007).

14.4 IMAGING TOOLS

The ACR-EULAR 390 classification describes ultrasonography, computed tomography (CT), and magnetic resonance imaging (MRI) as diagnostic tools for establishing an early diagnosis.

14.5 GENERAL GOALS OF TREATMENT

The treatment of rheumatoid arthritis aims to relieve symptoms, prevent joint destruction, maintain joint function, and preserve quality of life. In the past, rheumatologists and physicians usually followed the classical pyramid approach till the development of biological DMARDs (bDMARDs) for treatment and, afterward now following the inverted-pyramid approach while keeping these objectives in mind (Figure 14.1).

Earlier, the bottom of the pyramid is made up of early patient education, occupational and physical therapy, and the use of high doses of Aspirin. Physical therapists can design exercise programs that maintain or increase range of motion while limiting disuse atrophy. Historically; the pyramid approach has advocated an initial trial of nonsteroidal anti-inflammatory drugs (NSAIDs) with or without low-dose corticosteroids (e.g., prednisolone 5–7 mg/day), and has reserved the use of remitting agents, like conventional DMARDs (csDMARDs) for late in the course of the disease. Many previous studies indicated that in many patients the course of rheumatoid arthritis is progressive and destructive, thus warranting a more aggressive approach to treatment (Mitchell et al., 1986; Pincus et al., 1984; Pincus and Callahan, 1986). On the basis of such data, many rheumatologists supported intervention with potent anti-rheumatic agents, singly or in combination, much earlier than previously recommended. csDMARDs were introduced within the first several months of diagnosis, before extensive joint damage occurred. This classical pyramid approach to treatment may improve functional outcomes and survival rates and was followed till the last decade (Chatzidionysiou et al., 2021).

TNF inhibitors, one of the first bDMARDs developed in 1998 and signaled a new era in the arsenal of RA treatments (Bulpitt, 1999). Subsequent expansion in the number of agents and targets of these agents not only provided further therapeutic options for patients but also informed our understanding of the diseases. Interestingly, distinct targetable nodes within the complex aberrant immune response are emerging: IL-6 receptor (IL-6R) inhibitors, co-stimulation blockade, and anti-CD20 are all effective in RA. Indeed, the concept of molecular disease

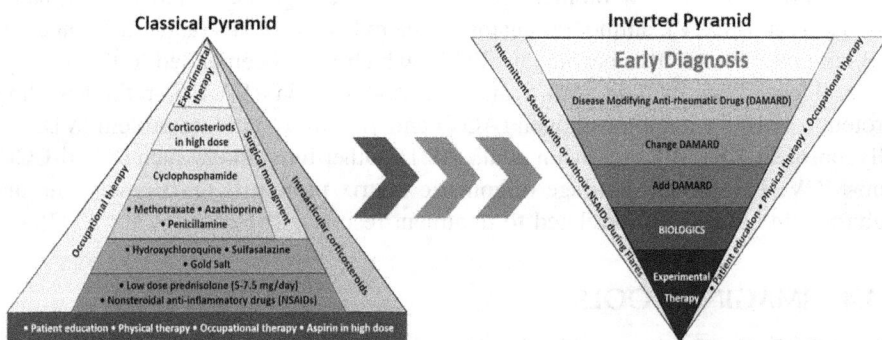

"Classical Pyramid" & "Inverted Pyramid" Treatment Approach of Rheumatoid Arthritis

FIGURE 14.1 Treatment approach of rheumatoid arthritis.

taxonomy, in which diseases can be regrouped according to therapeutically relevant cytokine responses, is emerging (Barturen et al., 2018). This evolving concept is clearly reflected by fascinating developments in biomarker research.

In the past few years, elegant studies have defined distinct synovial pathological subtypes in RA that might represent discrete inherent divisions within the patient population, or temporally contingent 'snapshots' of an evolving synovial landscape (Orange et al., 2018; Orr et al., 2017). Cutting-edge single-cell technology is beginning to enhance the scope of this work and will clarify the relevance of tissue pathotypes (Stephenson et al., 2018). This powerful set of techniques remains at a fledgling stage in translational terms, although uptake and expertise are quickly advancing. Additionally, several ongoing clinical trials are utilizing this divergence in synovial pathology to stratify patients in an effort to achieve improved clinical outcomes [15 ISRCTN10618686]. Parallel studies using peripheral blood-derived cells and serum or plasma biomarkers are also now offering encouraging potential in defining immunologically discrete subgroups of patients with RA; for example, by using autoantibody sub-specificities and titers, proteomic or transcriptional signatures and epigenetic profiles. Taken together, it seems likely that embracing precision medicine principles will inform the development and use of current and next-generation rheumatic disease therapeutics.

In the past five years, the success of Janus kinase (JAK) inhibitors has progressed the field once again (Figure 14.2); these oral agents have equivalent efficacies to bDMARDs in the treatment of several rheumatic diseases and acceptable safety profiles (Winthrop, 2017). Ongoing development of other kinase-targeting agents, such as inhibitors of tyrosine-protein kinases TYK and BTK or inhibitors of RAR-related orphan receptor γ (RORγ)3 (Meier and McInnes, 2014), suggest that this field and concept is set to grow considerably. In contrast to the bDMARDs thus far developed, these small molecule inhibitors affect numerous cytokines and effector immune pathways through interference with a variety of intracellular signaling pathways upon which immune functions converge (Schwartz et al., 2017). Interestingly, this effect is reminiscent of the effects of methotrexate and other

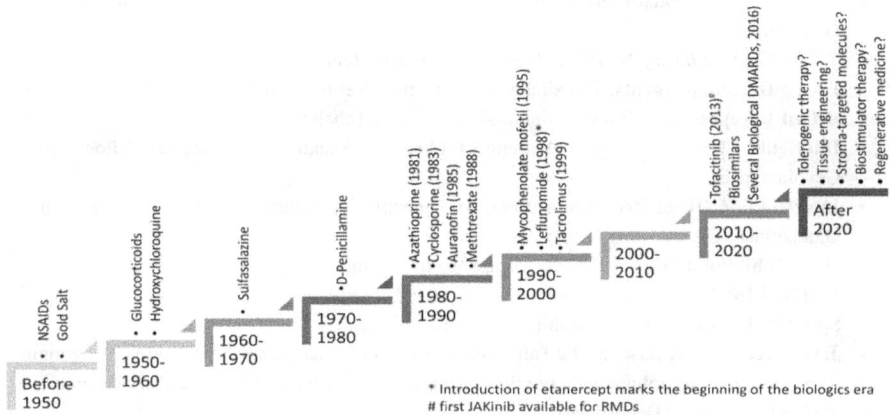

FIGURE 14.2 Drug discovery in rheumatic musculoskeletal diseases.

csDMARDs, which mediate at least some of their effects through the modulation of pivotal immune signaling pathways—the critical difference being that in the case of the latter, the intracellular target was not selected a priori for rheumatic disease application. Examining the immunological effects of well-established older drugs more closely might indirectly identify undiscovered mechanistically relevant pathways.

Finally, multi-omic technologies have become an integral component of modern-day molecular and translational biology (Tasaki et al., 2018). These methodologies produce vast quantities of data, which has prompted the proliferation of applied computational sciences within the field of rheumatology. Coordinating and gaining meaningful outputs from the analysis of big data necessitates the involvement of molecular biologists and bioinformaticians and the application of artificial intelligence. These techniques have gone some way toward answering the most fundamental questions, including what pathophysiological mechanisms underlie disease-specific differential joint patterns (Mizoguchi et al., 2018; Croft et al., 2019).

14.6   TREATMENT STRATEGIES FOR RA

The available current and evolving drugs for the treatment of RA are shown in Table 14.1.

TABLE 14.1

Treatment Modalities for RA

- **Non-steroidal anti-inflammatory drugs (NSAIDs)**
- **Corticosteroids**
- **Conventional Synthetic DMARDs**
  Methotrexate, Hydroxychloroquine, Sulfasalazine, Leflunomide
- **Other Immunomodulatory and Cytotoxic agents**
  Azathioprine, Cyclophosphamide, Cyclosporine A
- **Biological DMARDs as Targeted Therapy**
  - **Tumor Necrosis Factor Inhibitors:** Etanercept, Adalimumab, Infliximab, Certolizumab Pegol, Golimumab
  - **T-Cell Costimulatory Blocking Agents:** Abatacept, Belatacept
  - **B Cell Depleting Agents:** Rituximab, Ofatumumab, Veltuzumab, Ocrelizumab, Epratuzumab
  - **B-Cell Receptor Inhibitors:** Belimumab, Atacicept, Tabalumab
  - **Interleukin-1 (IL-1) Receptor Antagonist Therapy:** Anakinra, Canakinumab, Rilonacept, Gevokizumab
  - **Interleukin-6 (IL-6) Receptor Antagonist Therapy:** Tocilizumab, Sarilumab, Sirukumab, Olokizumab, Clazakizumab
  - **IL-17 inhibitors:** Ixekizumab, Secukinumab, Brodalumab
  - **IL 12/23 Inhibitor:** Ustekinumab
  - **Spleenic Tyrosine Kinase Inhibitor**: Fostamatinib
  - **Janus-Activated-Kinase (JAK) Inhibitors:** Tofacitinib, Baricitinib, Upadacitinib, Filgotinib
  - **Granulocyte-macrophage colony-stimulating factor inhibitor**: Mavrilimumab, Otilimab
  - **RANKL inhibitor**: Denosumab

TABLE 14.1 *(Continued)*
Treatment Modalities for RA

- **Biosimilars**
  - **Adalimumab:** Adalimumab – atto, Adalimumab – adbm, Adalimumab – adaz, Adalimumab – afzb, Adalimumab – bwwd, Adalimumab – fkjp
  - **Infliximab:** Infliximab – abda, Infliximab – axxq, Infliximab – dyyb, Infliximab – qbtx
  - **Etanercept:** Etanercept – szzs, Etanercept – ykro
- **Cell Therapy: Immunomodulation by Mesenchymal stem/stromal cells (MSCs)**
- **Plasma Cell Depletion**
- Epigenetic Factors in RA Therapy
  - **Polyphenols**
  - **DNMT and HDAC Inhibitors**
  - **Anti-Autophagy agents**
- **Reduction of joint stress** – Exercise, Yoga & Physical therapy
- **Surgical approaches** – Arthroplasty & Joint replacement, Arthrodesis, Synovectomy, Tendon release surgery, Tendon transfer surgery

14.7 EVOLVING STRATEGIES FOR RA TREATMENT

In the late 90s and early 2000s, NSAID therapies for treating arthritis were limited and lacked effectiveness on disease progression, though effective at relieving pain and inflammation associated with RA, chronic use of NSAIDs can result in cardiovascular and gastrointestinal (GI) toxicities such as acute coronary syndrome or stomach ulcers. Therefore, historically considered a first-line treatment option for RA, nonsteroidal anti-inflammatory drugs (NSAIDs) have been replaced by conventional and recently biological DMARDs that provide joint protective effects (Fitzgerald, 2004).

14.8 NON-STEROIDAL ANTI-INFLAMMATORY DRUGS

The most often used medications for treating symptoms are NSAIDs. NSAIDs are effective anti-inflammatory and analgesic drugs by virtue of their ability to inhibit the biosynthesis of prostaglandins at the level of the cyclooxygenase enzyme. However, many of the adverse effects of NSAIDs are also related to inhibition of prostaglandin production, making their use problematic in some patient populations. Understanding the biology of prostaglandins as it relates to gastrointestinal, renal, and cardiovascular physiology, as well as the pharmacologic properties of specific NSAIDs, is critical for health professionals to use these drugs safely. Recognizing co-morbid conditions and concurrent medications that may raise the risk of NSAIDs in particular patients is crucial. Using the lowest dose of a medication with a short half-life only when necessary is most likely the safest treatment approach for patients with risk factors for NSAID toxicity. For cost and safety reasons, patients with mild to moderate pain should try acetaminophen as their first line of treatment. However, switching to treatment with NSAIDs may offer more speedy and effective relief if patients have moderate to severe symptoms or if there is evidence of inflammation (Crofford, 2013).

14.9 CORTICOSTEROIDS

Glucocorticoids (GCs), which were first used to treat rheumatoid arthritis (RA) in the late 1940s, presently represent a significant part of the therapeutic approaches for RA. Although GCs are still frequently prescribed medications, there is debate about their toxicity, making it hard to reach a consensus regarding their use in RA. Therefore, the most recent recommendations from the American College of Rheumatology (ACR), and the European League Against Rheumatism (EULAR) on the management of early arthritis and RA support the use of GCs as an adjunct therapy to conventional synthetic DMARDs, at the lowest effective dose and for the shortest period of time and not recommended for long term use. However, the recommendations on dose regimens and routes of administration remain relatively vague. Indeed, numerous items, such as the benefit/risk ratio of low- and very-low-dose GCs and the optimal duration of GCs as bridging therapy, still be on the research focus, and future studies are required to guide the next recommendations for RA (Hua et al., 2020).

14.10 CONVENTIONAL SYNTHETIC DMARDS

Methotrexate (MTX), sulfasalazine, hydroxychloroquine, and leflunomide are the most popular conventional DMARDs. Much less frequently used drugs include azathioprine, Cyclophosphamide, Cyclosporine A, and others. These conventional synthetic DMARDs (csDMARDs) are also known as traditional DMARDs and are still in use. Despite the development of targeted therapies, conventional synthetic disease-modifying antirheumatic drugs remain the cornerstone of the treatment of rheumatoid arthritis (RA). Methotrexate is considered the "anchor drug" due to its high efficacy as monotherapy and in combination with other conventional and targeted agents. Due to its efficacy and safety profile, flexibility to administration, and low price, the 2021 ACR guideline for the treatment of RA accepted methotrexate as a first-line treatment for RA both as monotherapy as well as in combination with other molecules. Leflunomide and sulfasalazine are considered second-line drugs for RA because of their safety profile, whereas hydroxychloroquine is primarily used in combination with other csDMARDs in certain conditions.

DMARDs use is encouraged in all treatment phases either in combination with targeted agents or with other csDMARDs. Combining different csDMARDs is especially attractive in lower-income settings given the evidence proving (almost) equal efficacy and safety of the csDMARD combination approach compared to the combination of targeted agents with a csDMARD (Radu and Bungau, 2021).

14.11 BIOLOGICAL AGENTS

14.11.1 TNF INHIBITORS (TNFi)

Tumor necrosis factor plays an integral role in inflammatory cascade including that involved in RA. High levels of TNF-α have been found in the synovium and synovial fluid of RA patients (Di Giovine et al., 1988). Therefore, TNF forms an important target for symptom relief in RA treatment (Bullock et al., 2018; Singh et al. 2016; Bae and Lee, 2018; Radner and Aletaha, 2015). Five TNF-inhibitory drugs have been approved by the FDA and EMA; these include (Atiqi et al., 2020)

- Infliximab, a chimeric mouse–human monoclonal antibody (mAb)
- Etanercept, a soluble human dimeric TNF-receptor fusion protein first approved anticytokine drug for the treatment of RA. It has also shown its long-term safety and efficacy profile in different clinical trials. It has also shown its role in reducing the radiological progression of disease. There are also a few biosimilars such as Etanercept-szzs and etanercept-ykro available in the market for use. It is given through a subcutaneous route on a twice weekly schedule (Radu and Bungau, 2021).
- Adalimumab and Golimumab, fully human monoclonal antibody and Certolizumab, a PEGylated, Fab' only recombinant humanized antibody (Bullock et al., 2018; Radner and Aletaha, 2015; Mitoma et al., 2018; Moots et al., 2017). There also many approved biosimilars of Adalimumab are available for the treatment of RA.

The advent of TNFi has led to enhanced treatment efficacy and better disease outcomes in RA. However, the associated adverse reactions limit its use, such as an increased risk of infections, hepatotoxicity, hematological changes, and neurological disorders (Bullock et al., 2018; Subedi et al., 2019).

14.11.2 INTERLEUKIN INHIBITORS

Interleukins (IL) are pro-inflammatory cytokines that play a role in RA by starting and maintaining synovial inflammation and associated tissue destruction (Ramírez and Cañete, 2018). The main IL involved in RA are IL-1 and IL-6 and thus their inhibition forms a precise target for RA therapy. The first drug that was approved for the target was Anakinra, a recombinant human interleukin-1 receptor antagonist (Ramírez and Cañete, 2018; Cohen et al., 2002; Mejbri et al., 2020). Canakinumab, a human monoclonal antibody, is a recent addition to the armory, it specifically binds to IL-1ß (Ridker et al., 2017). The IL-1 and IL-6 inhibitors have shown potential, but their efficacy has been found to be lesser than TNFi (Cohen et al., 2002; Abramson, and Amin, 2002; Curtis, and Singh, 2011). They also have a widespread adverse effect profile including urinary and respiratory tract infections, neutropenia, or erythema at the injection site (Fleischmann et al. 2021; Maini et al., 2006).

For IL-6, Tocilizumab is a recombinant humanized monoclonal antibody directed against soluble and membrane-bound interleukin 6 receptors, or Sarilumab, a mAb directed against IL-6 receptor (Raimondo et al., 2017; Sheppard et al., 2017). Furthermore, members of the interleukin 17 (IL-17) family, consisting of six structurally related cytokines, have received more attention (Secukinumab) as potential triggers in autoimmune diseases and playing a relevant role in inflammation, among others (i.e., IL-21, IL-12/23) (McGeachy et al., 2019).

14.11.3   Co-stimulation Blockers

The blockade of T-cell co-stimulation poses to be another great treatment strategy in RA (Mackie et al., 2005). Abatacept is one of the first drugs approved which acts as a selective co-stimulation modulator (Rubbert-Roth et al., 2020; Blair and Deeks, 2017). Structurally, Abatacept is a fusion protein derived by assembly of the Fc region of human IgG_1 and the antigen of the extracellular domain of cytotoxic T-lymphocyte. It specifically binds to the co-stimulatory molecules CD80 and CD86 and thereby blocks interaction with CD28 on T-cells thus helping the ability to selectively modulate and inhibit T-cell activation (Blair and Deeks, 2017; Pombo-Suarez and Gomez-Reino, 2019). It also has an extended effect on Tregs, monocytes, osteoclasts, and B-cells (Bonelli and Scheinecker, 2018). The limited data available suggests promising results, presenting it as a great treatment alternative for RA patients showing an inadequate response to at least one of the agents used in DMARD therapy (Blair and Deeks, 2017; Pombo-Suarez and Gomez-Reino, 2019). Adverse effect profile limits the use and includes nasopharyngitis, headaches and nausea, hepatic disorders, and infections but usually clinical benefit outweighs the risk of adverse effects (Kremer et al., 2005; Szekanecz and Koch, 2016).

14.11.4   CXCL Chemokine Inhibitors

Chemokines are chemotactic cytokines that direct leukocyte recruitment in physiological and pathological processes including those in RA. Increased levels of these cytokines have been seen at sites of inflammation like synovia (Szekanecz and Koch, 2016; Hughes and Nibbs, 2018). Furthermore, these cytokines also direct cell proliferation, cell differentiation, and angiogenic activities. Imbalances or malfunction in the chemokine network thus predispose to the risk of failing immunological assembly opening doors for autoimmune diseases like RA (Elemam et al., 2020). Recent studies have demonstrated a significant role of chemokines in migration of Th1 cells into the synovium. Animal studies have shown promising results of chemokine receptor inhibitors demonstrating a suppressing effect on inflammatory Th1 cells, resulting in decreased synovitis (Szekanecz and Koch, 2016; Elemam et al., 2020). However, the results have not yet been mirrored in human trials with no clinically relevant improvement shown to date (Szekanecz and Koch, 2016). Further studies are warranted to explore this domain and bring the theoretical possibility to life for human benefit.

14.11.5   Anti-B-Cell-Agents

B-cells fundamentally contribute to the pathogenesis of RA through their antibody-dependent and independent functions. They also play an integral role in the secretion of important cytokines and directing the orchestra of inflammatory cells. By virtue of all these functions, the B-cells play a pivotal role in disease pathogenesis. Therefore, their depletion can be an effective treatment strategy (Marston et al., 2010). Various mechanisms have been sought to aid B-cell depletion including but not limited to apoptosis, complement-dependent cytotoxicity, and mediation of antibody-dependent cellular cytotoxicity (Clark and Ledbetter, 2005; Emery et al., 2014; Geh and Gordon, 2018; Giltiay et al., 2017; Milani and Castillo, 2009: Payandeh et al., 2019) which has led to the rise of drugs like Rituximab, Ofatumumab, Veltuzumab or Ocrelizumab, acting as CD20 Abs, and Epratuzumab, targeting CD22. Another potential target from B-cells is the plasma membrane-embedded CD79, which acts as a target protein for pre-plasma cells and B-cells. Inhibiting the CD79 halts the BCR signaling pathway, leading to the depletion of B-cells and germinal centers. Furthermore, CD40/ CD154 forms another potential target (Table 14.1). Stopping the complex formation not only helps attenuate T-cell co-stimulation and B-cell stimulation but also aids the conversion of CD4+ T-cells to Tregs (Li et al., 2013; Lai et al., 2019; Huang and Pope, 2009). The complex formation of TLR 7 and 9 plays an integral role in to inducing B-cell activation and hence can be targeted to inhibit binding between BCR and TLRs (Liu and Davidson 2011; Navarra et al., 2011) (Table 14.1). Another potent target is the inhibition of the transmembrane protein system of B-cell activating factor (BAFF) and a proliferation-inducing ligand (APRIL) (Kaegi et al., 2020; Vincent et al., 2013)

Recent developments have also seen the development of small-molecule inhibitors like Fostamatinib (Table 14.1). Fostamatinib inhibits spleen tyrosine kinase (Syk), a vital non-receptor-type protein tyrosine kinase (PTK) that aids the activation of downstream MAPKs and the PI3K signaling pathway, helping the process of inflammation (Pine et al., 2007).

The use of anti-B-cell agents is also limited by various adverse effects including infections, flushing, nausea, and pruritus (Emery et al., 2014; Giltiay et al., 2017). Due to the involvement of B-cells at various levels and the possibility of different targets, the anti-B-cell agents have shown great efficacy. However, individual differences have been seen in immunogenic and anatomical (synovial) heterogeneity. It is thus believed that a synovial-rich pathotype is more likely to respond to B-cell targeting than others (Barnas et al., 2019).

14.12 SYNTHETIC AGENTS

14.12.1 JANUS-ACTIVATED-KINASE (JAK) INHIBITORS

JAK signaling has been identified as an important pathway regulating the immune response. Many cytokines, interferons, and growth factors act through JAK signaling pathway and contribute to the pathogenesis of RA (Fragoulis et al., 2019; Morinobu, 2020). The JAK/STAT signaling pathway is dysregulated in patients with RA, which leads to continuous activation and thus increased levels of pro-inflammatory proteins in the inflamed synovial tissue.

The past decade has seen the evolution of many drugs targeting the JAK signaling pathway (Table 14.1). Instead of targeting extracellular proteins like biological agents, these suppress intracellular proteins (Hodge et al., 2016). The JAK family comprises four members (JAK1, JAK2, JAK3, tyrosine kinase 2 (TYK2)) exerting their effect through type I and type II receptors (Fragoulis et al., 2019). Tofacitinib is a drug that targets all JAKs (JAK1, JAK2, JAK3, and TYK2 (minimally)) acting as a competitive inhibitor of the ATP binding site of JAK thus reducing the mounted immune response (Hodge et al., 2016). Other agents like Baricitinib (JAK1/ JAK2), Upadacitinib, (JAK1), or Filgotinib (JAK1) only target specific members of the JAK family, reducing adverse effects (Fragoulis et al., 2019). The current recommendations by 2021 ACR guideline JAK inhibitors should be used when csDMARDs fail to control RA progression as higher compliance is observed with monotherapy of JAK inhibitors than with multiple therapies with csDMARDs (Radu and Bungau, 2021). Therefore, JAK inhibitors offer a bright perspective to exploit for the treatment of RA.

14.12.2 Cell Therapy: Immunomodulation by Mesenchymal Stem/Stromal Cells (MSCs)

Therapy using MSCs has a high potential for success, owing to the cells' features of self-renewal, tissue regeneration, and the ability to modulate the immune response (Lopez-Santalla et al., 2020; Luque-Campos et al., 2019). MSC immunomodulatory actions include cell-cell interaction and the synthesis of soluble factors such as IL-1, Indoleamine 2,3-dioxygenase, transforming growth factor ß (TGF-ß), prostaglandin E2, and others. MSCs may move to inflammatory areas and decrease pro-inflammatory cytokine release as well as the proliferation rate of B- and T-cells when activated (Lopez-Santalla et al., 2020; Luque-Campos et al., 2019; Liu et al., 2020). Furthermore, MSCs can direct the development of immune-suppressive cells such as monocytes, dendritic cells, macrophages, myeloid-suppressor cells, and neutrophils, making them a promising candidate for treating autoimmune diseases such as RA (Lopez-Santalla et al., 2020; Luque-Campos et al., 2019). Underlining MSCs immune-modulating properties, studies have shown that the expression of BAFF (B-Cell-Activating Factor) and APRIL (A proliferation-inducing ligand) cytokines can be significantly decreased after MSC transplantation (Gowhari Shabgah et al., 2020), while memory regulatory T cells (Tregs) level can be increased (Luque-Campos et al., 2019). Therefore, MSCs provide an interesting area of exploitation to help patients with RA.

14.12.3 Plasma Cell Depletion

B-cells not only play a pivotal role in inflammatory processes but after being differentiated into plasma cells, also synthesize pathogenic auto-antibodies, which often mediate autoimmune diseases (Hofmann et al., 2018; Wu et al., 2018]. Auto-immune diseases including RA can thus benefit from the elimination of Plasma Cells (PCs) (Hofmann et al., 2018; Smolen et al., 2020). It is, however, important to differentiate between short and long-lived PCs. Short-lived plasmablasts are essentially progenitors of mature plasma cells, living only as long as B-cells are active, but long-lived plasma cells may exist in bone marrow and inflammatory sites for months or even years without needing to interact with B- or T-cells. This context explains why B-cell targeted therapy has no effect on mature plasma cells and highlights the need for plasma cell-directed treatment techniques. Immuno-ablative treatment with anti-thymocyte globulin (ATG) for stem cell transplantation, as well as proteasome inhibitors, are now among the most promising medicines for successfully depleting mature plasma cells. The proteasome serves an important function in the breakdown of regulatory proteins, making it a critical pillar in controlling cellular activities. Inhibiting the proteasome with medicines arrests growth and initiates pro-apoptotic processes, contributing to PC apoptosis and depletion (Mohty, 2007; Hiepe et al., 2015).

14.13 COMBINATIONAL THERAPY

Combination treatment in RA refers to the administration of biological medicines in conjunction with DMARDs, such as MTX. When DMARDs are either poorly tolerated by RA patients or do not show any response and DMARDs monotherapy is ineffective, clinical guidelines propose a combinational treatment with both of them. These guidelines were developed after clinical trials showed that concomitant use of biologics and DMARDs, such as TNFi and MTX, resulted in a considerably greater response than using one of them alone (Smolen et al., 2020; Smolen et al., 2017; Gabay et al., 2015; Teitsma et al., 2016). Furthermore, in patients who did not respond to MTX alone, tocilizumab in conjunction with MTX showed greater benefits than tocilizumab alone (Teitsma et al., 2016). However, the choice of combinational treatment has to be individualized as per the response of patients and the severity of the disease (Smolen et al., 2020; Gabay et al., 2015).

14.14 EPIGENETIC FACTORS IN RA THERAPY

14.14.1 POLYPHENOLS

Over the last decade, epigenetic research has grown in prominence and therapeutic relevance. It is primarily concerned with changes in gene expression and cell phenotypes that are unrelated to changes in DNA sequence, which adds novel quality and a whole new dynamic to the gene expression overview. DNA methylation, chromatin remodeling, post-translational histone modifications, and non-coding RNAs (Li et al., 2007; Zhang and Cao, 2019; Araki et al., 2009) are crucial in regulating gene expression in medicine and numerous processes such as cell proliferation and differentiation, development, cardiovascular diseases, diabetes, autoimmune diseases, and cancer (de la Calle-Fabregat et al., 2021; Nair et al., 2021; Tsai et al., 2021; Chang et al., 2022). In addition to autoimmune illnesses like RA, epigenetic changes have been demonstrated to enhance inflammation in tissues by activating the pro-inflammatory transcription factor nuclear factor kappa B (NF-B) (Ai et al., 2018; Brondello et al., 2019; Buhrmann et al., 2011; Buhrmann et al., 2010; Buhrmann et al., 2013; Csaki et al., 2009; Loh et al., 2019; Mobasheri et al., 2012). Biological components in the diet (polyphenols) have also been shown to possess anti-inflammatory effects through epigenetic mechanisms (Shakibaei et al., 2013; Diomede et al., 2021; Patra et al., 2021; Zhang et al., 2021). Curcumin (diferuloylmethane) is a natural polyphenolic molecule found as a primary component of turmeric (Curcuma Longa) that is utilized as a spice and has extensive anti-inflammatory action and demonstrated advantages in the treatment of autoimmune illnesses, including RA (Kunnumakkara et al., 2017). Curcumin possesses potent anti-inflammatory, antioxidant, and anti-carcinogenic characteristics (Buhrmann et al., 2021a, 2021b; Buhrmann et al., 2014; Buhrmann et al., 2020; Satoskar et al., 1986; Shakibaei et al., 2014; Toden et al., 2015a, 2015b; Zhai et al., 2020) and is a natural inhibitor of the pro-inflammatory transcription factor NF-B, which regulates inflammatory cytokines and proteins during OA and RA (Buhrmann et al., 2010; Buhrmann et al., 2020a, 2020b; Chandran and Goel, 2012). Pilot clinical trial has shown that curcumin can significantly improve the American College of Rheumatology (ACR) Disease Activity Score (DAS). Furthermore, curcumin treatment has been shown to significantly reduce joint stiffness and swelling in patients with RA (Shakibaei et al., 2007; Hanai et al., 2006).

14.14.2   DNMT AND HDAC INHIBITORS

DNA methyltransferase (DNMT) and Histone deacetylase (HDAC) inhibitors have been studied for decades but were recently rediscovered for the treatment of inflammatory illnesses such as RA. DNA methylation and histone acetylation anomalies have been found to be prevalent in RA, presumably contributing to its pathophysiology (Daskalakis et al., 2018; Nakano et al., 2013; Vojinovic and Damjanov, 2011). The enzymes DNMT and HDACs belong to a family of key epigenetic regulators and inhibiting them has the ability to cure pathological processes (Lyko, 2018). Inhibiting DNMT reactivates genes that have been silenced by methylation and restore their normal function, whereas HDAC inhibitors enhance acetylation, resulting in increased DNA transcription activity, decreased cell proliferation, and the initiation of cell death (Castillo-Aguilera et al., 2017; Van Veggel et al., 2018). Studies and clinical studies with the HDAC inhibitor Givinostat have already demonstrated considerable benefits in pathological situations, such as decreased pain and inflammation. HDAC inhibitors, thus represent another promising treatment strategy for RA. The adverse effects of HDAC inhibitors include nausea, gastrointestinal and respiratory disturbances, and fatigue (Vojinovic and Damjanov, 2011; Göschl et al., 2020).

14.14.3   ANTI-AUTOPHAGY AGENTS

Several studies have shown that autophagy and autophagy-related proteins are important participants in immune control and play an important role in autoimmune illnesses such as RA. Furthermore, ablation of these autophagy-related proteins in mice results in an improvement in RA illness and the avoidance of joint degeneration (Wu and Adamopoulos, 2017).

Because autophagy contributes to the clearance of intracellular microorganisms, the generation of pro-inflammatory cytokines, antigen presentation, and lymphocyte dissemination, its regulation is being investigated as an additional target in RA treatment (van Loosdregt et al., 2016). Various therapies are used to modulate autophagy. For example, the autophagy-modulating medicines CQ and HCQ have been demonstrated to be effective in therapeutic applications by suppressing the lysosome, suppressing T-cell activity, and creating apoptosis resistance (Wu and Adamopoulos, 2017; Nirk et al., 2020). Rapamycin is another anti-autophagy agent that acts by activating autophagy and simultaneously inhibiting mTOR, which is activated in various inflammatory diseases (Suto and Karonitsch, 2020).

14.15 CONCLUSION

Rheumatoid arthritis (RA) is a well-known multisystem auto-immune poly-articular disease that leads to deformities of joints due to the progressive destruction of articular cartilage causing chronic disability. Early diagnosis and therapeutic interventions are key steps to prevent serious destruction of joints and loss of vital physical functions. We now have a better understanding of the disease mechanisms because of developments in the area of molecular medicine, which can further aid in the development of more efficient treatment strategies. Old therapeutic approaches have been improved, while new ones have also evolved. Despite these advances, many patients still have insufficient control of their RA or face side effects that are difficult to tolerate. As our understanding of RA grows and we appreciate the mechanisms that cause individual variation in RA symptoms and treatment effects in patients, RA therapies will become more precise, either through improved administration methods or with more individualized targeted therapies. We have included an outline of the most recent biologics/biosimilars, focused small molecule medications, and intriguing compounds under development, as well as developing safety signals related to more recent therapeutic choices. Future researches are still needed to aid clinicians in instructing them on the best ways to treat RA.

REFERENCES

Abramson, S. B., & Amin, A. (2002). Blocking the effects of IL-1 in rheumatoid arthritis protects bone and cartilage. *Rheumatology, 41*(9), 972–980. 10.1093/rheumatology/41.9.972

Ai, R., Laragione, T., Hammaker, D., Boyle, D. L., Wildberg, A., Maeshima, K., Palescandolo, E., Krishna, V., Pocalyko, D., Whitaker, J. W., Bai, Y., Nagpal, S., Bachman, K. E., Ainsworth, R. I., Wang, M., Ding, B., Gulko, P. S., Wang, W., & Firestein, G. S. (2018). Comprehensive epigenetic landscape of rheumatoid arthritis fibroblast-like synoviocytes. *Nature communications, 9*(1), 1921. 10.1038/s41467-018-04310-9

Aletaha, D., Neogi, T., Silman, A. J., Funovits, J., Felson, D. T., Bingham, C. O., 3rd, Birnbaum, N. S., Burmester, G. R., Bykerk, V. P., Cohen, M. D., Combe, B., Costenbader, K. H., Dougados, M., Emery, P., Ferraccioli, G., Hazes, J. M., Hobbs, K., Huizinga, T. W., Kavanaugh, A., Kay, J., ... & Hawker, G. (2010). 2010 Rheumatoid arthritis classification criteria: an American College of Rheumatology/European League Against Rheumatism collaborative initiative. *Arthritis and rheumatism, 62*(9), 2569–2581. 10.1002/art.27584

Araki, Y., Wang, Z., Zang, C., Wood, W. H., 3rd, Schones, D., Cui, K., Roh, T. Y., Lhotsky, B., Wersto, R. P., Peng, W., Becker, K. G., Zhao, K., & Weng, N. P. (2009). Genome-wide analysis of histone methylation reveals chromatin state-based regulation of gene transcription and function of memory CD8+ T cells. *Immunity, 30*(6), 912–925. 10.1016/j.immuni.2009.05.006

Atiqi, S., Hooijberg, F., Loeff, F. C., Rispens, T., & Wolbink, G. J. (2020). Immunogenicity of TNF-inhibitors. *Frontiers in immunology*, *11*, 312. 10.3389/fimmu.2020.00312

Bae, S. C., & Lee, Y. H. (2018). Comparative efficacy and safety of biosimilar-infliximab and originator-infliximab in combination with methotrexate in patients with active rheumatoid arthritis: a meta-analysis of randomized controlled trials. *International journal of rheumatic diseases*, *21*(5), 922–929. 10.1111/1756-185X.13305

Barnas, J. L., Looney, R. J., & Anolik, J. H. (2019). B cell targeted therapies in autoimmune disease. *Current opinion in immunology*, *61*, 92–99. 10.1016/j.coi.2019.09.004

Barturen, G., Beretta, L., Cervera, R., Van Vollenhoven, R., & Alarcón-Riquelme, M. E. (2018). Moving towards a molecular taxonomy of autoimmune rheumatic diseases. [Corrigendum: (2018). *Nat Rev Rheumatol.* 14(3), 180. 10.1038/nrrheum.2018.23]. *Nature reviews. Rheumatology*, *14*(2), 75–93. 10.1038/nrrheum.2017.220

Blair, H. A., & Deeks, E. D. (2017). Abatacept: a review in rheumatoid arthritis. *Drugs*, *77*(11), 1221–1233. 10.1007/s40265-017-0775-4

Bonelli, M., & Scheinecker, C. (2018). How does abatacept really work in rheumatoid arthritis? *Current opinion in rheumatology*, *30*(3), 295–300. 10.1097/BOR.0000000000000491

Brondello, J. M., Djouad, F., & Jorgensen, C. (2019). Where to stand with stromal cells and chronic synovitis in rheumatoid arthritis? *Cells*, *8*(10), 1257. 10.3390/cells8101257

Buhrmann, C., Brockmueller, A., Harsha, C., Kunnumakkara, A. B., Kubatka, P., Aggarwal, B. B., & Shakibaei, M. (2021a). Evidence that tumor microenvironment initiates epithelial-to-mesenchymal transition and Calebin A can suppress it in colorectal cancer cells. *Frontiers in pharmacology*, *12*, 699842. 10.3389/fphar.2021.699842

Buhrmann, C., Brockmueller, A., Mueller, A. L., Shayan, P., & Shakibaei, M. (2021b). Curcumin attenuates environment-derived osteoarthritis by Sox9/NF-kB signaling axis. *International journal of molecular sciences*, *22*(14), 7645. 10.3390/ijms2214 7645

Buhrmann, C., Honarvar, A., Setayeshmehr, M., Karbasi, S., Shakibaei, M., & Valiani, A. (2020a). Herbal remedies as potential in cartilage tissue engineering: an overview of new therapeutic approaches and strategies. *Molecules*, *25*(13), 3075. 10.3390/molecules25133075

Buhrmann, C., Kraehe, P., Lueders, C., Shayan, P., Goel, A., & Shakibaei, M. (2014). Curcumin suppresses crosstalk between colon cancer stem cells and stromal fibroblasts in the tumor microenvironment: potential role of EMT. *PLoS one*, *9*(9), e107514. 10.1371/journal.pone.0107514

Buhrmann, C., Mobasheri, A., Busch, F., Aldinger, C., Stahlmann, R., Montaseri, A., & Shakibaei, M. (2011). Curcumin modulates nuclear factor kappaB (NF-kappaB)-mediated inflammation in human tenocytes in vitro: role of the phosphatidylinositol 3-kinase/Akt pathway. *The journal of biological chemistry*, *286*(32), 28556–28566. 10.1074/jbc.M111.256180

Buhrmann, C., Mobasheri, A., Matis, U., & Shakibaei, M. (2010). Curcumin mediated suppression of nuclear factor-κB promotes chondrogenic differentiation of mesen-chymal stem cells in a high-density co-culture microenvironment. *Arthritis research & therapy*, *12*(4), R127. 10.1186/ar3065

Buhrmann, C., Shayan, P., Aggarwal, B. B., & Shakibaei, M. (2013). Evidence that TNF-β (lymphotoxin α) can activate the inflammatory environment in human chondrocytes. *Arthritis research & therapy*, *15*(6), R202. 10.1186/ar4393

Buhrmann, C., Shayan, P., Banik, K., Kunnumakkara, A. B., Kubatka, P., Koklesova, L., & Shakibaei, M. (2020b). Targeting NF-κB signaling by Calebin A, a compound of turmeric, in multicellular tumor microenvironment: potential role of apoptosis induction in CRC cells. *Biomedicines*, *8*(8), 236. 10.3390/biomedicines8080236

Bullock, J., Rizvi, S. A. A., Saleh, A. M., Ahmed, S. S., Do, D. P., Ansari, R. A., & Ahmed, J. (2018). Rheumatoid arthritis: a brief overview of the treatment. *Medical principles and practice: International journal of the Kuwait University, Health Science Centre*, 27(6), 501–507. 10.1159/000493390

Bulpitt K. J. (1999). Biologic therapies in rheumatoid arthritis. *Current rheumatology reports*, 1(2), 157–163. 10.1007/s11926-999-0013-5

Castillo-Aguilera, O., Depreux, P., Halby, L., Arimondo, P. B., & Goossens, L. (2017). DNA methylation targeting: the DNMT/HMT crosstalk challenge. *Biomolecules*, 7(1), 3. 10.3390/biom7010003

Chandran, B., & Goel, A. (2012). A randomized, pilot study to assess the efficacy and safety of curcumin in patients with active rheumatoid arthritis. *Phytotherapy research: PTR*, 26(11), 1719–1725. 10.1002/ptr.4639

Chang, C., Xu, L., Zhang, R., Jin, Y., Jiang, P., Wei, K., Xu, L., Shi, Y., Zhao, J., Xiong, M., Guo, S., & He, D. (2022). MicroRNA-mediated epigenetic regulation of rheumatoid arthritis susceptibility and pathogenesis. *Frontiers in immunology*, 13, 838884. 10.3389/fimmu.2022.838884

Chatzidionysiou, K., Liapi, M., Tsakonas, G., Gunnarsson, I., & Catrina, A. (2021). Treatment of rheumatic immune-related adverse events due to cancer immunotherapy with immune checkpoint inhibitors-is it time for a paradigm shift? *Clinical rheumatology*, 40(5), 1687–1695. 10.1007/s10067-020-05420-w

Clark, E. A., & Ledbetter, J. A. (2005). How does B cell depletion therapy work, and how can it be improved? *Annals of the rheumatic diseases*, 64 (Suppl 4), iv77–iv80. 10.1136/ard. 2005.042507

Cohen, S., Hurd, E., Cush, J., Schiff, M., Weinblatt, M. E., Moreland, L. W., Kremer, J., Bear, M. B., Rich, W. J., & McCabe, D. (2002). Treatment of rheumatoid arthritis with anakinra, a recombinant human interleukin-1 receptor antagonist, in combination with methotrexate: results of a twenty-four-week, multicenter, randomized, double-blind, placebo-controlled trial. *Arthritis and rheumatism*, 46(3), 614–624. 10.1002/art.10141

Crofford L. J. (2013). Use of NSAIDs in treating patients with arthritis. *Arthritis research & therapy*, 15(Suppl 3), S2. 10.1186/ar4174

Croft, A. P., Campos, J., Jansen, K., Turner, J. D., Marshall, J., Attar, M., Savary, L., Wehmeyer, C., Naylor, A. J., Kemble, S., Begum, J., Dürholz, K., Perlman, H., Barone, F., McGettrick, H. M., Fearon, D. T., Wei, K., Raychaudhuri, S., Korsunsky, I., Brenner, M. B., ... & Buckley, C. D. (2019). Distinct fibroblast subsets drive inflammation and damage in arthritis. *Nature*, 570(7760), 246–251. 10.1038/s41586-019-1263-7

Csaki, C., Mobasheri, A., & Shakibaei, M. (2009). Synergistic chondroprotective effects of curcumin and resveratrol in human articular chondrocytes: inhibition of IL-1beta-induced NF-kappaB-mediated inflammation and apoptosis. *Arthritis research & therapy*, 11(6), R165. 10.1186/ar2850

Curtis, J. R., & Singh, J. A. (2011). Use of biologics in rheumatoid arthritis: current and emerging paradigms of care. *Clinical therapeutics*, 33(6), 679–707. 10.1016/j.clinthera.2011.05.044

Daskalakis, M., Brocks, D., Sheng, Y. H., Islam, M. S., Ressnerova, A., Assenov, Y., Milde, T., Oehme, I., Witt, O., Goyal, A., Kühn, A., Hartmann, M., Weichenhan, D., Jung, M., & Plass, C. (2018). Reactivation of endogenous retroviral elements via treatment with DNMT- and HDAC-inhibitors. *Cell cycle (Georgetown, Tex.)*, 17(7), 811–822. 10.1080/15384101.2018.1442623

de la Calle-Fabregat, C., Niemantsverdriet, E., Cañete, J. D., Li, T., van der Helm-van Mil, A. H. M., Rodríguez-Ubreva, J., & Ballestar, E. (2021). Prediction of the progression of undifferentiated arthritis to rheumatoid arthritis using DNA methylation profiling. *Arthritis & rheumatology*, 73(12), 2229–2239. 10.1002/art.41885

Di Giovine, F. S., Nuki, G., & Duff, G. W. (1988). Tumour necrosis factor in synovial exudates. *Annals of the rheumatic diseases*, 47(9), 768–772. 10.1136/ard.47.9.768

Diomede, F., Fonticoli, L., Guarnieri, S., Della Rocca, Y., Rajan, T. S., Fontana, A., Trubiani, O., Marconi, G. D., & Pizzicannella, J. (2021). The effect of liposomal curcumin as an anti-inflammatory strategy on lipopolysaccharide E from *Porphyromonas gingivalis* treated endothelial committed neural crest derived stem cells: morphological and molecular mechanisms. *International journal of molecular sciences*, *22*(14), 7534. 10.3390/ijms22147534

Elemam, N. M., Hannawi, S., & Maghazachi, A. A. (2020). Role of chemokines and chemokine receptors in rheumatoid arthritis. *ImmunoTargets and therapy*, *9*, 43–56. 10.2147/ITT.S243636

Emery, P., Rigby, W., Tak, P. P., Dörner, T., Olech, E., Martin, C., Millar, L., Travers, H., & Fisheleva, E. (2014). Safety with ocrelizumab in rheumatoid arthritis: results from the ocrelizumab phase III program. *PLoS one*, *9*(2), e87379. 10.1371/journal.pone.0087379

Fitzgerald G. A. (2004). Coxibs and cardiovascular disease. *The New England journal of medicine*, *351*(17), 1709–1711. 10.1056/NEJMp048288

Fleischmann, R., Genovese, M. C., Maslova, K., Leher, H., Praestgaard, A., & Burmester, G. R. (2021). Long-term safety and efficacy of sarilumab over 5 years in patients with rheumatoid arthritis refractory to TNF inhibitors. *Rheumatology*, *60*(11), 4991–5001. 10.1093/rheumatology/keab355

Fragoulis, G. E., McInnes, I. B., & Siebert, S. (2019). JAK-inhibitors. New players in the field of immune-mediated diseases, beyond rheumatoid arthritis. *Rheumatology*, *58*(Suppl 1), i43–i54. 10.1093/rheumatology/key276

Gabay, C., Riek, M., Scherer, A., Finckh, A., & SCQM collaborating physicians (2015). Effectiveness of biologic DMARDs in monotherapy versus in combination with synthetic DMARDs in rheumatoid arthritis: data from the Swiss Clinical Quality Management Registry. *Rheumatology*, *54*(9), 1664–1672. 10.1093/rheumatology/kev019

Geh, D., & Gordon, C. (2018). Epratuzumab for the treatment of systemic lupus erythematosus. *Expert review of clinical immunology*, *14*(4), 245–258. 10.1080/1744666X.2018.1450141

Giltiay, N. V., Shu, G. L., Shock, A., & Clark, E. A. (2017). Targeting CD22 with the monoclonal antibody epratuzumab modulates human B-cell maturation and cytokine production in response to Toll-like receptor 7 (TLR7) and B-cell receptor (BCR) signaling. *Arthritis research & therapy*, *19*(1), 91. 10.1186/s13075-017-1284-2

Göschl, L., Preglej, T., Boucheron, N., Saferding, V., Müller, L., Platzer, A., Hirahara, K., Shih, H. Y., Backlund, J., Matthias, P., Niederreiter, B., Hladik, A., Kugler, M., Gualdoni, G. A., Scheinecker, C., Knapp, S., Seiser, C., Holmdahl, R., Tillmann, K., Plasenzotti, R., ... & Bonelli, M. (2020). Histone deacetylase 1 (HDAC1): a key player of T cell-mediated arthritis. *Journal of autoimmunity*, *108*, 102379. 10.1016/j.jaut.2019.102379

Gowhari Shabgah, A., Shariati-Sarabi, Z., Tavakkol-Afshari, J., Ghasemi, A., Ghoryani, M., & Mohammadi, M. (2020). A significant decrease of BAFF, APRIL, and BAFF receptors following mesenchymal stem cell transplantation in patients with refractory rheumatoid arthritis. *Gene*, *732*, 144336. 10.1016/j.gene.2020

Hanai, H., Iida, T., Takeuchi, K., Watanabe, F., Maruyama, Y., Andoh, A., Tsujikawa, T., Fujiyama, Y., Mitsuyama, K., Sata, M., Yamada, M., Iwaoka, Y., Kanke, K., Hiraishi, H., Hirayama, K., Arai, H., Yoshii, S., Uchijima, M., Nagata, T., & Koide, Y. (2006). Curcumin maintenance therapy for ulcerative colitis: randomized, multicenter, double-blind, placebo-controlled trial. *Clinical gastroenterology and hepatology: the official clinical practice journal of the American Gastroenterological Association*, *4*(12), 1502–1506. 10.1016/j.cgh.2006.08.008

Hiepe, F., Alexander, T., & Voll, R. E. (2015). Plasmazellen [Plasma cells]. *Zeitschrift fur Rheumatologie*, *74*(1), 20–25. 10.1007/s00393-014-1438-4

Hodge, J. A., Kawabata, T. T., Krishnaswami, S., Clark, J. D., Telliez, J. B., Dowty, M. E., Menon, S., Lamba, M., & Zwillich, S. (2016). The mechanism of action of tofacitinib – an oral Janus kinase inhibitor for the treatment of rheumatoid arthritis. *Clinical and experimental rheumatology*, *34*(2), 318–328.

Hofmann, K., Clauder, A. K., & Manz, R. A. (2018). Targeting B cells and plasma cells in autoimmune diseases. *Frontiers in immunology*, *9*, 835. 10.3389/fimmu.2018.00835

Hua, C., Buttgereit, F., & Combe, B. (2020). Glucocorticoids in rheumatoid arthritis: current status and future studies. *RMD open*, *6*(1), e000536. 10.1136/rmdopen-2017-000536

Huang, J., Fu, X., Chen, X., Li, Z., Huang, Y., & Liang, C. (2021). Promising therapeutic targets for treatment of rheumatoid arthritis. *Frontiers in immunology*, *12*, 686155. 10.3389/fimmu.2021.686155

Huang, Q. Q., & Pope, R. M. (2009). The role of toll-like receptors in rheumatoid arthritis. *Current rheumatology reports*, *11*(5), 357–364. 10.1007/s11926-009-0051-z

Hughes, C. E., & Nibbs, R. J. B. (2018). A guide to chemokines and their receptors. *The FEBS journal*, *285*(16), 2944–2971. 10.1111/febs.14466

ISRCTN registry. Stratification of biologic therapies for rheumatoid arthritis by pathobiology. http://www.isrctn.com/ISRCTN10618686. [Last accessed on 14 Oct. 2022)

Kaegi, C., Steiner, U. C., Wuest, B., Crowley, C., & Boyman, O. (2020). Systematic review of safety and efficacy of atacicept in treating immune-mediated disorders. *Frontiers in immunology*, *11*, 433. 10.3389/fimmu.2020.00433

Kremer, J. M., Dougados, M., Emery, P., Durez, P., Sibilia, J., Shergy, W., Steinfeld, S., Tindall, E., Becker, J. C., Li, T., Nuamah, I. F., Aranda, R., & Moreland, L. W. (2005). Treatment of rheumatoid arthritis with the selective costimulation modulator abatacept: twelve-month results of a phase IIb, double-blind, randomized, placebo-controlled trial. *Arthritis and rheumatism*, *52*(8), 2263–2271. 10.1002/art.21201

Kunnumakkara, A. B., Bordoloi, D., Padmavathi, G., Monisha, J., Roy, N. K., Prasad, S., & Aggarwal, B. B. (2017). Curcumin, the golden nutraceutical: multitargeting for multiple chronic diseases. *British journal of pharmacology*, *174*(11), 1325–1348. 10.1111/bph.13621

Lai, J. H., Luo, S. F., & Ho, L. J. (2019). Targeting the CD40-CD154 signaling pathway for treatment of autoimmune arthritis. *Cells*, *8*(8), 927. 10.3390/cells8080927

Li, B., Carey, M., & Workman, J. L. (2007). The role of chromatin during transcription. *Cell*, *128*(4), 707–719. 10.1016/j.cell.2007.01.015

Li, R., Wang, T., Bird, S., Zou, J., Dooley, H., & Secombes, C. J. (2013). B cell receptor accessory molecule CD79α: characterisation and expression analysis in a cartilaginous fish, the spiny dogfish (Squalus acanthias). *Fish & shellfish immunology*, *34*(6), 1404–1415. 10.1016/j.fsi.2013.02.015

Liu, H., Li, R., Liu, T., Yang, L., Yin, G., & Xie, Q. (2020). Immunomodulatory effects of mesenchymal stem cells and mesenchymal stem cell-derived extracellular vesicles in rheumatoid arthritis. *Frontiers in immunology*, *11*, 1912. 10.3389/fimmu.2020.01912

Liu, Z., & Davidson, A. (2011). BAFF inhibition: a new class of drugs for the treatment of autoimmunity. *Experimental cell research*, *317*(9), 1270–1277. 10.1016/j.yexcr.2011.02.005

Loh, C., Park, S. H., Lee, A., Yuan, R., Ivashkiv, L. B., & Kalliolias, G. D. (2019). TNF-induced inflammatory genes escape repression in fibroblast-like synoviocytes: transcriptomic and epigenomic analysis. *Annals of the rheumatic diseases*, *78*(9), 1205–1214. 10.1136/annrheumdis-2018-214783

Lopez-Santalla, M., Fernandez-Perez, R., & Garin, M. I. (2020). Mesenchymal stem/stromal cells for rheumatoid arthritis treatment: an update on clinical applications. *Cells*, *9*(8), 1852. 10.3390/cells9081852

Luque-Campos, N., Contreras-López, R. A., Jose Paredes-Martínez, M., Torres, M. J., Bahraoui, S., Wei, M., Espinoza, F., Djouad, F., Elizondo-Vega, R. J., & Luz-Crawford, P. (2019). Mesenchymal stem cells improve rheumatoid arthritis progression by controlling memory T cell response. *Frontiers in immunology*, *10*, 798. 10.33 89/fimmu.2019.00798

Lyko, F. (2018). The DNA methyltransferase family: a versatile toolkit for epigenetic regulation. *Nature reviews. Genetics*, *19*(2), 81–92. 10.1038/nrg.2017.80

Mackie, S. L., Vital, E. M., Ponchel, F., & Emery, P. (2005). Co-stimulatory blockade as therapy for rheumatoid arthritis. *Current rheumatology reports*, *7*(5), 400–406. 10. 1007/s11926-005-0029-4

Maini, R. N., Taylor, P. C., Szechinski, J., Pavelka, K., Bröll, J., Balint, G., Emery, P., Raemen, F., Petersen, J., Smolen, J., Thomson, D., Kishimoto, T., & CHARISMA Study Group (2006). Double-blind randomized controlled clinical trial of the interleukin-6 receptor antagonist, tocilizumab, in European patients with rheumatoid arthritis who had an incomplete response to methotrexate. *Arthritis and rheumatism*, *54*(9), 2817–2829. 10. 1002/art.22033

Marston, B., Palanichamy, A., & Anolik, J. H. (2010). B cells in the pathogenesis and treatment of rheumatoid arthritis. *Current opinion in rheumatology*, *22*(3), 307–315. 10.1097/BOR.0b013e3283369cb8

McGeachy, M. J., Cua, D. J., & Gaffen, S. L. (2019). The IL-17 family of cytokines in health and disease. *Immunity*, *50*(4), 892–906. 10.1016/j.immuni.2019.03.021

Meier, F. M., & McInnes, I. B. (2014). Small-molecule therapeutics in rheumatoid arthritis: scientific rationale, efficacy and safety. *Best practice & research. Clinical rheumatology*, *28*(4), 605–624. 10.1016/j.berh.2014.10.017

Mejbri, M., Theodoropoulou, K., Hofer, M., & Cimaz, R. (2020). Interleukin-1 blockade in systemic juvenile idiopathic arthritis. *Paediatric drugs*, *22*(3), 251–262. 10.1007/s402 72-020-00392-5

Milani, C., & Castillo, J. (2009). Veltuzumab, an anti-CD20 mAb for the treatment of non-Hodgkin's lymphoma, chronic lymphocytic leukemia and immune thrombocytopenic purpura. *Current opinion in molecular therapeutics*, *11*(2), 200–207.

Mitchell, D. M., Spitz, P. W., Young, D. Y., Bloch, D. A., McShane, D. J., & Fries, J. F. (1986). Survival, prognosis, and causes of death in rheumatoid arthritis. *Arthritis and rheumatism*, *29*(6), 706–714. 10.1002/art.1780290602

Mitoma, H., Horiuchi, T., Tsukamoto, H., & Ueda, N. (2018). Molecular mechanisms of action of anti-TNF-α agents – comparison among therapeutic TNF-α antagonists. *Cytokine*, *101*, 56–63. 10.1016/j.cyto.2016.08.014

Mizoguchi, F., Slowikowski, K., Wei, K., Marshall, J. L., Rao, D. A., Chang, S. K., Nguyen, H. N., Noss, E. H., Turner, J. D., Earp, B. E., Blazar, P. E., Wright, J., Simmons, B. P., Donlin, L. T., Kalliolias, G. D., Goodman, S. M., Bykerk, V. P., Ivashkiv, L. B., Lederer, J. A., Hacohen, N., ... & Brenner, M. B. (2018). Functionally distinct disease-associated fibroblast subsets in rheumatoid arthritis. *Nature communications*, *9*(1), 789. 10.1038/s41467-018-02892-y

Mobasheri, A., Henrotin, Y., Biesalski, H. K., & Shakibaei, M. (2012). Scientific evidence and rationale for the development of curcumin and resveratrol as nutraceutricals for joint health. *International journal of molecular sciences*, *13*(4), 4202–4232. 10.3390/ ijms13044202

Mohty M. (2007). Mechanisms of action of antithymocyte globulin: T-cell depletion and beyond. *Leukemia*, *21*(7), 1387–1394. 10.1038/sj.leu.2404683

Moots, R. J., Xavier, R. M., Mok, C. C., Rahman, M. U., Tsai, W. C., Al-Maini, M. H., Pavelka, K., Mahgoub, E., Kotak, S., Korth-Bradley, J., Pedersen, R., Mele, L., Shen, Q., & Vlahos, B. (2017). The impact of anti-drug antibodies on drug concentrations and clinical outcomes in rheumatoid arthritis patients treated with adalimumab, etanercept, or infliximab: results from a multinational, real-world clinical practice, non-interventional study. *PLoS one*, *12*(4), e0175207. 10.1371/journal.pone.0175207

Morinobu A. (2020). JAK inhibitors for the treatment of rheumatoid arthritis. *Immunological medicine*, *43*(4), 148–155. 10.1080/25785826.2020.1770948

Morozzi, G., Fabbroni, M., Bellisai, F., Cucini, S., Simpatico, A., & Galeazzi, M. (2007). Low serum level of COMP, a cartilage turnover marker, predicts rapid and high ACR70 response to adalimumab therapy in rheumatoid arthritis. *Clinical rheumatology*, *26*(8), 1335–1338. 10.1007/s10067-006-0520-y

Mun, S., Lee, J., Park, M., Shin, J., Lim, M. K., & Kang, H. G. (2021). Serum biomarker panel for the diagnosis of rheumatoid arthritis. *Arthritis research & therapy*, *23*(1), 31. 10.1186/s13075-020-02405-7

Nair, N., Barton, A., & Wilson, A. G. (2021). Cell-specific epigenetic drivers of pathogenesis in rheumatoid arthritis. *Epigenomics*, *13*(7), 549–560. 10.2217/epi-2020-0380

Nakano, K., Boyle, D. L., & Firestein, G. S. (2013). Regulation of DNA methylation in rheumatoid arthritis synoviocytes. *Journal of immunology*, *190*(3), 1297–1303. 10.4049/jimmunol.1202572

Navarra, S. V., Guzmán, R. M., Gallacher, A. E., Hall, S., Levy, R. A., Jimenez, R. E., Li, E. K., Thomas, M., Kim, H. Y., León, M. G., Tanasescu, C., Nasonov, E., Lan, J. L., Pineda, L., Zhong, Z. J., Freimuth, W., Petri, M. A., & BLISS-52 Study Group (2011). Efficacy and safety of belimumab in patients with active systemic lupus erythematosus: a randomised, placebo-controlled, phase 3 trial. *Lancet*, *377*(9767), 721–731. 10.1016/S0140-6736(10)61354-2

Nirk, E. L., Reggiori, F., & Mauthe, M. (2020). Hydroxychloroquine in rheumatic autoimmune disorders and beyond. *EMBO molecular medicine*, *12*(8), e12476. 10.15252/emmm.202012476

Orange, D. E., Agius, P., DiCarlo, E. F., Robine, N., Geiger, H., Szymonifka, J., McNamara, M., Cummings, R., Andersen, K. M., Mirza, S., Figgie, M., Ivashkiv, L. B., Pernis, A. B., Jiang, C. S., Frank, M. O., Darnell, R. B., Lingampali, N., Robinson, W. H., Gravallese, E., Accelerating Medicines Partnership in Rheumatoid Arthritis and Lupus Network, … Donlin, L. T. (2018). Identification of three rheumatoid arthritis disease subtypes by machine learning integration of synovial histologic features and RNA sequencing data. *Arthritis & rheumatology*, *70*(5), 690–701. 10.1002/art.40428

Orr, C., Vieira-Sousa, E., Boyle, D. L., Buch, M. H., Buckley, C. D., Cañete, J. D., Catrina, A. I., Choy, E. H. S., Emery, P., Fearon, U., Filer, A., Gerlag, D., Humby, F., Isaacs, J. D., Just, S. A., Lauwerys, B. R., Le Goff, B., Manzo, A., McGarry, T., McInnes, I. B., … & Tas, S. W. (2017). Synovial tissue research: a state-of-the-art review. [Corrigendum: (2017). *Nature reviews. Rheumatology*, *13*(10), 630. 10.1038/nrrheum.2017.161; Corrigendum: (2017), *Nature reviews. Rheumatology*, *14*(1), 60. 10.1038/nrrheum. 2017.206]. *Nature reviews. Rheumatology*, *13*(8), 463–475. 10.1038/nrrheum.2017.115

Patra, S., Pradhan, B., Nayak, R., Behera, C., Das, S., Patra, S. K., Efferth, T., Jena, M., & Bhutia, S. K. (2021). Dietary polyphenols in chemoprevention and synergistic effect in cancer: clinical evidences and molecular mechanisms of action. *Phytomedicine: international journal of phytotherapy and phytopharmacology*, *90*, 153554. 10.1016/j.phymed.2021.153554

Payandeh, Z., Bahrami, A. A., Hoseinpoor, R., Mortazavi, Y., Rajabibazl, M., Rahimpour, A., Taromchi, A. H., & Khalil, S. (2019). The applications of anti-CD20 antibodies to treat various B cells disorders. *Biomedicine & pharmacotherapy [Biomedecine & pharmacotherapie]*, *109*, 2415–2426. 10.1016/j.biopha.2018.11.121

Pincus, T., & Callahan, L. F. (1986). Taking mortality in rheumatoid arthritis seriously – predictive markers, socioeconomic status and comorbidity. *The journal of rheumatology*, *13*(5), 841–845.

Pincus, T., Callahan, L. F., Sale, W. G., Brooks, A. L., Payne, L. E., & Vaughn, W. K. (1984). Severe functional declines, work disability, and increased mortality in seventy-five rheumatoid arthritis patients studied over nine years. *Arthritis and rheumatism, 27*(8), 864–872. 10.1002/art.1780270805

Pine, P. R., Chang, B., Schoettler, N., Banquerigo, M. L., Wang, S., Lau, A., Zhao, F., Grossbard, E. B., Payan, D. G., & Brahn, E. (2007). Inflammation and bone erosion are suppressed in models of rheumatoid arthritis following treatment with a novel Syk inhibitor. *Clinical immunology, 124*(3), 244–257. 10.1016/j.clim.2007.03.543

Pombo-Suarez, M., & Gomez-Reino, J. J. (2019). Abatacept for the treatment of rheumatoid arthritis. *Expert review of clinical immunology, 15*(4), 319–326. 10.1080/1744666X.2019.1579642

Radner, H., & Aletaha, D. (2015). Anti-TNF in rheumatoid arthritis: an overview. *Wiener medizinische Wochenschrift (1946), 165*(1-2), 3–9. 10.1007/s10354-015-0344-y

Radu, A. F., & Bungau, S. G. (2021). Management of rheumatoid arthritis: an overview. *Cells, 10*(11), 2857. 10.3390/cells10112857

Raimondo, M. G., Biggioggero, M., Crotti, C., Becciolini, A., & Favalli, E. G. (2017). Profile of sarilumab and its potential in the treatment of rheumatoid arthritis. *Drug design, development and therapy, 11*, 1593–1603. 10.2147/DDDT.S100302

Ramírez, J., & Cañete, J. D. (2018). Anakinra for the treatment of rheumatoid arthritis: a safety evaluation. *Expert opinion on drug safety, 17*(7), 727–732. 10.1080/14740338.2018.1486819

Ridker, P. M., Everett, B. M., Thuren, T., MacFadyen, J. G., Chang, W. H., Ballantyne, C., Fonseca, F., Nicolau, J., Koenig, W., Anker, S. D., Kastelein, J. J. P., Cornel, J. H., Pais, P., Pella, D., Genest, J., Cifkova, R., Lorenzatti, A., Forster, T., Kobalava, Z., Vida-Simiti, L., ...CANTOS Trial Group (2017). Antiinflammatory therapy with Canakinumab for atherosclerotic disease. *The New England journal of medicine, 377*(12), 1119–1131. 10.1056/NEJMoa1707914

Rubbert-Roth, A., Enejosa, J., Pangan, A. L., Haraoui, B., Rischmueller, M., Khan, N., Zhang, Y., Martin, N., & Xavier, R. M. (2020). Trial of Upadacitinib or Abatacept in rheumatoid arthritis. *The New England journal of medicine, 383*(16), 1511–1521. 10.1056/NEJMoa2008250

Satoskar, R. R., Shah, S. J., & Shenoy, S. G. (1986). Evaluation of anti-inflammatory property of curcumin (diferuloylmethane) in patients with postoperative inflammation. *International journal of clinical pharmacology, therapy, and toxicology, 24*(12), 651–654.

Schwartz, D. M., Kanno, Y., Villarino, A., Ward, M., Gadina, M., & O'Shea, J. J. (2017). JAK inhibition as a therapeutic strategy for immune and inflammatory diseases. [Corrigendum: *Nature reviews. Drug discovery, 17*(1), 78. 10.1038/nrd.2017.267]. *Nature reviews. Drug discovery, 16*(12), 843–862. 10.1038/nrd.2017.201

Shakibaei, M., Buhrmann, C., Kraehe, P., Shayan, P., Lueders, C., & Goel, A. (2014). Curcumin chemosensitizes 5-fluorouracil resistant MMR-deficient human colon cancer cells in high density cultures. *PLoS one, 9*(1), e85397. 10.1371/journal.pone.0085397

Shakibaei, M., John, T., Schulze-Tanzil, G., Lehmann, I., & Mobasheri, A. (2007). Suppression of NF-kappaB activation by curcumin leads to inhibition of expression of cyclo-oxygenase-2 and matrix metalloproteinase-9 in human articular chondrocytes: implications for the treatment of osteoarthritis. *Biochemical pharmacology, 73*(9), 1434–1445. 10.1016/j.bcp.2007.01.005

Shakibaei, M., Mobasheri, A., Lueders, C., Busch, F., Shayan, P., & Goel, A. (2013). Curcumin enhances the effect of chemotherapy against colorectal cancer cells by inhibition of NF-κB and Src protein kinase signaling pathways. *PLoS one, 8*(2), e57218. 10.1371/journal.pone.0057218

Shapiro S. C. (2021). Biomarkers in rheumatoid arthritis. *Cureus*, *13*(5), e15063. 10.7759/cureus.15063

Sheppard, M., Laskou, F., Stapleton, P. P., Hadavi, S., & Dasgupta, B. (2017). Tocilizumab (Actemra). *Human vaccines & immunotherapeutics*, *13*(9), 1972–1988. 10.1080/21645515.2017.1316909

Singh, J. A., Saag, K. G., Bridges, S. L., Jr, Akl, E. A., Bannuru, R. R., Sullivan, M. C., Vaysbrot, E., McNaughton, C., Osani, M., Shmerling, R. H., Curtis, J. R., Furst, D. E., Parks, D., Kavanaugh, A., O'Dell, J., King, C., Leong, A., Matteson, E. L., Schousboe, J. T., Drevlow, B., ... & McAlindon, T. (2016). 2015 American College of Rheumatology guideline for the treatment of rheumatoid arthritis. *Arthritis & rheumatology*, *68*(1), 1–26. 10.1002/art.39480

Smolen, J. S., Landewé, R. B. M., Bijlsma, J. W. J., Burmester, G. R., Dougados, M., Kerschbaumer, A., McInnes, I. B., Sepriano, A., van Vollenhoven, R. F., de Wit, M., Aletaha, D., Aringer, M., Askling, J., Balsa, A., Boers, M., den Broeder, A. A., Buch, M. H., Buttgereit, F., Caporali, R., Cardiel, M. H., ... & van der Heijde, D. (2020). EULAR recommendations for the management of rheumatoid arthritis with synthetic and biological disease-modifying antirheumatic drugs: 2019 update. *Annals of the rheumatic diseases*, *79*(6), 685–699. 10.1136/annrheumdis-2019-216655

Smolen, J. S., Landewé, R., Bijlsma, J., Burmester, G., Chatzidionysiou, K., Dougados, M., Nam, J., Ramiro, S., Voshaar, M., van Vollenhoven, R., Aletaha, D., Aringer, M., Boers, M., Buckley, C. D., Buttgereit, F., Bykerk, V., Cardiel, M., Combe, B., Cutolo, M., van Eijk-Hustings, Y., ... & van der Heijde, D. (2017). EULAR recommendations for the management of rheumatoid arthritis with synthetic and biological disease-modifying antirheumatic drugs: 2016 update. *Annals of the rheumatic diseases*, *76*(6), 960–977. 10.1136/annrheumdis-2016-210715

Stephenson, W., Donlin, L. T., Butler, A., Rozo, C., Bracken, B., Rashidfarrokhi, A., Goodman, S. M., Ivashkiv, L. B., Bykerk, V. P., Orange, D. E., Darnell, R. B., Swerdlow, H. P., & Satija, R. (2018). Single-cell RNA-seq of rheumatoid arthritis synovial tissue using low-cost microfluidic instrumentation. *Nature communications*, *9*(1), 791. 10.1038/s41467-017-02659-x

Subedi, S., Gong, Y., Chen, Y., & Shi, Y. (2019). Infliximab and biosimilar infliximab in psoriasis: efficacy, loss of efficacy, and adverse events. *Drug design, development and therapy*, *13*, 2491–2502. 10.2147/DDDT.S200147

Suto, T., & Karonitsch, T. (2020). The immunobiology of mTOR in autoimmunity. *Journal of autoimmunity*, *110*, 102373. 10.1016/j.jaut.2019.102373

Szekanecz, Z., & Koch, A. E. (2016). Successes and failures of chemokine-pathway targeting in rheumatoid arthritis. *Nature reviews. Rheumatology*, *12*(1), 5–13. 10.1038/nrrheum.2015.157

Tasaki, S., Suzuki, K., Kassai, Y., Takeshita, M., Murota, A., Kondo, Y., Ando, T., Nakayama, Y., Okuzono, Y., Takiguchi, M., Kurisu, R., Miyazaki, T., Yoshimoto, K., Yasuoka, H., Yamaoka, K., Morita, R., Yoshimura, A., Toyoshiba, H., & Takeuchi, T. (2018). Multi-omics monitoring of drug response in rheumatoid arthritis in pursuit of molecular remission. *Nature communications*, *9*(1), 2755. 10.1038/s41467-018-05044-4

Teitsma, X. M., Marijnissen, A. K., Bijlsma, J. W., Lafeber, F. P., & Jacobs, J. W. (2016). Tocilizumab as monotherapy or combination therapy for treating active rheumatoid arthritis: a meta-analysis of efficacy and safety reported in randomized controlled trials. *Arthritis research & therapy*, *18*(1), 211. 10.1186/s13075-016-1108-9

Toden, S., Okugawa, Y., Buhrmann, C., Nattamai, D., Anguiano, E., Baldwin, N., Shakibaei, M., Boland, C. R., & Goel, A. (2015a). Novel evidence for curcumin and boswellic acid-induced chemoprevention through regulation of miR-34a and miR-27a in colorectal cancer. *Cancer prevention research*, *8*(5), 431–443. 10.1158/1940-6207.CAPR-14-0354

Toden, S., Okugawa, Y., Jascur, T., Wodarz, D., Komarova, N. L., Buhrmann, C., Shakibaei, M., Boland, C. R., & Goel, A. (2015b). Curcumin mediates chemosensitization to 5-fluorouracil through miRNA-induced suppression of epithelial-to-mesenchymal transition in chemoresistant colorectal cancer. *Carcinogenesis*, *36*(3), 355–367. 10.1093/carcin/bgv006

Tsai, C. Y., Hsieh, S. C., Liu, C. W., Lu, C. H., Liao, H. T., Chen, M. H., Li, K. J., Wu, C. H., Shen, C. Y., Kuo, Y. M., & Yu, C. L. (2021). The expression of non-coding RNAs and their target molecules in rheumatoid arthritis: a molecular basis for rheumatoid pathogenesis and its potential clinical applications. *International journal of molecular sciences*, *22*(11), 5689. 10.3390/ijms22115689

van Loosdregt, J., Rossetti, M., Spreafico, R., Moshref, M., Olmer, M., Williams, G. W., Kumar, P., Copeland, D., Pischel, K., Lotz, M., & Albani, S. (2016). Increased autophagy in CD4$^+$ T cells of rheumatoid arthritis patients results in T-cell hyperactivation and apoptosis resistance. *European journal of immunology*, *46*(12), 2862–2870. 10.1002/eji.201646375

Van Veggel, M., Westerman, E., & Hamberg, P. (2018). Clinical pharmacokinetics and pharmacodynamics of panobinostat. *Clinical pharmacokinetics*, *57*(1), 21–29. 10.1007/s40262-017-0565-x

Vincent, F. B., Saulep-Easton, D., Figgett, W. A., Fairfax, K. A., & Mackay, F. (2013). The BAFF/APRIL system: emerging functions beyond B cell biology and autoimmunity. *Cytokine & growth factor reviews*, *24*(3), 203–215. 10.1016/j.cytogfr.2013.04.003

Vojinovic, J., & Damjanov, N. (2011). HDAC inhibition in rheumatoid arthritis and juvenile idiopathic arthritis. *Molecular medicine*, *17*(5–6), 397–403. 10.2119/molmed.2011.00030

Winthrop K. L. (2017). The emerging safety profile of JAK inhibitors in rheumatic disease. [Corrigendum: *Nature reviews. Rheumatology*, *13*(5), 320. 10.1038/nrrheum.2017.51]. *Nature reviews. Rheumatology*, *13*(4), 234–243. 10.1038/nrrheum.2017.23

Wu, D. J., & Adamopoulos, I. E. (2017). Autophagy and autoimmunity. *Clinical immunology*, *176*, 55–62. 10.1016/j.clim.2017.01.007

Wu, H., Deng, Y., Feng, Y., Long, D., Ma, K., Wang, X., Zhao, M., Lu, L., & Lu, Q. (2018). Epigenetic regulation in B-cell maturation and its dysregulation in autoimmunity. *Cellular & molecular immunology*, *15*(7), 676–684. 10.1038/cmi.2017.133

Zhai, K., Brockmüller, A., Kubatka, P., Shakibaei, M., & Büsselberg, D. (2020). Curcumin's beneficial effects on neuroblastoma: mechanisms, challenges, and potential solutions. *Biomolecules*, *10*(11), 1469. 10.3390/biom10111469

Zhang, Q., & Cao, X. (2019). Epigenetic regulation of the innate immune response to infection. *Nature reviews. Immunology*, *19*(7), 417–432. 10.1038/s41577-019-0151-6

Zhang, S., Li, L., Chen, W., Xu, S., Feng, X., & Zhang, L. (2021). Natural products: the role and mechanism in low-density lipoprotein oxidation and atherosclerosis. *Phytotherapy research: PTR*, *35*(6), 2945–2967. 10.1002/ptr.7002

15 Toxicology and Risk Factors of Nanomedicine Uses

Hitesh Chopra and Kunal Sharma

15.1 INTRODUCTION

Nanoparticles, which range in size from 1 to 100 nm, are the subject of research and manipulation within the field of nanotechnology (Yadav et al. 2022). As a result of their enhanced relative surface area and quantum effects, nanoparticles are gaining popularity for use in a wide range of fields (Bhattacharya et al., 2022; Yousaf et al., 2022). Over the last decade, nanotechnology has come to the forefront of the scientific community owing to its widespread potential applications in fields as diverse as biology (Yadav et al., 2023), electronics (Jindal et al., 2022), aircraft, and computing (Yadav et al., 2024). Nanotechnology has lately found a new home in the subject of nanomedicine, (Yadav et al., 2023a, 2023b) which focuses on the improvement of human health and wellbeing via the detection, treatment, and prevention of human illnesses like cancer using nanotechnology (Chopra et al., 2022; Chopra et al., 2021). Nanoparticles are widely used in the field of nanomedicine as a means of transporting therapeutic agents (Yadav et al., 2022). Polymers, inorganic nanoparticles, and metallic nanoparticles are all examples of possible classifications based on their physicochemical properties (Chopra et al., 2022). Polymers, such as polysaccharide chitosan nanoparticles (CS-NPs), (Yadav et al., 2022) are advantageous in drug delivery due to their ability to facilitate protein and drug conjugation (Divya & Jisha, 2018). The polymer-protein conjugates enhance protein stability while lowering immunogenicity, in contrast to the polymer-drug conjugates, which increase permeability and retention effects. Poly-(lactic-co-glycolic acid) (PLGA) polymeric nanoparticles have recently been used as a nanocarrier for medication transport across the blood-brain barrier, assuring the safety of therapy due to their biocompatibility and biodegradability. Inorganic ceramic nanoparticles, such as silica, titania, and alumina, are appealing for drug delivery in cancer therapy because of their porosity nature. However, their limited use is due to the fact that they are not biodegradable. Due to their capacity to stable nanoparticles and excellent optical/chemical characteristics, silver nanoparticles (AgNP) (Srivastava et al., 2012) are being investigated as antibacterial agents for the treatment of infectious disorders (Bedlovičová et al., 2020; Mathur et al., 2018). However, nanoparticles made of superparamagnetic iron oxide (Panda et al.

DOI: 10.1201/9781003348672-15

2021; Mudgal et al, 2023a, 2023b), gold shell, and titanium dioxide (TiO2) are frequently utilized to improve contrast in MRI scans and transport chemotherapy drugs to tumors. Due to their high electrical conductivity and strength, as well as the numerous attachment sites on fullerenes that are important for tissue binding, carbon nanoparticles (composed of fullerenes and nanotubes) are the most preferred material used for drug administration.

The use of nanoparticles for the discovery of disease biomarkers has advanced proteomics and genomics and has improved in vivo and ex vivo diagnostic applications (Amri et al., 2021; Saha et al., 2020; Pallares et al., 2019; Zhang et al., 2021). Streptadivin-coated fluorescent polystyrene nanospheres are a promising new method for detecting epidermal growth factor receptors (EGFR) in human cancer cells, making them a promising candidate for use as a biomarker (Bhalgat et al., 1998). There was also the development of a nanoparticle-based test for the detection of prostate-specific antigen (PSA) in serum, which might be up to six orders of magnitude more sensitive than the conventional assay (Nam et al., 2003). Small particle size, the capacity to coat surfaces in a variety of ways, and increased stability are just a few of the physicochemical benefits that have helped nanoparticles rise to prominence in the field of molecular diagnostics and imaging (Medina et al., 2007).

Another area where nanotechnology has been put to use is in molecular imaging techniques including magnetic resonance imaging, fluorescence imaging, computed tomography imaging, and ultrasound. Gadolinium-based paramagnetic nanoparticles have been produced to improve the imaging of fibrin in atherosclerotic plaques over traditional contrast agents (Aime et al., 2009; Wang et al., 2010; Flacke et al., 2001). Thus, vulnerable plaques may now be identified at an earlier stage. Nanoparticles have also been proven to improve the drug's solubility, stability, and absorption, in addition to enhancing its targeted specificity (Yadav et al., 2023). Nanoparticle formulations delivering anti-cancer medications including paclitaxel, 5-fluorouracil, and doxorubicin have been shown to be more effective drug delivery methods, increasing the cytotoxic effects of the drug while decreasing non-specific targeting of normal cells.

15.2   NANOPARTICLE-BASED TOXICITY

Nanotechnology is gaining popularity in the medical field, although its applications are restricted because of worries about toxicity and the potential for adverse effects (Lanone & Boczkowski, 2006). Scientists have established a branch called nanotoxicology to study the possible risks associated with employing nanoparticles. While nanoparticles offer many potential applications in nanomedicine, their physical properties, such as their small size, large surface area, and malleable chemical composition/structure, have also been associated with more severe toxicological repercussions (Zielińska et al., 2020). Since the surface area of nanoparticles increases as their size decreases, the smaller the particle, the greater its hazardous effects (Oberdörster et al., 2005). The size and surface area of nanoparticles are considered key characteristics since they significantly and directly affect their toxicity. However, there are other factors than particle size that affect

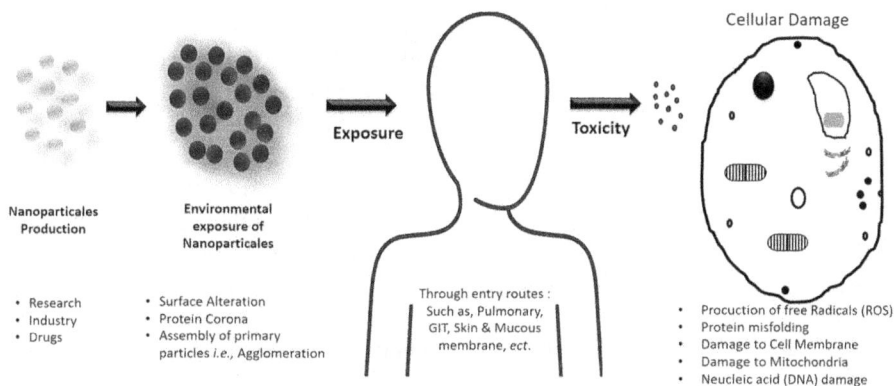

Cellular Damage

Exposure

Toxicity

Nanoparticales
Production

Environmental
exposure of
Nanoparticales

Through entry routes :
Such as, Pulmonary,
GIT, Skin & Mucous
membrane, *ect.*

• Research
• Industry
• Drugs

• Surface Alteration
• Protein Corona
• Assembly of primary
  particles *i.e.,* Agglomeration

• Procuction of free Radicals (ROS)
• Protein misfolding
• Damage to Cell Membrane
• Damage to Mitochondria
• Neucleic acid (DNA) damage

FIGURE 15.1 Toxicological impact of nanoparticles.

nanotoxicity. For instance, studies using carbon nanofibers, SWCNTs, and MWCNTs have shown that particle shape and size affect the toxicity of high-aspect-ratio carbon materials (Salesa et al., 2021). Adsorption of ions and biomolecules onto the nanoparticle surface also adds to nanoparticle-induced toxicity (Li et al., 2015), since it modifies the cellular responses elicited (as shown in Figure 15.1).

Humans may be exposed to nanoparticles via a variety of routes, including inhalation, injection, oral consumption, and skin contact. The respiratory, digestive, circulatory, and central neurological systems are especially susceptible to nanoparticles (Medina et al., 2007). In vivo studies (Morimoto et al., 2013; Dreher, 2004) have shown that long-term exposure to carbon nanotubes causes dose-dependent interstitial inflammation and epithelioid granulomatous lesions in the lungs. It has also been shown that ceramic nanoparticles, which are often used for drug delivery, exhibit oxidative stress/cytotoxic activity in the lungs, liver, heart, and brain and have teratogenic/carcinogenic effects (Singh et al., 2016).

It has been shown that intravenous injection of nanoparticles may enter the systemic circulation, where they can damage the lungs and perhaps even the central nervous system. Platelet aggregation and a rise in vascular thrombosis in the carotid artery of rats were seen in in vitro investigations using engineered carbon nanoparticles and nanotubes (Radomski et al., 2005). According to research using cell models of human kidneys and lungs, SWCNTs promote cell apoptosis and decrease cell adhesion by upregulating genes involved in cell death and downregulating genes related with cell proliferation and survival (Cui et al., 2005; Alazzam et al., 2010). Over the course of 20 days, Wistar rats administered 20 mg/kg TiO2NPs intraperitoneally every two days showed accumulation in their liver, lungs, and brains, with an increase in their aspartate aminotransferase/alanine aminotransferase ratio (AST/ALT ratio) suggesting subacute toxicity. TiO2NPs may translocate and biodistribute to other organs, producing toxicity (Younes et al., 2015). Injected rats exhibited pathological abnormalities in the liver and reduced neuro-behavioral function (as indicated by a raised concerned index).

When given in a single dosage of 500 mg/kg, nanoparticles of titanium dioxide (TiO2), zinc oxide (ZnO), or aluminum oxide (Al2O3) were found in the central nervous system. Axillary toxicity produced by the buildup of these nanoparticles in the brain resulted in abnormalities in neurotransmitter metabolism and, ultimately, brain damage (Shrivastava et al., 2014). When tested on rat astrocytes, different-sized TiO2 nanoparticles were shown to decrease cell survival rates in a dose-dependent manner, causing pathological effects such as cellular edema, brain tissue necrosis, and disruption of the blood-brain barrier. In addition, nano-manganese dioxide (MnO2) was shown to reduce learning capacity in rats by disrupting dopaminergic neuronal activity and activating astrocytes (Liu et al., 2013).

Using cosmetics or wound dressings containing nanomaterials is one of the most prevalent ways that nanoparticles are absorbed via the skin (Zou et al., 2022). It has been claimed that sunscreens containing titanium dioxide (TiO2) may go through the skin's epidermis and into the hair follicles (Lademann et al., 1999). Acticoat, a wound dressing coated with nanocrystalline silver, may now be used in the treatment of burn patients. Although multiple trials have indicated that Acticoat is safe for use on burn patients, a patient with 30% burns who were treated with an Acticoat silver-coated dressing reported having silver poisoning (Trop et al., 2006). Negative effects and worries about nanoparticle buildup in many organs have prevented nanomedicine from reaching its full potential in molecular diagnostics and as medication delivery systems. The development and use of nanoparticles in the area of nanomedicine may be aided by a deeper understanding of the processes of nanotoxicity.

15.3   MECHANISM OF NANOTOXICITY

During the last several years, there has been a dramatic uptick in the usage and study of nanomaterials for cutting-edge biological applications. The potential dangers of nanomaterials to people and the environment have slowed their widespread adoption. Groups with weakened immune systems, fewer defense mechanisms, and less capacity for self-repair, such as the young, the pregnant, and the elderly, are more vulnerable to the adverse effects of nanomaterial exposure. Size, surface, shape, charges, functional groups, chemical composites, activation by ultraviolet (UV) radiation, aggregation and dissolution, and contact with cells are only some of the intrinsic features of nanoparticles that might influence their nanotoxicity. Nanoparticles' cytotoxicity, genotoxicity, and immunotoxicity have not been thoroughly elucidated, nor have their exact mechanisms and consequences. However, certain overarching processes are explored further below, including the overproduction of reactive oxygen species (ROS), inflammation, a failure to degrade or self-degrade, and a shift in cellular shape and the cytoskeleton network. Long-term nanotoxicity studies, in addition to improving nanoparticle qualities to minimize and even eliminate toxicity, are necessary for the safe and well-controlled usage of nanomaterials for the benefit of humanity.

15.3.1   AN EXCESS OF REACTIVE OXYGEN SPECIES

A major mechanism of nanotoxicity is the production of reactive oxygen species (ROS). Most cell types are able to withstand brief elevations in ROS that occur under normal conditions. However, ROS may be damaging if present in large amounts or if their levels are artificially elevated over an extended period of time. When cells are exposed to nanoparticles, they develop an excess of reactive oxygen species (ROS), leading to oxidative stress. Signal transmission may be disrupted and made dysfunctional by reactive oxygen species (ROS) interacting with cellular macromolecules such as functional proteins and DNA. The inability of cells that overproduce ROS to preserve their normal physiological activities increases the risk of pathologies including cancer, fibrosis, and a host of other diseases. Nanoparticles of many different types, but notably those made of metals and carbon, have been shown to induce reactive oxygen species (ROS). Among these nanomaterials, quantum dots and carbon nanotubes have been widely documented to exhibit nanotoxicity owing to the overproduction of reactive oxygen species (ROS) they produce (Horie & Tabei, 2021; Yu et al., 2020).

15.3.2 Nanotoxicity Induced by Inflammation

The immune system functions as the body's first line of defense against pathogens, tumors, and other harmful external substances. Many immunological responses, such as boosting or dampening, are altered after exposure to nanoparticles. Toxic effects on the immune system from exposure to nanoparticles are linked to their ability to produce reactive oxygen species (ROS). The mitochondria of phagocytic cells have been found to create reactive oxygen species (ROS) in response to nanoparticle exposure, activating the inflammasomes (Sun et al., 2013; Müllebner et al., 2018). It is now well established that ROS produced by phagocytes can cause damage to human tissues and play a role in the inflammatory response. Chronic inflammation has been linked to several forms of cell death and has been established as a major contributor to toxicity. Induced apoptosis and autophagy are among the outcomes of producing pro-inflammatory cytokines including TNF-a, IL-1, and IL-8. Studies have shown that lipid-based nanoparticles might trigger hyper-sensitivity responses and even anaphylaxis in certain people (Moghimi, 2021; Alsaleh & Brown, 2020).

15.3.3 Degradation of Nanoparticles

Some nanoparticles are quickly broken down in the microenvironment of the human body, whereas others are either non-degradable or slowly degradable, leading to accumulation in organs or cells and perhaps having a harmful impact in the long run. Nanoparticles' ability to interact or interfere with many biological systems is a key cause for worry. Nanoparticles' large surface area, compact size, and high local charge densities make them able to interact readily with their surrounding biological molecules. Surface charges on nanoparticles, for instance, may encourage their binding of serum enzymes, resulting in a so-called protein corona, which in turn may alter enzymatic regulatory mechanisms.

One of the key modes of action of biodegradable nanoparticles is the intracellular toxic impact they have. Nanoparticle instability may result in the release of hazardous components and a shift in the body's microenvironment.

Nanoparticles may often be taken in by cells through endocytic pathways. Endosomes (pH6) and lysosomes (pH4.5) have pH values that are much lower than the external environment (pH7). Some nanoparticles are degradable and shed their coating on the surface due to the local pH shift and the presence of degradative enzymes in the cells, such as cathepsin L. Research has demonstrated, for instance, that certain iron oxide nanoparticles undergo acid etching in the acidic environment of the endosomes, generating free ions, which causes a reduction in particle size, the loss of magnetic function, and even consequences on cell homeostasis. Hydrogen peroxide and hypochlorous acid, both byproducts of phagocytes, have been discovered to acid etch quantum dots at amounts important to physiology.

15.3.4 ABNORMALITIES IN CELL MORPHOLOGY AND THE CYTOSKELETON

Nanoparticles of certain sizes may change cellular shape and/or functional components such as the cytoskeleton network, mitochondria, and synaptic apparatus, albeit the exact process is yet unknown. It seems to reason that for a cell to carry out its intended tasks, its constituent parts must be in proper working order. Cell shape, motility, division, cell-extracellular matrix sticky contact, and the creation of neural architecture are all greatly influenced by the cytoskeleton. If the cytoskeleton is deformed, the cell will lose some of its ability to operate. Neurotoxicity may be induced by a number of mechanisms, including damage to cytoskeletal proteins like tubulin and actin, dissolution of synaptic proteins, and impairment of mitochondrial function(Akter et al., 2017; Xu et al., 2013; Gurunathan, et al., 2019).

15.4 MODELS FOR TOXICITY EVALUATION

15.4.1 INVITRO MODELS

15.4.1.1 Stem Cell Technology

The toxicity of therapies for several common diseases and conditions, such as those affecting the cardiovascular system, the nervous system, the eyes, the bones, and the immune system, are now evaluated using cell-based evaluations (Buzhor et al., 2014). Toxicology testing may make use of a wide range of stem cell types, including those isolated from fibromatosis (Wang et al., 2018; Kouroupis et al., 2019), mesenchymal (Pang, 2020; Horie et al., 2016), cardiac (51,52 Rikhtegar et al., 2019; Thomson et al., 1998), and embryonic (Horie et al., 2016; Rikhtegar et al., 2019). First described in 1998 (Thomson et al., 1998), human ESC research demonstrates that cells isolated from early human embryos are pluripotent and capable of developing into a wide range of cell types. In light of this, human ESCs may be a viable cell source for future applications in tissue engineering. Using human embryonic stem cells (ESCs) for toxicological research or testing is controversial due to ethical and religious considerations (Volarevic et al., 2018; Kugler et al., 2017). The use of human embryos in ESC research is controversial from an ethical standpoint (Niemiec & Howard, 2020). To help researchers sidestep potential moral minefields, several have turned their focus to non-traditional stem cell sources (Afshar et al., 2020).

Directly produced from either skin or blood cells, induced pluripotent stem cells (iPSCs) are multipotent stem cells that have the potential to circumvent ethical concerns about scientific publishing (Afshar et al., 2020). The initial iPSC approach was developed by Shinya Yamanaka's group in 2006 (Takahashi & Yamanaka, 2006), and it included the use of four encoding transcription factors to transform adult mice fibroblasts into pluripotent stem cells through reprogramming. These four proteins, collectively known as the "Yamanaka factors," may be used to reprogram and differentiate somatic cells from mice or humans into iPSCs. The iPSCs have the ability to self-renew and can be differentiated into any other cell type. This means that iPSCs may be used for a wide variety of purposes, including tissue healing and safety evaluation, without raising any ethical issues (Peng et al., 2018; Labusca et al., 2018). Some research has effectively integrated genetically diverse iPSCs into cardiotoxicity testing (Luz & Tokar, 2018), a key area in the advancement of toxicity testing employing iPSCs. Recent research has shown that iPSCs, as a cell-based in vitro model, may be used to determine the safety of tailored NPs (Handral et al., 2016). To examine NP toxicity, hepatocyte-like cells (HLCs) derived from induced pluripotent stem cells (iPSCs) are one example of a potential replacement in vitro hepatotoxicity paradigm. The hepatotoxicity of silver NPs (AgNPs) may be evaluated using HLCs generated from iPSCs (Gao et al., 2021). Comparatively, human-induced pluripotent stem cell-derived cardiomyocytes (hiPSC-CMs) may be used to study ZnO NPs' toxicity for cardiac safety assessment (Li et al., 2020). Therefore, iPSCs not only serve as testing platforms for NP toxicity evaluations but also play a role in preclinical drug toxicology investigations.

15.4.1.2   Bioengineering of Tissues

Tissue engineering integrates the study of engineering, materials, medicine, and biology (Garrod & Chau, 2016). The biochemical and physicochemical aspects of many biological tissues may now be modified with the help of tissue engineering. Tissue engineering using scaffolds is a typical method for creating functional tissues for medical or research purposes. One of the most well-known approaches to imitating the physicochemical features of the extracellular matrix is the use of chitosan-based polymers (ECM). Three-dimensional (3D) scaffolds have the potential to improve tissue replacement by creating a favorable environment for cell adhesion and proliferation, which in turn may promote cell differentiation. Smart materials and 3D printing methods each have special features that may be used to determine the final 3D scaffold's form, allowing for highly individualized scaffold designs. 3D scaffolds may be molded to closely resemble tissue (Bezek et al., 2020).

The long-term objective of this method is to replace animal testing with toxicity evaluations performed on biopolymer-based 3D organ models. Cell development and differentiation in 3D organ structure models need the integration of synthetic or natural biological materials and stem cells to offer cell-to-cell contacts and proper cell signaling pathways and allow growth in all directions. When it comes to designing cell-based screening systems in 3D models, the thermally sensitive characteristics, shape memory, and self-healing processes of synthetic materials are considered to be significant elements. Several reports over the last decade have shown that tissue engineering synthetic materials may influence stem cell development by altering their characteristics in 3D culture settings via external stimulation (Dawson et al., 2008).

As an alternative to toxicity evaluation through animal testing, 3D culture settings have been developed via tissue engineering (Movia et al., 2020; Schmidt et al., 2020). Studies of biological processes, disease causes, medication development, and toxicity testing (Kapałczyńska et al., 2018) often use conventional two-dimensional (2D) cell cultures. However, there are many factors that prevent 2D cultures from being a perfect representation of the in vivo environment, including the absence of tissue-tissue interfaces (Jensen & Teng, 2020), the presence of natural barriers, hypoxic gradients, and tight cell-cell junctions that reduce the efficacy of drug diffusion (Koti et al., 2020). Growing cells in 3D overcomes the constraints of 2D culture techniques by simulating the circumstances of tissues. The three most common approaches to generating 3D culture models for scientific study are scaffold-based methods, cell spheroids grown on gel-like substances, and scaffold-free cell cultures in suspension (Kapałczyńska et al., 2018).

15.4.2 IN-SILICO

When it comes to computer simulations and the assessment of chemical-biomolecule interactions based on 3D structural information, molecular docking studies are a viable technique. Docking studies are a kind of molecular modeling that may be used to foretell how tiny molecules (like medicines or NPs) will interact with big macromolecules (e.g., proteins or enzymes). First, a docking study generates every potential conformation and orientation for each ligand, based on the geometry of the designated binding site in the protein structure. In the second phase, scoring functions are run to provide a rough prediction of the protein's affinity for the docked ligand and the orientations in which the ligand may form stable connections with the protein. Docking scores, computed by the scoring functions, are then used to rank each ligand that has been correctly fitted into its binding site, ultimately leading to the identification of the highest affinity ligand for the target protein. In docking, a high score indicates that the molecule has strong hydrogen bonds, electrostatic interactions, and hydrophobic interactions with the target ligand, making it a suitable candidate for binding. The crystal structure of the protein is taken from the RCSB protein databank, and the docking procedure inserts the stiff chemical compounds into the active site. Typically, the search strategies used have a direct bearing on the precision and velocity of the docking conformation. Every docking program uses a different conformational search methodology, such as the GA (Spiegel & Durrant, 2020), MC (Zhang et al., 2020), or IC (Rarey et al., 1999).

When a ligand docks to a protein, the resulting protein-ligand complex may either stimulate or inhibit the target protein's biological activity, depending on the experimental conditions. Over the last several years, scientists have been using molecular docking to determine the likelihood that bioactive chemicals would bind to a target protein at a certain position. Some recent research has used docking techniques to study the binding conformations of ligands for toxicity evaluations rather than relying on animal models. As a result, NPs' chemical interactions with target enzymes may be investigated using the docking technique. This has shed light on a putative process by which the geometric structures of the protein-NP complex are created.

Nanotoxicity evaluations may be conducted with less time, money, and effort thanks to this computational method (Rarey, Kramer & Lengauer, 1999). Quantitative structure-activity relationship (QSAR) modeling is a powerful tool for predicting the biological activity or toxicity of chemicals using quantitative statistics and expertize in machine learning. Once upon a time, a century ago to be exact, Crum-Brown and Fraser (Brown & Fraser, 1868) introduced the idea of QSAR and established that chemical composition is related to physiological activity. Subsequently, in 1962 (Hansch et al., 1962), Corwin Hansch presented the first simple chemical compounds as a reaction to the free energy connection model. The QSAR model's overarching goal is to characterize a useful function that exhibits a rational connection between chemical structure and biological activity. This might help summarize physiochemical and biological data, which could be used to foretell toxicity consequences or design optimal nanomaterials.

In the current age of computational nanotoxicology, MD modeling has matured into a frequently utilized tool for investigating chemical and physical characteristics. The experimental data from methods like X-ray crystallography and nuclear magnetic resonance (NMR) spectroscopy may be supplemented with MD simulations to better understand the atomic mobility of the resulting 3D structures. Modern MD simulations not only offer the thermodynamic and kinetic parameters of the material systems at the atomic level but also help with understanding the time-dependent behavior of the physical motions of atoms and molecules. This means that MD simulations may provide rich data on the conformational changes of macromolecules and NPs.

Toxicology prediction models useful for NP design and development may be generated utilizing computational approaches, like as MD simulations. Traditional methods of assessing toxicity, such as cell-based or animal assays, are fraught with ethical concerns, budgetary difficulties, and extended testing times. As a result, computational toxicology is frequently used in the field of biomedicine to predict the adverse effects of hazardous substances on a broad range of organisms. This approach provides another means of investigating the hazards of chemicals. Recently, researchers in the fields of computational toxicology and nanotoxicology have used MD simulations to investigate potential toxicity pathways. An increase in toxicity might occur, for instance, if NPs become aggregated or agglomerated either during production or when embedded in a polymer matrix (Zare, 2016). This may cause intracellular reactive oxygen species (ROS) to be produced (Fu et al., 2014), which in turn can promote apoptosis. Agglomeration of titanium dioxide (TiO_2) NPs, for instance, has been found to induce toxicity reactions in cell-based and animal investigations. Large TiO_2 NP agglomerates promoted more potent biological effects, including DNA damage, GSH depletion, and inflammation, than tiny NP agglomerates did (Murugadoss et al., 2020). Therefore, it is crucial to evaluate the toxicity of NPs by analyzing their aggregation with other NPs.

15.5   RISK FACTORS FOR USING NANOMEDICINES

Experts were divided on whether or not these nanomedicines posed a threat to the environment, but most agreed that they did (as environmental concentrations, and therefore exposure, would be low). The conventional wisdom among industry professionals was that pharmaceutical companies adhere to good manufacturing procedures (GMP) and that the high cost of nanomedicines would lead to less waste. Medicines are designed to either kill cancer cells or to influence specific biochemical pathways; as a result, they can influence similar biological pathways in non-target organisms. However, experts have noted that any risks or hazards associated with medicine use will be local, occurring in hospital wastewater. Oestrogens and anti-cancer medications were used as examples to back up the specialists' claims. Many professionals have speculated that nanomedicines pose no immediate danger to the environment because of their small size and high degree of diluting power. A large number of specialists, however, responded with more caution (and thought). As a result, a health risk researcher has discovered pharmaceutical industry contamination.

It has been widely agreed upon by experts that nanotechnology-based medical devices pose no threat to the surrounding ecosystem since the nanoparticles used in their construction are contained inside larger, non-nanomaterial casings. In a classification paradigm for nanomaterials proposed by Hansen et al., 2008, consumer items in which nanoparticles are suspended in solids are deemed to have no exposure. Both Weil, in her study of 22 companies in the US Midwest, (Weil, 2013; Capon et al., 2015), in their survey of Australian scientists, representatives of business and government, and laypeople, indicated a belief that embedded or bound nanomaterials would not cause damage or raise less worries. However, it has been noted by certain specialists that exposure might occur due to normal wear and use. Reports have surfaced about the potential dangers to human health posed by the fragmentation of medical implants such artificial hip joints, and fresh pathways of their harmful consequences have been revealed (Bhabra et al., 2009; Sood et al., 2011).

Interestingly, several nanomedicine developers and regulatory agency representatives have brought up the idea of "safer-by-design" or "benign-by-design" concerns while making new medical treatments and devices (Rycroft et al., 2018). Unprompted concerns about potential dangers to human health posed by nanomedicine reveal how abstract the idea of environmental risk assessment might seem (except for specialist eco-toxicologists). In any case, it was encouraging to learn that health and safety concerns have become commonplace and regular at all stages of a product's value chain, notwithstanding the possibility of naivete and overconfidence on the part of academics working on nanomedicine development. Nonetheless, our findings reveal a sizable knowledge gap concerning environmental legislation and a lack of orientation toward an ecological approach. Consequently, this paper's major takeaway is a plea for improved methods of communication and debate to bridge this knowledge gap and bring light to the environmental concerns related to the risk assessment of nanomedicines and pharmaceuticals more generally. Since social scientists are aware of the subjective character of risk and that risk can never be negated, funding bodies may mandate more cross-disciplinary work, including social scientists (such as how EPSRC financed the grand challenge for nanotechnology for health care). It is helpful to include stakeholders in research subjects, and the EPSRC's policy of sponsoring a public engagement exercise prior to the grand challenge call to identify and prioritize the funding areas in nanomedicine is one such technique (Jones, 2008).

Guidance documents on risk assessment state that risk assessment is a scientific process, but risk perception is not unidimensional because risk is not an "objective" fact described solely by the probability of harm. Risk is a multidimensional socially constructed concept and is dependent on many factors. The European Medicines Agency (EMA) conducted research to determine what factors impact medicinal assessors' view of risks and benefits when making judgments on the authorization of medical goods. However, despite the positivist philosophy's assumption of science's objectivity, scientific "facts" are sometimes disputed, such as the relationship between dietary fat and cholesterol and coronary heart disease (Garrety, 1997) and the latest discussion about glyphosphate's carcinogenic potential (Tarone, 2018). Furthermore, academics in the social sciences have shown how both local and global societal interests may shape research and its conclusions (Jasanoff, 1987, Stirling, 2007). Furthermore, Stirling (Stirling, 2007) has stated why risk assessment, a reductive approach, is not scientifically based nor logical under contexts of uncertainty, ambiguity, and ignorance. Because of this, anticipatory risk governance has to be conceived of before any technological or commercial endeavors ever begin.

Research on nano-security has blossomed during the last two decades. The safety of nanoparticles is unclear, and several studies contradict one another (Krug, 2014). Several nanomaterials were found to pass through the lungs and gastrointestinal system, but only a fraction of them made it into circulation and were carried to secondary target organs. Most nanoparticles are eliminated by lung macrophage uptake or via feces (Borm et al., 2006).

Experts on nanotoxicology say they can characterize and evaluate the toxicological risk of carbon nanotubes and fullerenes using a set of criteria that has been effective in the past (Aschberger et al., 2010; Fatkhutdinova et al., 2015; Oberdörster et al., 2015). These standards were developed in response to the researchers' most frequent errors: (1) poor characterization, which may usually be traced back to the supplier; for example, if the particle size claimed by the supplier is wrong, it will lead to large mistakes in future studies; (2) inadequate testing for contamination of the studied nanomaterial. In most instances, the samples were not handled in a sterile manner, which might have introduced contamination, such as endotoxins, which would have the same response as inflammatory mediators if used in assays analyzing the inflammatory processes. Consequently, false positives are achieved; (3) solvent and dispersant interactions with the test system are ignored; (4) no control tests are conducted, leading to insufficient findings.

While most studies fail to show a toxicological impact owing to experimental mistakes, the majority of papers nevertheless include terms related to "the toxicological effect" as keywords (Krug & Nau, 2017). Determining the safety of nanoparticles is hindered by a lack of conclusive and verifiable evidence. Animal testing, for instance, cannot adequately assess the toxicological risk of NMs to the environment and human health, nor can it establish a suitable dose (Henschler, 1973). It has also been inferred that labs might benefit from a standardization approach and quality control to cut down on unnecessary repetition. This behavior, once easy to prevent, is now pervasive. As epidemiological investigations become more uniform, labs will need to choose a sample for universal modeling to enable comparability of assessment criteria. Results analysis should be performed by trained professionals in compliance with Good Laboratory Practices. Although they are meant to ensure the safety of NMs, it seems that in most instances the Standard Operating Procedure is not followed.

According to nanotoxicologists' evaluations, not all nanomaterials are made in the same manner, which indicates that there might be variations in biological reactions even when there are only minor variances in the materials' characteristics (Costa & Fadeel, 2016). Concerns regarding potential hazardous effects on human health and the environment have been prompted by the exponential increase in the number of nanomaterials(Ray et al., 2009). Medical gadgets, pharmaceuticals, and personal care items are a major source of worry because of their constant and prolonged interaction with living systems.

However, it is still challenging to foresee the bioavailability, biodistribution, degradation, elimination, and biological activity of nanostructures despite a decade's worth of research on nanotoxicity (Zhou et al., 2019). However, there are already well-established protocols for ensuring worker safety in the industrial, commercial, and healthcare sectors. Knowing the full extent of the toxicological processes and interactions of novel NMs is, thus, important. Nanoparticle-cell interactions, endocytosis, and intracellular traffic are just a few of the areas that may be elucidated by these types of investigations (Behzadi et al., 2017; Panariti et al., 2012). To evaluate chemical or pharmaceutical safety, researchers might use in vitro and in vivo biological models. In vitro models rely heavily on isolated cells and may be utilized in test tubes with the chemical under investigation. In turn, in vivo models are used on living creatures to track any changes in their growth, reproduction, death, etc. that may serve as toxicity markers. Metabolomics and transcriptomics are beginning to be used together in nanotoxicity research (Shin et al., 2018). Nanomaterials testing should be reevaluated with the goal of developing a reliable strategy for identifying nanotoxicity. Consequently, nano-ecotoxicological sciences are beginning to take into account and actively implement the methods of biological systems.

15.6 CONCLUSION

In this chapter, we've tried to give you a bird's-eye view of nanotoxicity from all angles. Looking back, there is a clear deficiency in comprehensive knowledge of toxicity and its influence on the human world, despite the availability of various research and reviews in literature. As noted previously, the toxicity of the nanomaterials relies on multiple physicochemical parameters, and modification of any single parameter would affect the toxicity pattern and result in a distinct physiological endpoint. There is little to no association between in vitro, in vivo, and in silico data for many nanomaterials. As a result, throughout the course of the last several decades, there has been an increasing desire for nanomaterial toxicity libraries. The prevention and prediction of the toxicity of a number of newly developed nanomaterials may be greatly aided by combining the various toxicity assaying approaches and creating a center for emphasizing the possible toxicity of the materials. Therefore, comprehensive research is needed to standardize the sizes of the various nanomaterials that are mass-produced and used in industries. Toxicology is the study of the causes, effects, and prevention of poisoning in both animals and people, and this will help us better grasp these topics.

REFERENCES

Afshar, L., Aghayan, H. R., Sadighi, J., Arjmand, B., Hashemi, S. M., Basiri, M., Samani, R. O., Ashtiani, M. K., Azin, S. A., Hajizadeh-Saffar, E., Gooshki, E. S., Hamidieh, A. A., Rezania Moallem, M. R., Azin, S. M., Shariatinasab, S., Soleymani-Goloujeh, M., & Baharvand, H. (2020). Ethics of research on stem cells and regenerative medicine: ethical guidelines in the Islamic Republic of Iran. *Stem cell research & therapy*, *11*(1), 396. 10.1186/s13287-020-01916-z

Aime, S., Castelli, D. D., Crich, S. G., Gianolio, E., & Terreno, E. (2009). Pushing the sensitivity envelope of lanthanide-based magnetic resonance imaging (MRI) contrast agents for molecular imaging applications. *Accounts of chemical research*, *42*(7), 822–831. 10.1021/ar800192p

Akter, M., Sikder, M. T., Rahman, M. M., Ullah, A. K. M. A., Hossain, K. F. B., Banik, S., Hosokawa, T., Saito, T., & Kurasaki, M. (2017). A systematic review on silver nanoparticles-induced cytotoxicity: physicochemical properties and perspectives. *Journal of advanced research*, *9*, 1–16. 10.1016/j.jare.2017.10.008

Alazzam, A., Mfoumou, E., Stiharu, I., Kassab, A., Darnel, A., Yasmeen, A., Sivakumar, N., Bhat, R., & Al Moustafa, A. E. (2010). Identification of deregulated genes by single wall carbon-nanotubes in human normal bronchial epithelial cells. *Nanomedicine: Nanotechnology, biological medicine*, *6*(4), 563–569. 10.1016/j.nano.2009.12.005.

Alsaleh, N. B., & Brown, J. M. (2020). Engineered nanomaterials and type I allergic hypersensitivity reactions. *Frontiers in immunology*, *11*, 222. 10.3389/fimmu.2020.00222

Amri, C., Shukla, A. K., & Lee, J. H. (2021). Recent advancements in nanoparticle-based optical biosensors for circulating cancer biomarkers. *Materials*, *14*(6), 1339. 10.3390/ma14061339

Aschberger, K., Johnston, H. J., Stone, V., Aitken, R. J., Tran, C. L., Hankin, S. M., Peters, S. A., & Christensen, F. M. (2010). Review of fullerene toxicity and exposure – appraisal of a human health risk assessment, based on open literature. *Regulatory toxicology and pharmacology: RTP*, *58*(3), 455–473. 10.1016/j.yrtph.2010.08.017

Bedlovičová, Z., Strapáč, I., Baláž, M., & Salayová, A. (2020). A brief overview on antioxidant activity determination of silver nanoparticles. *Molecules*, *25*(14), 3191. 10.3390/molecules25143191

Behzadi, S., Serpooshan, V., Tao, W., Hamaly, M. A., Alkawareek, M. Y., Dreaden, E. C., Brown, D., Alkilany, A. M., Farokhzad, O. C., & Mahmoudi, M. (2017). Cellular uptake of nanoparticles: journey inside the cell. *Chemical society reviews*, *46*(14), 4218–4244. 10.1039/c6cs00636a

Bezek, L. B., Cauchi, M. P., De Vita, R., Foerst, J. R., & Williams, C. B. (2020). 3D printing tissue-mimicking materials for realistic transseptal puncture models. *Journal of the mechanical behavior of biomedical materials*, *110*, 103971. 10.1016/j.jmbbm.2020. 103971

Bhabra, G., Sood, A., Fisher, B., Cartwright, L., Saunders, M., Evans, W. H., Surprenant, A., Lopez-Castejon, G., Mann, S., Davis, S. A., Hails, L. A., Ingham, E., Verkade, P., Lane, J., Heesom, K., Newson, R., & Case, C. P. (2009). Nanoparticles can cause DNA damage across a cellular barrier. *Nature nanotechnology*, *4*(12), 876–883. 10.1038/nnano.2009.313

Bhalgat, M. K., Haugland, R. P., Pollack, J. S., Swan, S., & Haugland, R. P. (1998). Green- and red-fluorescent nanospheres for the detection of cell surface receptors by flow cytometry. *Journal of immunological methods*, *219*(1–2), 57–68. 10.1016/s0022-1759(98)00121-5

Bhattacharya, T., Soares, G. A. B. E., Chopra, H., Rahman, M. M., Hasan, Z., Swain, S. S., & Cavalu, S. (2022). Applications of phyto-nanotechnology for the treatment of neurodegenerative disorders. *Materials*, *15*(3), 804. 10.3390/ma15030804

Borm, P. J., Robbins, D., Haubold, S., Kuhlbusch, T., Fissan, H., Donaldson, K., Schins, R., Stone, V., Kreyling, W., Lademann, J., Krutmann, J., Warheit, D., & Oberdorster, E. (2006). The potential risks of nanomaterials: a review carried out for ECETOC. *Particle and fibre toxicology*, *3*, 11. 10.1186/1743-8977-3-11

Brown, A. C., & Fraser, T. R. (1868). On the connection between chemical constitution and physiological action; with special reference to the physiological action of the salts of the ammonium bases derived from Strychnia, Brucia, Thebaia, Codeia, Morphia, and Nicotia. *Journal of anatomy and physiology*, *2*(2), 224–242.

Buzhor, E., Leshansky, L., Blumenthal, J., Barash, H., Warshawsky, D., Mazor, Y., & Shtrichman, R. (2014). Cell-based therapy approaches: the hope for incurable diseases. *Regenerative medicine*, *9*(5), 649–672. 10.2217/rme.14.35

Capon, A., Gillespie, J., Rolfe, M., & Smith, W. (2015). Perceptions of risk from nanotechnologies and trust in stakeholders: a cross sectional study of public, academic, government and business attitudes. *BMC public health*, *15*, 424. 10.1186/s12889-015-1795-1

Chopra, H., Bibi, S., Singh, I., Hasan, M. M., Khan, M. S., Yousafi, Q., Baig, A. A., Rahman, M. M., Islam, F., Emran, T. B., & Cavalu, S. (2022). Green metallic nanoparticles: biosynthesis to applications. *Frontiers in bioengineering and biotechnology*, *10*, 874742. 10.3389/fbioe.2022.874742

Chopra, H., Dey, P. S., Das, D., Bhattacharya, T., Shah, M., Mubin, S., Maishu, S. P., Akter, R., Rahman, M. H., Karthika, C., Murad, W., Qusty, N., Qusti, S., Alshammari, E. M., Batiha, G. E., Altalbawy, F. M. A., Albooq, M. I. M., & Alamri, B. M. (2021). Curcumin nanoparticles as promising therapeutic agents for drug targets. *Molecules*, *26*(16), 4998. 10.3390/molecules26164998

Costa, P.M., & Fadeel, B. (2016). Emerging systems biology approaches in nanotoxicology: towards a mechanism-based understanding of nanomaterial hazard and risk. *Toxicology and applied pharmacology*, *299*, 101–111. 10.1016/j.taap.2015.12.014.

Cui, D., Tian, F., Ozkan, C. S., Wang, M., & Gao, H. (2005). Effect of single wall carbon nanotubes on human HEK293 cells. *Toxicology letters*, *155*(1), 73–85. 10.1016/j.toxlet.2004.08.015

Dawson, E., Mapili, G., Erickson, K., Taqvi, S., & Roy, K. (2008). Biomaterials for stem cell differentiation. *Advanced drug delivery reviews*, *60*(2), 215–228. 10.1016/j.addr.2007.08.037

Divya, K., & Jisha, M.S. (2018). Chitosan nanoparticles preparation and applications. *Environmental chemistry letters*, 16, 101–112.

Dreher K. L. (2004). Health and environmental impact of nanotechnology: toxicological assessment of manufactured nanoparticles. *Toxicological sciences: An official journal of the society of toxicology*, *77*(1), 3–5. 10.1093/toxsci/kfh041

Fatkhutdinova, L. M., Khaliullin, T. O., & Shvedova, A. A. (2015). Carbon nanotubes exposure risk assessment: from toxicology to epidemiologic studies (overview of the current problem). *Nanotechnologies in Russia*, *10*(5), 501–509. 10.1134/s1995078015030064

Flacke, S., Fischer, S., Scott, M. J., Fuhrhop, R. J., Allen, J. S., McLean, M., Winter, P., Sicard, G. A., Gaffney, P. J., Wickline, S. A., & Lanza, G. M. (2001). Novel MRI contrast agent for molecular imaging of fibrin: implications for detecting vulnerable plaques. *Circulation*, *104*(11), 1280–1285. 10.1161/hc3601.094303

Fu, P. P., Xia, Q., Hwang, H. M., Ray, P. C., & Yu, H. (2014). Mechanisms of nanotoxicity: generation of reactive oxygen species. *Journal of food and drug analysis*, *22*(1), 64–75. 10.1016/j.jfda.2014.01.005

Gao, X., Li, R., Sprando, R.L., Yourick, J.J. (2021). Concentration-dependent toxicogenomic changes of silver nanoparticles in hepatocyte-like cells derived from human induced pluripotent stem cells. *Cell biology and toxicology*, *37*(2), 245–259. 10.1007/s10565-020-09529-1

Garrety K. (1997). Social worlds, actor-networks and controversy: the case of cholesterol, dietary fat and heart disease. *Social studies of science*, *27*(5), 727–773. 10.1177/03 0631297027005002

Garrod, M., & Chau, D. Y. (2016). An overview of tissue engineering as an alternative for toxicity assessment. *Journal of pharmacy & pharmaceutical sciences: A publication of the Canadian Society for Pharmaceutical Sciences, Societe canadienne des sciences pharmaceutiques*, *19*(1), 31–71. 10.18433/J35P6P

Gurunathan, S., Jeyaraj, M., Kang, M. H., & Kim, J. H. (2019). Mitochondrial peptide humanin protects silver nanoparticles-induced neurotoxicity in human neuroblastoma cancer cells (SH-SY5Y). *International journal of molecular sciences*, *20*(18), 4439. 10.3390/ijms20184439

Handral, H. K., Tong, H. J., Islam, I., Sriram, G., Rosa, V., & Cao, T. (2016). Pluripotent stem cells: an *in vitro* model for nanotoxicity assessments. *Journal of applied toxicology*, *36*, 1250–1258. 10.1002/jat.3347

Hansch, C., Maloney, P. P., Fujita, T., & Muir, R. M. (1962). Correlation of biological activity of phenoxyacetic acids with hammett substituent constants and partition coefficients. *Nature*, *194*, 178–180. 10.1038/194178b0

Hansen, S. F., Michelson, E. S., Kamper, A., Borling, P., Stuer-Lauridsen, F., & Baun, A. (2008). Categorization framework to aid exposure assessment of nanomaterials in consumer products. *Ecotoxicology*, *17*(5), 438–447. 10.1007/s10646-008-0210-4

Henschler, D. (1973). Toxicological problems relating to changes in the environment. *Angewandte Chemie (International Edition in English)*, *12*, 274–283. 10.1002/anie.197302741

Horie, M., & Tabei, Y. (2021). Role of oxidative stress in nanoparticles toxicity. *Free radical research*, *55*(4), 331–342. 10.1080/10715762.2020.1859108

Horie, S., Masterson, C., Devaney, J., & Laffey, J. G. (2016). Stem cell therapy for acute respiratory distress syndrome: a promising future? *Current opinion in critical care*, *22*(1), 14–20. 10.1097/MCC.0000000000000276

Jasanoff, S. (1987). Contested boundaries in policy-relevant science. *Social studies of science*, *17*, 195–230. 10.1177/030631287017002001

Jensen, C., & Teng, Y. (2020). Is it time to start transitioning from 2D to 3D cell culture? *Frontiers in molecular biosciences*, *7*, 33. 10.3389/fmolb.2020.00033

Jones, R. (2008). When it pays to ask the public. *Nature nanotechnology*, *3*, 578–579. 10.1038/nnano.2008.288

Kapałczyńska, M., Kolenda, T., Przybyła, W., Zajączkowska, M., Teresiak, A., Filas, V., Ibbs, M., Bliźniak, R., Łuczewski, Ł., & Lamperska, K. (2018). 2D and 3D cell cultures – a comparison of different types of cancer cell cultures. *Archives of medical science: AMS*, *14*(4), 910–919. 10.5114/aoms.2016.63743

Koti, P., Nath, S., Blell, J., Boyer, C., & Redwan I. N. (2020). *Comparing drug response in 2D cultures and 3D bioprinted tumoroids*, by Cellink lifesciences. Viewed 11 December 2022, https://www.cellink.com/global/wp-content/uploads/sites/7/2020/06/AppNote_3DCellCulture_-Part-3-_052020V1-1.pdf

Kouroupis, D., Sanjurjo-Rodriguez, C., Jones, E., & Correa, D. (2019). Mesenchymal stem cell functionalization for enhanced therapeutic applications. *Tissue engineering. Part B, Reviews, 25*(1), 55–77. 10.1089/ten.TEB.2018.0118

Krug, H. F. (2014). Nanosafety research – are we on the right track? *Angewandte Chemie (International edition in English), 53*(46), 12304–12319. 10.1002/anie.201403367

Krug, H. F., & Nau, K. (2017). Reliability for nanosafety research – considerations on the basis of a comprehensive literature review. *ChemBioEng Reviews,* 4(6), 331. 10.1002/cben.201700013

Kugler, J., Huhse, B., Tralau, T., Luch, A. (2017). Embryonic stem cells and the next generation of developmental toxicity testing. *Expert opinion on drug metabolism and toxicology, 13*(8), 833–841. 10.1080/17425255.2017.1351548

Labusca, L., Herea, D. D., & Mashayekhi, K. (2018). Stem cells as delivery vehicles for regenerative medicine-challenges and perspectives. *World journal of stem cells, 10*(5), 43–56. 10.4252/wjsc.v10.i5.43

Lademann, J., Weigmann, H., Rickmeyer, C., Barthelmes, H., Schaefer, H., Mueller, G., & Sterry, W. (1999). Penetration of titanium dioxide microparticles in a sunscreen formulation into the horny layer and the follicular orifice. *Skin pharmacology and applied skin physiology, 12*(5), 247–256. 10.1159/000066249

Lanone, S., & Boczkowski, J. (2006). Biomedical applications and potential health risks of nanomaterials: molecular mechanisms. *Current molecular medicine, 6*(6), 651–663. 10.2174/156652406778195026

Li, X., Liu, W., Sun, L., Aifantis, K.E., Yu, B., Fan, Y., Feng, Q., Cui, F. & Watari, F. (2015). Effects of physicochemical properties of nanomaterials on their toxicity. *Journal of biomedical materials research – Part A, 103*(7), 2499–2507. 10.1002/jbm.a.35384

Li, Y., Li, F., Zhang, L., Zhang, C., Peng, H., Lan, F., Peng, S., Liu, C., & Guo, J. (2020). Zinc oxide nanoparticles induce mitochondrial biogenesis impairment and cardiac dysfunction in human iPSC-derived cardiomyocytes. *International journal of nano-medicine, 15*, 2669–2683. 10.2147/IJN.S249912

Liu, Y., Xu, Z., & Li, X. (2013). Cytotoxicity of titanium dioxide nanoparticles in rat neuroglia cells. *Brain injury, 27*(7–8), 934–939. 10.3109/02699052.2013.793401

Luz, A. L., & Tokar, E. J. (2018). Pluripotent stem cells in developmental toxicity testing: A review of methodological advances. *Toxicological sciences: an official journal of the Society of Toxicology, 165*(1), 31–39. 10.1093/toxsci/kfy174

Mathur, P., Jha, S., Ramteke, S., & Jain, N. K. (2018). Pharmaceutical aspects of silver nanoparticles. *Artificial cells, nanomedicine, and biotechnology, 46*(1), 115–126. 10.1080/21691401.2017.1414825

Medina, C., Santos-Martinez, M. J., Radomski, A., Corrigan, O. I., & Radomski, M. W. (2007). Nanoparticles: pharmacological and toxicological significance. *British journal of pharmacology, 150*(5), 552–558. 10.1038/sj.bjp.0707130

Moghimi, S. M. (2021). Allergic reactions and anaphylaxis to LNP-based COVID-19 vaccines. *Molecular therapy: The journal of the American Society of Gene Therapy, 29*(3), 898–900. 10.1016/j.ymthe.2021.01.030

Morimoto, Y., Horie, M., Kobayashi, N., Shinohara, N., & Shimada, M. (2013). Inhalation toxicity assessment of carbon-based nanoparticles. *Accounts of chemical research, 46*(3), 770–781. 10.1021/ar200311b

Movia, D., Bruni-Favier, S., & Prina-Mello, A. (2020). *In vitro* alternatives to acute inhalation toxicity studies in animal models – a perspective. *Frontiers in bioengineering and biotechnology, 8*, 549. 10.3389/fbioe.2020.00549

Müllebner, A., Dorighello, G. G., Kozlov, A. V., & Duvigneau, J. C. (2018). Interaction between mitochondrial reactive oxygen species, heme oxygenase, and nitric oxide synthase stimulates phagocytosis in macrophages. *Frontiers in medicine, 4*, 252. 10.3389/fmed.2017.00252

Murugadoss, S., Brassinne, F., Sebaihi, N., Petry, J., Cokic, S. M., Van Landuyt, K. L., Godderis, L., Mast, J., Lison, D., Hoet, P. H., & van den Brule, S. (2020). Agglomeration of titanium dioxide nanoparticles increases toxicological responses in vitro and in vivo. *Particle and fibre toxicology, 17*(1), 10. 10.1186/s12989-020-00341-7

Nam, J. M., Thaxton, C. S., & Mirkin, C. A. (2003). Nanoparticle-based bio-bar codes for the ultrasensitive detection of proteins. *Science, 301*(5641), 1884–1886. 10.1126/science.1 088755

Niemiec, E., & Howard, H. C. (2020). Ethical issues related to research on genome editing in human embryos. *Computational and structural biotechnology journal, 18*, 887–896. 10.1016/j.csbj.2020.03.014

Oberdörster, G., Castranova, V., Asgharian, B., & Sayre, P. (2015). Inhalation exposure to carbon nanotubes (CNT) and carbon nanofibers (CNF): methodology and dosimetry. *Journal of toxicology and environmental health. Part B, Critical reviews, 18*(3–4), 121–212. 10.1080/10937404.2015.1051611

Oberdörster, G., Oberdörster, E., & Oberdörster, J. (2005). Nanotoxicology: an emerging discipline evolving from studies of ultrafine particles. *Environmental health perspectives, 113*(7), 823–839. 10.1289/ehp.7339

Pallares, R. M., Thanh, N. T., & Su, X. (2019). Sensing of circulating cancer biomarkers with metal nanoparticles. *Nanoscale.* 10.1039/c9nr03040a.

Panariti, A., Miserocchi, G., & Rivolta, I. (2012). The effect of nanoparticle uptake on cellular behavior: disrupting or enabling functions? *Nanotechnology, science and applications, 5*, 87–100. 10.2147/NSA.S25515

Pang, L. (2020). Toxicity testing in the era of iPSC: a perspective regarding the use of patient-specific iPSC-CMs for cardiac safety evaluation. *Current opinion in toxicology, 23–24.* 10.1016/j.cotox.2020.04.001

Peng, B. Y., Dubey, N. K., Mishra, V. K., Tsai, F. C., Dubey, R., Deng, W. P., & Wei, H. J. (2018). Addressing stem cell therapeutic approaches in pathobiology of diabetes and its complications. *Journal of diabetes research, 2018*, 7806435. 10.1155/2018/ 7806435

Radomski, A., Jurasz, P., Alonso-Escolano, D., Drews, M., Morandi, M., Malinski, T., & Radomski, M. W. (2005). Nanoparticle-induced platelet aggregation and vascular thrombosis. *British journal of pharmacology, 146*(6), 882–893. 10.1038/sj.bjp. 0706386

Rarey, M., Kramer, B., & Lengauer, T. (1999). The particle concept: placing discrete water molecules during protein-ligand docking predictions. *Proteins, 34*(1), 17–28.

Ray, P. C., Yu, H., & Fu, P. P. (2009). Toxicity and environmental risks of nanomaterials: challenges and future needs. *Journal of environmental science and health. Part C, Environmental carcinogenesis & ecotoxicology reviews, 27*(1), 1–35. 10.1080/105905 00802708267

Rikhtegar, R., Pezeshkian, M., Dolati, S., Safaie, N., Afrasiabi Rad, A., Mahdipour, M., Nouri, M., Jodati, A. R., & Yousefi, M. (2019). Stem cells as therapy for heart disease: iPSCs, ESCs, CSCs, and skeletal myoblasts. *Biomedicine & pharmacotherapy = Biomedicine & pharmacotherapie, 109*, 304–313. 10.1016/j.biopha.2018.10.065

Rycroft, T., Trump, B., Poinsatte-Jones, K., & Linkov, I. (2018). Nanotoxicology and nanomedicine: making development decisions in an evolving governance environment. *Journal of nanoparticle research, 20*(2). 10.1007/s11051-018-4160-3

Saha, A., Ben Halima, H., Saini, A., Gallardo-Gonzalez, J., Zine, N., Viñas, C., Elaissari, A., Errachid, A., & Teixidor, F. (2020). Magnetic nanoparticles fishing for biomarkers in artificial saliva. *Molecules, 25*(17), 3968. 10.3390/molecules25173968

Salesa, B., Assis, M., Andrés, J., & Serrano-Aroca, Á. (2021). Carbon nanofibers versus silver nanoparticles: time-dependent cytotoxicity, proliferation, and gene expression. *Biomedicines, 9*(9), 1155. 10.3390/biomedicines9091155

Schmidt, K., Berg, J., Roehrs, V., Kurreck, J., & Al-Zeer, M. A. (2020). 3D-bioprinted HepaRG cultures as a model for testing long term aflatoxin B1 toxicity *in vitro*. *Toxicology reports*, *7*, 1578–1587. 10.1016/j.toxrep.2020.11.003

Shin, T. H., Lee, D. Y., Lee, H. S., Park, H. J., Jin, M. S., Paik, M. J., Manavalan, B., Mo, J. S., & Lee, G. (2018). Integration of metabolomics and transcriptomics in nanotoxicity studies. *BMB reports*, *51*(1), 14–20. 10.5483/bmbrep.2018.51.1.237

Shrivastava, R., Raza, S., Yadav, A., Kushwaha, P., & Flora, S. J. (2014). Effects of sub-acute exposure to TiO_2, ZnO and Al_2O_3 nanoparticles on oxidative stress and histological changes in mouse liver and brain. *Drug and chemical toxicology*, *37*(3), 336–347. 10.3109/01480545.2013.866134

Singh, D., Singh, S., Sahu, J., Srivastava, S., & Singh, M. R. (2016). Ceramic nanoparticles: Recompense, cellular uptake and toxicity concerns. *Artificial cells, nanomedicine, and biotechnology*, *44*(1), 401–409. 10.3109/21691401.2014.955106

Sood, A., Salih, S., Roh, D., Lacharme-Lora, L., Parry, M., Hardiman, B., Keehan, R., Grummer, R., Winterhager, E., Gokhale, P. J., Andrews, P. W., Abbott, C., Forbes, K., Westwood, M., Aplin, J. D., Ingham, E., Papageorgiou, I., Berry, M., Liu, J., Dick, A. D., … & Case, C. P. (2011). Signalling of DNA damage and cytokines across cell barriers exposed to nanoparticles depends on barrier thickness. *Nature nanotechnology*, *6*(12), 824–833. 10.1038/nnano.2011.188

Spiegel, J. O., & Durrant, J. D. (2020). AutoGrow4: an open-source genetic algorithm for de novo drug design and lead optimization. *Journal of cheminformatics*, *12*(1), 25. 10.1186/s13321-020-00429-4

Stirling A. (2007). Risk, precaution and science: towards a more constructive policy debate. Talking point on the precautionary principle. *EMBO reports*, *8*(4), 309–315. 10.1038/sj.embor.7400953

Sun, B., Wang, X., Ji, Z., Li, R., and Xia, T. (2013), NLRP3 inflammasome activation induced by engineered nanomaterials. *Small*, *9*, 1595–1607. 10.1002/smll.201201962

Takahashi, K., & Yamanaka, S. (2006). Induction of pluripotent stem cells from mouse embryonic and adult fibroblast cultures by defined factors. *Cell*, *126*(4), 663–676. 10.1016/j.cell.2006.07.024

Tarone, R. E. (2018). On the International Agency for Research on Cancer classification of glyphosate as a probable human carcinogen. *European journal of cancer prevention: The official journal of the European Cancer Prevention Organisation (ECP)*, *27*(1), 82–87. 10.1097/CEJ.0000000000000289

Thomson, J. A., Itskovitz-Eldor, J., Shapiro, S. S., Waknitz, M. A., Swiergiel, J. J., Marshall, V. S., & Jones, J. M. (1998). Embryonic stem cell lines derived from human blastocysts. *Science*, *282*(5391), 1145–1147. 10.1126/science.282.5391.1145

Trop, M., Novak, M., Rodl, S., Hellbom, B., Kroell, W., & Goessler, W. (2006). Silver-coated dressing acticoat caused raised liver enzymes and argyria-like symptoms in burn patient. *The journal of trauma*, *60*(3), 648–652. 10.1097/01.ta.0000208126.22089.b6

Volarevic, V., Markovic, B. S., Gazdic, M., Volarevic, A., Jovicic, N., Arsenijevic, N., Armstrong, L., Djonov, V., Lako, M., & Stojkovic, M. (2018). Ethical and safety issues of stem cell-based therapy. *International journal of medical sciences*, *15*(1), 36–45. 10.7150/ijms.21666

Wang, J. P., Yu, H. M., Chiang, E. R., Wang, J. Y., Chou, P. H., & Hung, S. C. (2018). Corticosteroid inhibits differentiation of palmar fibromatosis-derived stem cells (FSCs) through downregulation of transforming growth factor-β1 (TGF-β1). *PLoS one*, *13*(6), e0198326. 10.1371/journal.pone.0198326

Wang, X. F., Jin, P. P., Zhou, T., Zhao, Y. P., Ding, Q. L., Wang, D. B., Zhao, G. M., Jing-Dai, Wang, H. L., & Ge, H. L. (2010). MR molecular imaging of thrombus: development and application of a Gd-based novel contrast agent targeting to P-selectin. *Clinical and applied thrombosis/hemostasis: Official journal of the International Academy of Clinical and Applied Thrombosis/Hemostasis, 16*(2), 177–183. 10.1177/1076029608330470

Weil, V. (2013) Responsible management in private sector nano enterprises: conversations with lead technologists and managers. *NanoEthics 7*(3), 217–229. 10.1007/S11569-013-0180-8.

Xu, F., Piett, C., Farkas, S., Qazzaz, M., & Syed, N. I. (2013). Silver nanoparticles (AgNPs) cause degeneration of cytoskeleton and disrupt synaptic machinery of cultured cortical neurons. *Molecular brain, 6*, 29. 10.1186/1756-6606-6-29

Younes, N. R., Amara, S., Mrad, I., Ben-Slama, I., Jeljeli, M., Omri, K., El Ghoul, J., El Mir, L., Rhouma, K. B., Abdelmelek, H., & Sakly, M. (2015). Subacute toxicity of titanium dioxide (TiO$_2$) nanoparticles in male rats: emotional behavior and pathophysiological examination. *Environmental science and pollution research international, 22*(11), 8728–8737. 10.1007/s11356-014-4002-5

Yousaf, S., Chopra, H., Khan, M. A., Mustafa, F., Kamal, M. A., & Baig, A. A. (2022). Nanotechnology and its applications: insight into bacteriological interactions and bacterial gene transfer. In S. Gopi, P. Balakrishnan, N. M. Mubarak (eds.), *Nanotechnology for biomedical applications*. Singapore: Springer. pp. 479–497. 10.1007/978-981-16-7483-9_20

Yu, Z., Li, Q., Wang, J., Yu, Y., Wang, Y., Zhou, Q., & Li, P. (2020). Reactive oxygen species-related nanoparticle toxicity in the biomedical field. *Nanoscale research letters, 15*(1), 115. 10.1186/s11671-020-03344-7

Zare, Y. (2016). Study of nanoparticles aggregation/agglomeration in polymer particulate nanocomposites by mechanical properties. *Composites Part A: Applied science and manufacturing, 84*, 158–164. 10.1016/j.compositesa.2016.01.020

Zhang, Q., Jeppesen, D. K., Higginbotham, J. N., Graves-Deal, R., Trinh, V. Q., Ramirez, M. A., Sohn, Y., Neininger, A. C., Taneja, N., McKinley, E. T., Niitsu, H., Cao, Z., Evans, R., Glass, S. E., Ray, K. C., Fissell, W. H., Hill, S., Rose, K. L., Huh, W. J., Washington, M. K., ... & Coffey, R. J. (2021). Supermeres are functional extracellular nanoparticles replete with disease biomarkers and therapeutic targets. *Nature cell biology, 23*(12), 1240–1254. 10.1038/s41556-021-00805-8

Zhang, W., Bell, E. W., Yin, M., & Zhang, Y. E. (2020). Dock: blind protein-ligand docking by replica-exchange monte carlo simulation. *Journal of cheminformatics, 12*(1), 37. 10.1186/s13321-020-00440-9

Zhou, M., Ge, X., Ke, D. M., Tang, H., Zhang, J. Z., Calvaresi, M., Gao, B., Sun, L., Su, Q., & Wang, H. (2019). The bioavailability, biodistribution, and toxic effects of silica-coated upconversion nanoparticles in vivo. *Frontiers in chemistry, 7*, 218. 10.3389/fchem.2019.00218

Zielińska, A., Costa, B., Ferreira, M. V., Miguéis, D., Louros, J. M. S., Durazzo, A., Lucarini, M., Eder, P., Chaud, M. V., Morsink, M., Willemen, N., Severino, P., Santini, A., & Souto, E. B. (2020). Nanotoxicology and nanosafety: safety-by-design and testing at a glance. *International journal of environmental research and public health, 17*(13), 4657. 10.3390/ijerph17134657

Zou, Y., Xie, J., Zheng, S., Liu, W., Tang, Y., Tian, W., Deng, X., Wu, L., Zhang, Y., Wong, C.-W., Tan, D., Liu, Q., & Xie, X. (2022). Leveraging diverse cell-death patterns to predict the prognosis and drug sensitivity of triple-negative breast cancer patients after surgery. *International journal of surgery, 107*, 10693610.1016/j.ijsu.2022.106936

Panda, Sandip K., Aggarwal, I., Kumar, H., Prasad, L., Kumar, A., Sharma, A., Vo, D.-V. N., Van Thuan, D., & Mishra, V. (2021). Magnetite nanoparticles as sorbents for dye removal: a review. *Environmental chemistry letters, 19*, 2487–2525. 10.1007/s10311-020-01173-9

Jindal, S., Anand, R., Sharma, N., Yadav, N., Mudgal, D., Mishra, R., & Mishra, V. (2022). Sustainable approach for developing graphene-based materials from natural resources and biowastes for electronic applications. *ACS applied electronic materials*, *4*, 2146–2174. 10.1021/acsaelm.2c00097

Yadav, N., Mudgal, D., Anand, R., Jindal, S., & Mishra, V. (2022). Recent development in nanoencapsulation and delivery of natural bioactives through chitosan scaffolds for various biological applications. *International journal of biological macromolecules*, *220*, 537–572. 10.1016/j.ijbiomac.2022.08.098

Srivastava, A., Mishra, V., Singh, P., & Kumar, R. (2012). Coumarin-based polymer and its silver nanocomposite as advanced antibacterial agents: synthetic path, kinetics of polymerization, and applications. *Journal of applied polymer science*, *126*, 395–407. 10.1002/app.36999

Yadav, N., Gaikwad, R. P., Mishra, V., & Gawande, M. B. (2022). Synthesis and photocatalytic applications of functionalized carbon quantum dots. *Bulletin of the chemical society of Japan*, *95*, 1638–1679. 10.1246/bcsj.20220250

Yadav, N., Mudgal, D., Mishra, S., Sehrawat, H., Singh, N. K., Sharma, K., Sharma, P. C., Singh, J., & Mishra, V. (2023). Development of ionic liquid-capped carbon dots derived from *Tecoma stans* (L.) Juss. ex Kunth: combatting bacterial pathogens in diabetic foot ulcer pus swabs, targeting both standard and multi-drug resistant strains. *South African journal of botany*, *163*, 412–426. 10.1016/j.sajb.2023.10.063

Yadav, N., Mudgal, D., Mishra, A., Shukla, S., Malik, T., & Mishra, V. (2024). Harnessing fluorescent carbon quantum dots from natural resource for advancing sweat latent fingerprint recognition with machine learning algorithms for enhanced human identification. *PLOS One*, *19*, e0296270 10.1371/journal.pone.0296270

Mudgal, D, Singh, R. P., Yadav, N, Bharti, T, & Mishra, V. (2023). Exploring the catalytic efficiency of copper-doped magnetic carbon aerogel for the coupling reaction of isatin oxime with phenylboronic acid derivatives. *SynOpen*, *07*, 570–579. 10.1055/a-2182-7757

Mudgal, D., Yadav, N., Singh, J., Srivastava, G. K., & Mishra, V. (2023). Xanthan gum-based copper nano-magnetite doped carbon aerogel: a promising candidate for environmentally friendly catalytic dye degradation. *International journal of biological macromolecules*, *253*, 127491. 10.1016/j.ijbiomac.2023.127491

Yadav, N., Mudgal, D., & Mishra, V. (2023). In-situ synthesis of ionic liquid-based-carbon quantum dots as fluorescence probe for hemoglobin detection. *Analytica chimica acta*, *1272*, 341502. 10.1016/j.aca.2023.341502

Index

Note: **Bold** page numbers refer to tables and *italic* page numbers refer to figures.

For Product Safety Concerns and Information please contact our EU
representative GPSR@taylorandfrancis.com
Taylor & Francis Verlag GmbH, Kaufingerstraße 24, 80331 München, Germany

www.ingramcontent.com/pod-product-compliance
Lightning Source LLC
Chambersburg PA
CBHW060802220326
41598CB00022B/2521